THROUGH THE SHADOWLANDS

THROUGH THE SHADOWLANDS

A SCIENCE WRITER'S ODYSSEY
INTO AN ILLNESS
SCIENCE DOESN'T UNDERSTAND

JULIE REHMEYER

RODALE

RODALE *wellness*

Live happy. Be healthy. Get inspired.

Sign up today to get exclusive access to our authors, exclusive bonuses, and the most authoritative, useful, and cutting-edge information on health, wellness, fitness, and living your life to the fullest.

Visit us online at RodaleWellness.com
Join us at RodaleWellness.com/Join

Rodale books may be purchased for business or promotional use or for special sales. For information, please write to:
Trade Books/Special Markets Department, Rodale, Inc., 733 Third Avenue, New York, NY 10017

Printed in the United States of America
Rodale Inc. makes every effort to use acid-free ⊗, recycled paper ♲.

Book design by Christina Gaugler

Library of Congress Cataloging-in-Publication Data is on file with the publisher.

ISBN–13: 978-1-62336-765-7   hardcover

Distributed to the trade by Macmillan

2 4 6 8 10 9 7 5 3 1   hardcover

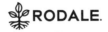

RODALE.

We inspire health, healing, happiness, and love in the world.
Starting with you.

To John Kadlecek
You are my treasure

CONTENTS

PART 4: EMERGENCE

PROLOGUE

The tent was possessed. Death Valley's wind breathed a wicked life into it, whipping it into a writhing demon intent on freeing itself from my grasp and flying off on some maniacal mission. Determined to put it up, I engulfed as much of the tent in my arms as I could, stomped on it with both feet, tugged on the strip of webbing holding a grommet, and strained to bend the tip of the tent pole toward the hole. I howled with effort and the sound tore away on the wind, just as the tent so wanted to.

I knew I was breaking my own cardinal rule: Stop When You're Tired. That rule had burned itself into my brain over the dozen years since I'd first developed the symptoms of chronic fatigue syndrome, the illness I had come to the desert attempting to outwit. Even mild exertion could leave me nearly paralyzed the next day, sometimes unable to turn over in bed.

Now I was spending all my strength wrestling with this nylon and fiberglass fiend. Before I left home, I'd made sure I was capable of setting up this borrowed hurricane-grade tent, but I hadn't counted on a hurricane-grade wind. I was miles up a jeep trail off a long dirt road in the middle of the godforsaken desert, alone except for my dog. Should I wake up crippled and call for help, my shouts would shred in the wind long before they reached a human ear.

On top of all that, I didn't even much believe in the mission that brought me to the desert in the first place. I had come to Death Valley on the theory that I needed to get clear of mold—from moldy buildings, from mold in the outside air, from mold in my belongings. Strangers on the Internet had told me there was a good chance that mold had triggered my illness and that by strictly avoiding it, I would eventually recover. I had never had any obvious reaction to mold in the past, but my Internet advisors told me that when I returned home after two weeks in the desert, the mold in my own house and belongings would likely make me dramatically sick. And then, at last, I would know what was doing me in.

This whole thing is probably a crock of shit, I'd thought, *but at least it'll make a good story.*

The truth was, though, that I was desperate to get better. Over the previous year, my health had deteriorated so much that I could barely work, often couldn't walk, couldn't even take care of myself. I had gone to the top specialists in the world, and I'd pretty much run out of medical options. I would soon run out of money, too, and I had little family to turn to. I was 39, and I had no idea what was going to happen to me. Consignment to a nursing home?

Without that level of desperation, I couldn't have brought myself to pursue a theory that so many scientists sneered at. I was a science writer and a mathematician, and science was my primary lens for viewing the world. Coming to Death Valley had unmoored me from both my physical and intellectual homes.

The wind tried again to rip the tent away as the last pole snicked into its grommet. *Thank god,* I thought, clutching the tent harder. I allowed myself only a moment to catch my breath, not wanting to let my exhaustion undo me. Then I began pounding stakes into the ground.

My two-year-old puppy, Frances, bounded up to me, her brown nose covered in fine tan sand, and then she ran off in pursuit of a fly. I smiled—she, clearly, wasn't a bit worried about the tent or the wind. I watched her leap and snap at the invisible insect. *At least I'm not completely alone,* I thought.

I plodded 50 feet to the car to gather essentials before I ran out of energy. As I reached toward the trunk, I stopped, arrested by the valley that surrounded me. Bands of red and blue and yellow and pink rippled through the mountains facing me, the peaks' geological story written on their naked flanks for all to read. The Panamint Mountains at my back were ever so slowly listing eastward like a great ship keeling over, the summits twisting higher as the valley floor sank. Salt flats shone white on the valley floor, the residue of millennia of rain that had run off the mountains and evaporated, carrying a load of salt and minerals to join the dried-up remains of Pleistocene lakes. Except for a few tiny cars inching along the road ten miles away, I saw no sign of a human being.

I felt myself expand into this great space, this emptiness. Despite the wind's immense swirl of energy, the land felt quiet, still, impassive. Everything fell away from me—my body, my pain and exhaustion, my fear, my strange experiment—and was replaced with a huge and ancient stillness. All the time, I thought, this place was here, whether I was pinned to my bed or bounding up a mountain trail. As I poured out into the valley, I felt the valley pouring into me, its enormous spaciousness filling my chest.

The wind buffeted me, and I staggered. I returned to my task, gathering a couple days' worth of food to take to the tent in case I couldn't make it back to the car the next day. Then I returned for my sleeping bag, pad, and Frances's blanket. All were new to me—one of the requirements of this experiment was that I leave all my own belongings behind, since everything I owned, on this theory, was contaminated with mold. The sleeping bag and pad I had borrowed from a friend, and the cheap blanket came from Target. I could only hope they were mold-free.

After the weeks of slow preparation, I had made it. It was only 6 p.m., but I was done for. I called Frances into the tent and curled up in my sleeping bag.

Before I left for Death Valley, I'd told friends that I felt like I was going to the desert to die. I fully expected to be breathing at the end of the trip, but I couldn't keep everything together as I had been doing for years, holding on to my responsibilities and dreams in spite of the barriers my illness threw in my path. Whether the experiment worked or didn't, the life I had lived was over. I was staring into a cavernous darkness, beyond any imagined future I could invent. I wrapped my arms around my dog and closed my eyes. *Okay,* I thought. *Whatever is next, okay.*

PART 1

DESCENT

CHAPTER 1

CONSTRUCTION AND DESTRUCTION

Summer 2000
12 years earlier

The cool mud squished between my fingers. It was so thick with chopped straw that I could pick it up by the handful to plaster the straw-bale wall of the house I was building. I mushed the mud into the bales with both hands, working it deep into the straw in a hypnotic, sensual cadence: Grab, mush. Grab, mush. Grab, mush.

The rhythm helped me ignore the exhaustion gnawing at me. A couple dozen friends had spent the day at our plaster party, helping us with the enormous job of mudding all the walls of the house my husband and I were building on our streamside land outside Santa Fe, New Mexico. All day, I hustled to keep everyone busy, teaching people to screen dirt and chop straw and mix mud, answering questions, running around with 35-pound buckets of mud in each hand to keep everyone supplied.

After all our friends had left, I gathered up the scraps of plaster left in various buckets and, despite my tiredness, gave myself this great pleasure of plastering a wall with my own hands. I reveled in the softness of the mud and the solidity of the bales—and the simplicity of a task with few decisions to make and no one else to satisfy.

I finished the wall faster than a crew of four of our friends would have. A couple years earlier, the Tewa Indian women who had taught me how to plaster had similarly outpaced me.

I stepped back from the wall, and a rush of awe filled me. That mud was now part of a wall that was destined, I hoped, to stand for decades, sheltering me from wind and cold. I imagined that someday my children would play in that spot, bumping against the wall, kept safe by its solidity. It seemed almost impossible that this seemingly endless series of mundane tasks would someday result in a *house*.

Once my job was done, my exhaustion wormed its way into my awareness—carrying my fear along with it. A couple of hours earlier, I had sent my husband, Geoff, inside for the evening, tired of telling him what to do. *Please spray out the mixer. Please gather and wash the buckets. Please put away the screen.* It was less painful to do it myself than to deal with his daze. Bits of Geoff's soul seemed to be disappearing, nibbled away by bipolar disorder. As hard as I was working to construct our house, I couldn't keep up with the destruction overtaking him—and us.

At one point recently, Geoff had come to me with eyes alight. "Look!" he said, handing me an eight-inch scrap of rebar, the material we had used to reinforce the concrete in our foundation. Rebar was ordinarily a dull, rusty brown rod, studded with bumps to help the concrete adhere to the steel—but the end of this piece was so smooth it felt soft against my finger, and blue and gray seemed to swirl inside the metal. Geoff held a file in his other hand, and metal dust lay at his feet. "It's so shiny!" he said, in a five-year-old's voice.

The wonder in his eyes nearly brought tears to mine. I hadn't seen a moment of joy in him for months. If a shiny bit of metal could bring that back to him, could remind him that life had pleasures that made the fight against the depression worth it, that he wasn't better off dead—well, it made me want to enshrine the thing on our mantelpiece.

At the same time, I wanted to bash the bit of rebar against his head: *You just spent an hour filing a piece of trash while I've been working my ass off building our house, and you have no clue that's a problem?*

Even as I felt my anger billowing outward, though, I knew the force fueling it was fear—and grief. I missed my husband. Less than two years earlier, Geoff had been my stronger half as we had hauled railroad ties and shoveled concrete to build a bridge across our stream that was sturdy enough to hold a concrete truck. Before that, we had turned ourselves into mathematicians together, spending hour after hour discussing mathematical puzzles in cafés as students at the Massachusetts Institute of Technology. I'd been dazzled by the way he could feel his way to the spine of a math problem and crack it; by the emotional maturity that helped him persist even when we were out of ideas; by his panther walk, honed by martial arts; and by the softness in his eyes whenever I was feeling down or discouraged.

If only I could talk to Geoff, the real Geoff, right now, I thought. *He'd help me figure out how to deal with this mess.* I counted the weeks since we'd last changed his medication, praying that the latest pills would bring him back to me.

I knew there was no point letting him see either my rage or my despair, so I forced myself to say, "That's so cool, Geoff!" The pitch of my voice rose against my will, assuming a singsong bounce. "Now, think you could give me a hand for a minute?"

As I cleaned up after the plaster party these months later, worry about Geoff's dissolution ate at my mind like acid. Would he ever be himself again? And even if he recovered, would our relationship recover too? Would we ever have the children I'd dreamed of? This house was supposed to be a jointly constructed container for our life as a couple and one day as a family. Instead, it was coming to be my personal burden. Our pain was getting built into it along with the straw and mud.

I pushed those worries aside, just as I had so many times before. Having finished plastering my wall, I went to rinse off my hands. As always, I was the dirtiest person on the building site at the end of the day. My arms seemed to have been dipped in chocolate up to the elbows, and I could feel dried mud cracking on my cheek. Bits of straw had cemented themselves to my legs. Long strands of blond hair straggled into my face, having snuck out of their braid. Most absurdly, two large, brown circles marked the front of my white T-shirt. *How,* I wondered, *do I always manage to brush my breasts against a freshly plastered wall?*

The next morning, Geoff and I awoke at dawn to make a run to town in Santa Fe, collecting supplies to keep the work going. I was exhausted, but then I was always exhausted, and I knew how to push through it.

When we got home, I stood and looked up the path to the house, sheltered by its great ponderosas. The slight slope felt like a mountain. My whole body ached, and earlier, just walking on the flat, even floors of Home Depot had hurt. When I groaned slightly at the first step, Geoff wrapped his arm around my waist and supported me up the slope. His brain might be dissolving, but his love for me still felt solid.

Even with Geoff's help, walking up that slope felt like a cruel thing to demand of my body. I wanted to sag out of my husband's embrace, to lie down in the pine needles, to feel my body melt into the soil. I just couldn't do this. I couldn't finish this house all by myself. I couldn't go teach my summer class at the college the next day. I couldn't keep Geoff from killing himself.

A worker we'd hired, Jessica, stood at the top of the slope, agape. "Were you up all night on a search?" she asked, her voice urgent and horrified. Geoff and I were both members of a search-and-rescue team, and over the previous couple of years, our pagers had often woken us in the night. We'd strap on our always-ready, fifty-pound rescue packs and hustle out the door to tromp through the wilderness hollering for some lost soul, often in the midst of a storm. But we'd both turned off our pagers many months ago, too busy with the work of building. Our backpacks were still packed, but they were buried under shovels and picks in a corner of the shed.

I stopped trudging up the path and looked at Jessica, astonished. *Yesterday's work isn't enough to explain my appearance?* I thought. *To look this bad, I'd also need to have been up all night searching?* But she had worked all day yesterday too, and she seemed fresh and ready for the day.

The pain and fatigue in my body spoke to me. It seemed to be saying something more than *Stop. Rest. Lie down.* A thought crept into my mind for the first time: Maybe I wasn't just tired. Maybe I was sick.

A COUPLE OF MONTHS LATER, in the fall, I noticed that when I walked from my office to the bathroom at St. John's College, where I taught mathematics and the classics, I sometimes trailed my hand along the wall, vaguely worried that I might pass out. My exhaustion got so extreme that, despite my scramble to get the house closed in before winter, I took whole days off from the physical labor of building. But even on my rest days, I dragged, and I felt no stronger when I got back to work. Geoff's parents heard the weary desperation in my voice and offered us money to hire more help. I gratefully accepted.

In the winter, I got worried enough to see my doctor about it. I'd been tired, I told her, really tired, all the time—chronically fatigued. Might I have chronic fatigue syndrome?

She looked up from her pad and into my eyes. "Are you under stress?" she asked in the gentlest tone imaginable, her face soft. I instantly knew I was going to cry, and I felt a blast of hatred toward her. *Why does she have to be so nice about it?* If she'd asked that with more detachment, perhaps I could have answered in kind. I felt as though a thin scab allowed me to function in the world, and she, with her wretched kindness, had ripped it right off. I knew she couldn't give me the motherly care that her tone promised. She could only remind me of what I lacked— my mother had died of cancer when I was 18.

I mumbled out a yes, mentioning the house and my husband. She handed me a tissue. "Sounds like you have good reason to be worn out," she said, in that same tender voice.

Then she asked if I was feeling depressed. I told her my therapist had said I wasn't, that my life was just falling apart, and that's different. The doctor offered me antidepressants anyway, but I declined them, mostly out of loyalty to my therapist.

I left her office with nothing that would help, but even so, I thought she was almost certainly right: I just needed to finish the house and get my life in order. I'd be fine.

In late 2001, three and a half years after Geoff and I began building, we—or really I—finally finished the house. I knew the house was more beautiful than I could have imagined when we started, but I could hardly see the lovely curves of the kiva fireplace or the swirling brown of the walnut counter. I saw the screws that protruded from the ceiling into the living room and the mar where the plaster had gotten wiped down with a dirty cloth while it was drying.

Whatever my therapist said, I was clearly depressed. Every time I drove along one leftward curve of the road as I came home, I had the urge to unbuckle my seatbelt, crank the steering wheel to the right, and tumble down the piñon-studded cliff beyond. I eventually decided to try antidepressants when my doctor suggested them to prevent the migraines that had been plaguing me. I kept secret my hope that the pills might also improve my mood and energy. I found that they did none of those things, but instead made my teeth chatter so hard it felt like my brain might rattle out of my skull. I declined the offer of a different flavor of antidepressant.

Geoff's mental state continued to be far worse than mine. He had lost his job and spent hours driving around aimlessly in his truck. His brown Toyota seemed to reflect his internal state: A missing screw left its license plate hanging askew, and the stickers declaring his ham radio call sign were crooked because of the medication-induced shake in his hands. My desperation to save him had withered. Now I just hoped I could save myself.

We agreed on the obvious: Our marriage was over. But Geoff insisted on moving into the house, setting up residence in the guest room. I feared I wouldn't be able to get him to leave, an uneasiness that mounted as he unpacked his library of math books, a residue of our former lives. The volumes formed a more impressive collection than most of our professors at MIT had had. I knew he'd read few of them, and now that we'd both left graduate school, he almost certainly never would. Had those thousands of dollars of math books been an early sign of his mania that I'd missed, a harbinger of the spending sprees to come?

Geoff's sister came to visit for Thanksgiving just after we'd moved into the house, and bless her heart, she found him a new place to live and helped him move out. By then, I couldn't feel enough to be heartbroken.

I set to work to rebuild my life. I was at my happiest coming out of a good class discussion—my life might be a mess, but at the college, I felt confident I was contributing to the world. I volunteered with Big Brothers Big Sisters. I forced myself to socialize, even though I often only wanted to curl up in bed. I started running, picking up again three years after running a marathon back when Geoff and I had first begun building. I rejoined the search-and-rescue team, though when my body slumped at the mere idea of carrying a loaded pack, I stuck to administration, eventually becoming president of the team.

I was coming back to life, but it was slow. Something had broken in me that I didn't know how to heal. At 30, how had I managed to make such a mess of my life? The easiest mistake to point to had been marrying Geoff. He'd already slid well into bipolar disorder by then, so what had I been thinking?

The memory of the morning of our wedding pricked me like an invisible pin stuck in a chair, and mentally I shifted this way and that, trying to find some position I could sit in unpoked. When Geoff and I got married, we were in the middle of building our house, and our wedding reception was our wall-raising. The morning of the ceremony, we carved out enough time to hike up our south hill and sit quietly together in the early morning light. We'd planned to say a few things about each other as part of the ceremony, but I'd been rushing all summer to get the house ready to stack the bales and hadn't yet found a moment to consider what I'd say. That half hour on the hilltop was my only time to do it.

We sat there together as the sky brightened behind us, looking out across the Rio Grande Valley. It was the first time I'd sat still in weeks. The early-morning chill seeped beneath my shell of determination, bringing a sudden, unwelcome awareness: I was terrified.

Already, then, I'd felt him slipping through my fingers, as though his illness were gelatinizing his very flesh, oozing him into a different world. *Oh god, what am I doing?*

I glanced over, and Geoff's face looked vague, lost, its edges blurred with insecurity. I no longer knew what was his illness and what was him—or even if the question made sense. I tried to blink my eyes clear as I wrapped my arms around my goosebump-covered knees and looked out across the valley.

Our little village snaked along the stream below, and the ribbon of green stretched out across the strange, eroded pink mud-hills called barrancas toward the Rio Grande. Georgia O'Keeffe's favorite mountain, Cerro Pedernal, poked up like a pig snout on the other side of the great valley where 35 million years before, the continent had been ripped open and wrenched apart, the wound slowly healing, slowly becoming this place where I was staking my tiny claim.

I reached back in my memories to remind myself that Geoff had once been Geoff, that I hadn't been crazy to fall in love with him. He'd caught my eye the first day of my first undergraduate class at MIT, a strapping 29-year-old man among the nerdy boys that surrounded me. We'd discovered we were in the wrong classroom and run down the hall together. Later, his voice had sliced through the testosterone-driven clamor of the math study group we both joined, saying as he often did, "Wait, guys, I think Julie's idea might work." Then his arms had wrapped around me for the first time, his scent had filled my nostrils, and I'd suddenly known that my life was about to change. And later, I had woken in the night, felt how graduate school was breaking me, and sobbed for hours in his arms so intensely I wondered if I might suffocate, while he massaged my face and stroked my hair.

Sitting on that rock on the hilltop years later, those times felt mythical, remote, like someone else's life. But I reminded myself that all that was real, as real as the pain that was ripping me apart as surely as the rift had split the continent.

I pulled the piñon-spiked air deep into my lungs, and the immensity of the world filled me, the forces so far beyond the hubbub of individual wanting and avoiding and trying to bring about, beyond my desire for a happy marriage, a healthy partner, and children playing in the stream. Clarity flowed from deep in the earth, up through the rock I was sitting on, searing my spine as it reached beyond me into the sky. It etched into my bones the knowledge of the beauty and wholeness of the world, even though—as I would eventually discover—I had no more power to heal my beloved than I had to close that great gash in the earth.

I looked at Geoff again, his familiar strong brow, his fluid body that could pick me up as if I were made of air: I loved him. We would join our lives together. And we would let the wind and the rain and the ice shape us, as it had the rock.

I took his hand and we walked down the hill together to meet our guests.

Remembering this two years later, living alone in the house we'd built, I thought, *Stupid! I was just too young and starry-eyed when we got married to know how terrible things could get.* My psyche seemed to have played a stunningly cruel trick on me, pouring that clarity into me the morning of our wedding and then snatching it away, leaving me surrounded by the shards of that world I had envisioned as whole and beautiful.

But that grim view provided me no peace or resolution, because it couldn't answer a basic question: If I couldn't trust a feeling like that clarity, then what the hell *could* I trust? As I went through my days, teaching my classes and living in my house, I felt disoriented, as if I were descending stairs and had lost the feeling of where the next step would be, my leg dangling in the air while my body still traveled downward, my foot seeking solid wood while my back braced to tumble, tumble, tumble.

Mostly I just tried to set these questions aside and build a new life for myself. My exhaustion was easing, but I couldn't exercise the way I used to. I had trained myself to run slowly when I was building up to the marathon, but now I wasn't just slow—my body plodded along like an old nag, inching forward joylessly and only when forced. I found it bizarre that all that labor of building could leave me out of shape, but so it seemed to be.

Perhaps, I thought, the problem was that, mysteriously, I had gained 40 pounds while building, despite eating the same way as ever and working like hell. I was running such short distances that I swallowed my pride and joined a group of couch potatoes training to run a 5K, only to find that I trailed the back of the pack week after week. Over months, I barely got faster or stronger. Nor did I lose any weight.

Still, gradually, gradually, I began to feel a bit of the pleasure in exercise I had before. I also found myself noticing the incredible blueness of the sky with a shock, as if I hadn't truly seen it in years. Sometimes as I drove home, I traced the voluptuous lines of the hills and marveled at this place I lived in. I still couldn't see a path from my broken-down life to the life I wanted to live, but I did feel like I was drifting in the right direction.

Then one Saturday morning in late 2002, about a year after finishing the house, I received a letter in my college mailbox informing me that my reappointment at the college had been denied. My knees went weak and I closed my eyes. Teaching had been the one thing I thought I was doing well, the thing I held on to amidst the devastation. I felt as though gravelly pavement were scouring the thin pink flesh just emerging from under warty scabs.

The first thought that went through my mind was, *Julie, this is the limit. You now have permission to kill yourself.* The thought washed over me like a warm shower, comforting and welcome.

But when, driving home, I reached the cliff that had drawn me for so long, I found to my surprise that I no longer felt tempted to crank the steering wheel over the edge. Time, it seemed, was healing me more than I had realized.

When I went to teach on Monday morning, I could barely look my colleagues or students in the eye. But when my students heard that I hadn't been reappointed, they gathered in a tight knot around me. "We're going to get this fixed!" they cried, full of the youthful power that had been ground to powder in me. I cried as they hugged me.

Over the coming weeks, I began recognizing other emotions mixed in with the shock and humiliation and fear that I expected: Relief. Excitement. Possibility. As much as I loved teaching, I felt like I never finished a thought of my own—my job, after all, was to help my students develop their thoughts in our discussions, not to run off with mine. Fantasizing about a career with my own ideas and creativity at its center made me tingly and nervous.

I appealed the reappointment decision and, gratifyingly, got my job back. But it was time to move on. I couldn't imagine spending the next 40 years of my life doing this. I felt hungry and trapped, like a dragon imprisoned in a cave, twisting up as I outgrew the space. Instead of slowly knitting myself together, it seemed to be time to blow my life up completely, to change everything, to see how I was out of my confinement.

And surely, in the process, I would leave the dregs of my exhaustion behind.

CHAPTER 2

CRIPPLED

Fall 2005

Blowing my life up sounded like a good idea, but I had to figure out what to do next.

I wasn't drawn to math research anymore. My experience in graduate school at MIT had been brutal, and I hadn't recovered from it. I also found that I was more drawn to the real world now than I had been in my early twenties. I wanted to become more fully baked, acquiring a browned crust where academia had left me white and squishy. My thoughts turned toward writing: Beginning in childhood, I'd been conceiving of books I'd like to write. I settled on writing about science, since that seemed to weave together many of my interests and talents. To get started, I decided to do a yearlong graduate program in science writing at the University of California, Santa Cruz.

The morning I left Santa Fe for Santa Cruz, my next-door neighbor brought me fresh milk from his goats. I wrapped my hands around the jar, a quart of my own beloved valley to fortify me for the trip, and then tucked it next to me in the car's console. I watched my house disappear behind the oaks and willows as I drove away pulling a U-Haul trailer, my heart simultaneously constricting and expanding. I felt as though I were ripping myself apart in leaving my house, but it was time to leave the agony of the past few years behind and build a new life. I wondered who

I would be when I drove a trailer in the other direction on this road and reunited with my house and land.

I felt like my body was finally coming back, so when I arrived in Santa Cruz, I decided not to buy a parking pass and to bike to class instead. Biking required climbing a brutally steep road through massive redwoods, emerging from the trees to find a view that stretched all the way across the Monterey Bay—well worth the sweat and pain, I figured. I started off so slow I half expected to be passed by a toddler on a tricycle. *That just means I'll improve more quickly,* I figured. *Plus, it gives me a bit more time to enjoy my ride.* At the end of the first quarter, though, another bicyclist flew past me and called out encouragements: "It's always hard the first few times you try it! You're doing great!" I smiled through gritted teeth: *First few times, huh? Why am I not getting faster?*

It was easy to push away those worries in my delight over graduate school. A fleet of top-notch writers devoted themselves to my learning, and as a grown-up, I was exempt from the angst of having my identity at stake. I spent half my time in class and half at internships with newspapers and magazines in the area, writing some science stories and some more general ones. I wrote a story about an Internet cable being installed in Monterey Bay that underwater robots would use to communicate with their scientist overlords to reveal the unexplored deep sea; I interviewed an 11-year-old girl who rescued herself and her two younger brothers after her uncle stabbed her parents and set their house ablaze; I walked through stubbly fields with farmers whose land would be ruined if neglected levees failed in an earthquake. I felt like I had a backstage pass to the entire world.

I went home to Santa Fe for winter break, and since I'd rented out my house, I stayed with my next-door neighbors in my own enchanted valley. I hiked up the stream to the first big waterfall, which had frozen into a fractal fantasyland of delicate pillars. Falling water flickered behind the ice like the royal occupants of a rococo ice palace. I felt my body realigning with the land, as though my feet were reaching down through the earth, my body stretching up along the waterfall and blending with the water, my fingers extending to the peaks of the mountains where the water first seeped out of the ground. When I visited my renters in my house, I was oddly pleased to see that they seemed to be camping out, their belongings strewn about in ragtag piles. It was easy to imagine sweeping them out of there and reoccupying it myself.

My love for my own house and land simultaneously grounded and ungrounded me. I was building a new life when I still didn't understand why my previous life had dissolved. I felt like a tree emerging from a tiny crack in a cliff. Would the next wind rip me out by the roots? And although I liked my classmates, instructors, and colleagues, I struggled against a relentless loneliness. Were these my people—or at least could they become so?

Still, when I got together with friends from the college in Santa Fe, I confidently reported that I was thrilled with my new life. My worries squirreled themselves into a corner of my mind, rarely emerging into consciousness. And in any case, the change felt irrevocable: I seemed to have stepped across a small crack, and now the Atlantic Ocean was opening up between me and my old colleagues, our two continents drifting inexorably apart.

The first day of classes after I returned to Santa Cruz after winter break, my legs screamed as I rode my bike up the hill. I tried standing up for better leverage, but it felt so hard that I sat down and shifted to the easiest gear, my legs spinning as I labored but barely moved. I found myself eyeing the hollows at the roots of trees, imagining curling up in them and sleeping. The ride didn't just feel hard, harder even than when I'd first arrived—it also felt in some indefinable way wrong, like I shouldn't ask this of my body.

Fuck this, I finally thought, turning my bike around to zoom back down the hill. My joy at the effortless speed temporarily soothed my shock and disappointment.

I tried biking another day with the same result, and then another. Never again did I ride up the hill. I didn't give up on exercise, but I scaled back, doing short runs instead. I couldn't come up with a reasonable explanation for what was happening to me. It didn't seem normal, but I didn't know of any disease whose only manifestation was an inability to exercise much. And as long as I didn't push it, I felt fine.

An old boyfriend visited for a few days in the spring, providing a longed-for respite from the loneliness. I took him up to campus, we ate at my favorite burrito joint, we rode a tandem bike across the Golden Gate

Bridge, and our bodies again fit together when we tangoed. Shortly before he left, though, we reenacted one of our old arguments, and I was forced to remember all the ways we weren't right for each other. After he left, I found that I could barely get out of bed. I shivered uncontrollably, and my back throbbed. My new therapist, Chris, suggested it could just be an odd emotional reaction to having spent time with my ex-boyfriend. *I'll just take good care of myself today,* I figured. But the next day, I had to call in sick to my internship. The third day, I staggered through classes in a daze and then went back to bed. I told people I had the flu, but it wasn't like any flu I'd ever experienced—no stuffy nose, no upset stomach, just pain and an exhaustion that pulverized my brain.

Over a week, the "flu" gradually faded away, and I dove back into my work and thought about it no further.

I finished the Santa Cruz program in June and moved to Berkeley to do an internship at the alumni magazine of the University of California, Berkeley, and to be with a new guy I'd met, William. William struck me as smart and grounded, less impressed with me than my previous partners had been. He seemed like someone with the strength to stand up to me.

After nine intensive months of graduate school, I figured I was finally really going to get into shape. I didn't know why I'd lost my ability to exercise in the spring, but now that the stress of graduate school was over, surely I could get through that strange glitch, whatever it was. I rode my bike in the Berkeley hills and delighted in how I could so quickly pedal from urban intensity into the wilderness of Tilden Park—and I was even getting a little bit faster. The day after a ride, though, I was always outrageously sore. William and I would laugh about my "Frankenstein walk." I "worked from home" on those days, though mostly I lay in bed, drifting in and out of sleep. I finally got worried enough to go see a doctor in Berkeley, but all she suggested was to test my thyroid, which turned out to be normal.

In the fall of 2006 I moved to Washington, DC, for a four-month internship at *Science News,* and by that time, I was forced to admit that something was wrong. I had to give up exercise entirely so I could do my work consistently, and I rested almost all the rest of the time. I went to a doctor a friend had recommended, and she put me on adrenal supplements, probiotics, and a near-vegan, grain-free diet. None of it made me feel any better—though as a side effect, I did steadily and happily lose the weight I had gained while building my house.

William invited me on a trip to Peru to celebrate the end of my internship in January. Visions of Machu Picchu dancing in my head, I got a hepatitis A vaccine for the trip on a Thursday evening in November. Twenty-four hours later, I felt anesthetized, as if some external force were shutting my brain down.

I made it home from work in a daze, fell asleep, and then slept through the weekend, finally forcing myself up on Sunday afternoon to get groceries. When I got out of bed, I staggered as if I'd powered up a mountain on my bike the day before rather than sleeping for 48 hours.

Wow, weird, I thought. *Maybe moving around will help.* I headed out to walk to the grocery store, just a half mile away, but soon, my walking deteriorated further and I stopped to rest, sprawling on a lawn to call William back in Berkeley. I laughed, telling him that my Frankenstein walk had turned into an old-lady shuffle. *Ha ha ha! I can't even stand up straight!* Laughing calmed me down, making it seem self-evident that this would pass, just as it always had after exercise.

But after chatting with William and resting another half hour, I knew I couldn't possibly walk to the store. It started not to seem so funny anymore. I had left my car in Berkeley and was getting around by foot and metro, so I called the family I rented a room from to ask for a ride. The mother agreed, but grudgingly. At the store, I used the shopping cart as a walker, and by the time I had finished checking out, I felt delirious with exhaustion. I seethed when my landlady didn't help lift the bags into the car, instead just watching me as I lifted each bag with two hands, quickly moved one hand to the side of the car to stabilize myself, then swung the bag into the car with a groan. After I got home and put my groceries away, I could only get up the stairs to my third-floor bedroom backward, on my butt, lifting myself a stair at a time. As I collapsed into bed, the fear I had been pushing aside flooded over me, and I sobbed into the pillow.

Something is really, really wrong with me.

I tried to calm down and think it through. It felt like a mash-up of that weird flu I'd had in Santa Cruz and my post-exercise pain and hob-bling, with extra intensity sprinkled on top like hot sauce. I already knew something was going wrong with my body, but this was a new and terrify-ing level. What the hell was I going to do? My thoughts started scrabbling toward solutions—Call my doctor! Find a specialist! Go to the emer-gency room!—but the mental effort of trying to figure it out made my brain hurt. I also recognized that the middle of a crisis wasn't a great time for strategizing. Surely my body would recover on its own, just as it had before, and then I'd work out my next steps.

And indeed, although I woke up Monday morning feeling far too ill to go to work, over the course of the day, my walking normalized and my strength returned. *Thank god,* I thought, *it's going away, just like I expected.*

It occurred to me that maybe this was all just a strange side effect of the vaccine, unrelated to the other ways my body had been struggling. I turned to Google and read that the hepatitis A vaccine was pretty benign, with no similar bad reactions. *Still,* I thought, *maybe I'm just special, giving the doctors a run for their money with my one-of-a-kind bodily freak-out.*

That evening, I had a phone call with my therapist, Chris, and I pre-sented the episode as concerning but not really a big deal. I heard the worry in his voice as he questioned me about it. "It's okay," I told him. "It's over. I'll talk to my doctor about it the next time I see her."

But it wasn't over. I woke up Tuesday feeling addled. I staggered out of bed and went down the stairs on my butt to get to the bathroom. My face in the mirror looked weirdly swollen. I butt-scooted my way back upstairs to bed and then slept through most of the day.

During a brief period of awakeness, I called my doctor's office—that seemed like a straightforward, reasonable step to take. But I was told I couldn't see her until the following week. Because my mother had been a Christian Scientist and had avoided doctors as the religion dictated, I had little experience with them, and I wasn't quite sure what doctor-oriented people even did in a situation like this. I'd never been to an emergency room and couldn't imagine going all by myself. Plus, how would I get there? I didn't have a car, the metro was too far away, I'd probably scare the hell out of a taxi driver in this state, and calling an ambulance seemed awfully histrionic. *This isn't precisely an emergency anyway, is it? It's not like I'm in immediate danger.*

The idea that my body would recover on its own was irresistibly alluring, so much nicer than getting all worked up about it. Nearly every health problem I'd ever had had gone away with nothing more than some good self-care.

My thoughts kept drifting to Majorca. Wasn't that where the composer Chopin had gone with his lover when his health was poor? Imagining it made my situation feel almost romantic. I fantasized about lying on some beach, having a buff male attendant wheel me about, bringing me delicious food and giving me massages. Surely that would fix me right up. I Googled to see if any such option existed, but all I found was a fancy medical spa in Mexico that charged $5,000 a week plus whatever their dubious-sounding treatments cost. I also read that Chopin and his lover had fled Majorca, frozen out by north winds and unsympathetic locals.

Okay, maybe not such a good plan.

Unsure of what else to do, I went back to sleep.

Wednesday morning, I felt better. I walked to the shower fluidly, grinning and swinging my arms with delight. After I got dressed, though, the bed seemed to be exerting an irresistible gravitational force. I lay down and then woke up several hours later, still exhausted. I sprawled in bed, limp as a fish.

I felt as though I could hear the tinkle of fantasies shattering as they fell to the ground. *This is seriously fucked up,* I thought. *Time to face it.*

I started by calling my boss and explaining that I was very ill and didn't know how long I'd be out. The warmth and concern in his voice— "You just take care of yourself, don't worry about us"—made my breath catch in my throat.

After I hung up the phone, I lay back in bed, smoothed my breathing, and evaluated the situation: Something was clearly wrong with my body on a level I'd never experienced. It had been five days, and I was no better. I was living in a city where I hardly knew anyone. I didn't have a car. I couldn't get to work. I couldn't cook for myself. I couldn't even get groceries. *This is not going to work.*

My first thought was to get help. I'd already called my one old friend who lived near DC, but she was busy with her three kids and her job. She might, if she was lucky, be able to come see me in a week or so. My only family, really, was my sister, who lived in Arkansas. I'd called her a couple of times and she talked sympathetically with me, but she never initiated a call herself, and caring for herself and her daughter seemed like as much as she could handle. William felt like a lifeline, and we talked frequently. I mentioned the possibility of him flying out to help, and he didn't refuse but certainly didn't jump at it either. I wondered what the cost of him coming would be, both financially and in relationship capital.

I want my mother, I thought. If my mother were alive, she would already be on an airplane to come help me. She would fly me home—I would *have* a home to go to, I thought, imagining the renters who occupied my own house—and she would ask me what I wanted her to cook for me. I'd tell her vegetable beef stew and homemade multigrain bread and caramel brownies (my new, useless diet be damned), and she'd bring them to me in bed. She would stroke my hair while I fell asleep with my head in her lap, and I would know without question that she'd help me figure out what to do.

Okay, Julie. Back to reality.

I felt as though my net of connections had frayed, and now I had fallen and was crashing through it. I couldn't quite believe it: Wasn't there someone, somewhere, who would come in and take care of me when I so obviously needed it?

My computer dinged with an e-mail from a coworker, Susan, who had heard I was ill and wrote to ask what she could do to help. She explained that she lived alone and whenever she had a crisis, friends and neighbors bailed her out. "So my deal with the universe is that I try to build up karma by picking up other folks' prescriptions, etc., in hopes that friends and strangers will keep stepping in to help me out." She offered to cook for me, clean my house, shop for groceries, or even to sleep on my couch to keep an eye on me. She closed her e-mail with, "Please, PLEASE call/e-mail me."

I sobbed.

Then I called Susan up: Could she help me make stew from the massive quantity of vegetables I had bought on Sunday and didn't have the strength to cook? "I'll come tonight," she said.

Then I tried to think. Clearly, I needed to get out of DC and go somewhere where I knew people and could get around. A cousin in Berkeley was going out of town for a week—perhaps, I thought, I could go back there, stay in her house (and hence not impose on William), and find a doctor. At least I'd have my car, and I'd be in a town I knew, and I'd be with my boyfriend again. The only problem was the stairs. My cousin's house was full of stairs, a full flight up the hill just to reach her front door, and more to get to a bedroom. I couldn't see how to manage that.

I talked about this with William, and he offered to let me stay with him for a bit while I sorted things out. I gratefully accepted. Surely I'd quickly figure out what was wrong with me and be able to make some long-term plan.

My boss agreed that I could do my internship from California, as I was capable. William had a friend in DC I'd met once who volunteered to come help me pack—that is, he volunteered to pack for me while I laid in bed and pointed. I found a not-too-horrendously expensive flight back to Berkeley for Saturday, and Susan agreed to take me to the airport.

On Saturday, I woke up and found that not only could I stay awake, not only could I walk, I could even carry things upstairs! I laughed with some embarrassment with Susan about it and imagined myself showing up in Berkeley feeling fine, William having a distant suspicion I'd made the whole thing up. Well, I figured, at least I'd get to go have a good time with my boyfriend, and then I could come back and finish my internship.

At the airport, I settled into a wheelchair, though the move seemed excessively cautious. I decided to walk through the metal detector to avoid an awkward pat-down, but when I stood up, I found I was staggering again. After I was wheeled to the gate, I walked slowly and carefully onto the airplane, found three blessedly empty seats in a back row, and stretched out. *It's okay, Julie*, I thought. *Sleep and you'll feel better.*

I was woken by a bumpy descent into Atlanta to find that I was desperately tired, more tired than I'd ever felt before, so tired I felt frantic. I waited for everyone else to exit the airplane, and when I got up to leave, I could hardly even stand, having to support myself on the seat backs. I lurched from one seat back to the next, groaning loudly. The flight attendant flapped her hands and clucked, "Be careful! Be careful! Be careful!" I didn't have the energy even to glare at her, so I kept my head down as I continued my lurch. Then the flight attendant declared the problem must be the weight of my backpack—though she didn't offer to help me with it.

At the end of the long trek out of the airplane, I was shocked to find no wheelchair. The flight attendant told me to wait and it would be along sometime soon. There was nowhere to sit. Perhaps, I suggested through gritted teeth, she might inquire about the wheelchair for me, since I was barely capable of standing. She reluctantly did so, and then she kept gibbering over me, this time insisting I put on my jacket. Finally, I lost my temper: "Look! I'm sick! The problem isn't the backpack or the jacket or anything else, I'm just sick!" She was silent.

By the time the wheelchair arrived, I barely made my connection. I had started shivering violently, though I wasn't cold. When we reached the gate, the wheelchair pusher said in her sweet-as-sugar-pie voice, "Honey, I'm so glad you made the flight. You're not feeling well and just want to be home." Teary, I gave her a $20 tip.

I staggered onto the next plane, not knowing that I could have ordered a special wheelchair that would fit in the aisle. I was so bent over that I could barely support myself on the tops of the seats and was tempted to lean down to the armrests. The other passengers openly stared. I collapsed into my seat and shivered. I pulled my pillow out of my backpack and buried my face in it, hoping no one could hear me crying.

By the time I arrived in San Francisco, I felt better, and I was even able to walk off the airplane without groaning, using the seat backs just for balance, with mincing steps. The wheelchair pusher wheeled me to the baggage carousel, where William was waiting for me, standing in his familiar blue jacket. I searched his face: What was he feeling, seeing me in a wheelchair? Could he handle this? But I couldn't read him. I saw the crinkles around his eyes, perhaps some anticipation, perhaps anxiety. I felt terribly small and low in the chair, so I struggled up to standing. William wrapped his arms around me, and I breathed his scent.

I'd made it home—or at least, as close to home as I was going to get.

CHAPTER 3

DOCTORS

A few days after I returned to Berkeley, William drove me to the office of the only neurologist I could find who had an appointment available in the next several weeks. I felt as though the signal to move was getting lost on its way from my brain to my legs, so a neurologist seemed to be the right choice. As we drove, I struggled with a feeling of unreality: I had never been seriously sick before, never gone to a doctor desperate to know what was wrong with me. Multiple sclerosis niggled at my mind. Or maybe Lou Gehrig's disease?

I felt my mother's horror projecting toward me from the grave. She would have hated to see me sick, but she also would have hated to see me going to a doctor. Christian Science was central to her conception of the world—including the religion's rejection of medicine. When her bowel became obstructed, she hesitantly saw a doctor and even agreed to surgery, but she would never have gone back if I hadn't insisted on it. She didn't even fully acknowledge she had cancer. "That's what *they* say," she would sniff.

My only significant experience with a doctor had been when I was 16 and a freshman in college. I developed a robin's-egg-size cyst next to my vagina, and the throbbing pain in my groin shooed me into the doctor's office fast. When the first doctor I went to refused to treat me without a parent's permission, I huffed out. I sure as hell didn't want to ask for my mother's permission—that was bound to be a battle. But even more, I was morally offended at the idea that I wasn't allowed to make decisions about my own body. The next doctor treated me without hesitation and told me I had to have surgery to cut open the cyst.

When I told my mother, she cried, "You're going to let them cut into your sacred body!" and then she refused to talk to me for several days. In the past, I had always scurried to appease her when she was upset, but this time, I felt a shocking urge to roll my eyes. Despite her histrionics, I knew the real problem wasn't the surgery—it was that I'd excluded her. If I'd included her in the decision-making process, I was pretty sure she'd have gone along with it. Anyway, I knew I'd already thought about the problem in the ways her Christian Science mindset dictated: I considered whether it had any emotional significance in my life (not hard to figure, given that I had just started having sex); I worked to unravel my own fear about it; I believed that internal psychological and spiritual work might cure it (though it hadn't, at least so far). But I didn't share any of that with her—*I am not interested in discussing my vagina with my mother, thank you.* And if she was upset about that, well, too bad.

A classmate took me to surgery and let me recover in her dorm room. The following day, my mother told me stiffly that a friend of hers had told her that she should apologize. "So I'm apologizing," she said, her voice flat. I had never heard her apologize before, and I felt pleased but uneasy: What did the word "apologize" mean, coming from her? I gradually realized that it was mostly an agreement not to discuss it again.

The surgery was, in my view, a smashing success. Within a day, I had no more pain, and within a couple of weeks, I was back to having sex. My mother might have argued that it didn't solve the problem on the real, spiritual level, that the cyst was a manifestation of deeper dynamics within myself that I hadn't addressed and that would thus crop up elsewhere in my life. But I wasn't so convinced of that. Having surgery directly addressed one important dynamic in my life: It established a needed boundary with my mother. The surgeon's knife that had sliced through my cyst had also sliced through an emotional cord binding us too tightly together. I figured I'd done the precise psychological and spiritual work the cyst was demanding of me, and I believed God himself would have approved.

As William and I drove to the neurologist's office these years later, though, I felt as though my mother were scolding me from the dead. I wanted to growl at her: *What the hell do you want me to do now, Ma? I've been trying to grow my way out of this illness psychologically and spiritually for years, and look where that's gotten me.* And you're *certainly not here to help. Am I really supposed to be this sick without getting care from a doctor?*

William's voice, tight and halting, interrupted my internal conversation. "Some of the possibilities we're facing," he said, "I'm not sure I can handle." He was looking straight ahead at the road, showing me only his hawkish profile.

The air in my lungs crystallized into frozen daggers and my mind turned to static. Dimly, I realized I was supposed to say something. "Okay," I mumbled.

I closed my eyes and let the static engulf me. *Do people really just decide they can't handle something? Wish I could decide that and escape whatever the hell this is. But yeah, I suppose we've only been together a few months, so what do I have a right to expect from him?* I felt as though the two feet between our shoulders were expanding as the whole world receded, leaving me hurtling through empty space.

I tried to picture asking my sister to take care of me. I couldn't imagine her saying no, but I couldn't imagine her managing to do it either.

There was no one else to ask.

I opened my eyes again and watched the shabby double-decker houses along Ashby Avenue glide past. I'd have to think about this at another time. *I'll figure it out. I always do.*

When we arrived at the neurologist's office, the closest parking place was a good hundred feet from the door. I used crutches, but I wasn't sure they helped. My feet seemed to be glued to the pavement. I leaned forward into the crutches and, using all my strength, pulled my leg up, embarrassed by the groan I couldn't suppress. Nothing happened. Suddenly, my foot popped from the ground and then crashed down again, a few inches forward. I panted, gathered my strength, repeated the effort. Each step got a little harder, each groan a little louder. I looked down, ignoring any gawking onlooker, and focused on my task. William ran ahead to open doors, but he couldn't do much to help me get my legs to move.

In the neurologist's office, I recited my story. The doctor listened impassively, his round, blank face revealing little. He had me move to the examining table and pushed down on my leg, telling me to resist. "Harder!" he cried. I pushed until tears sprang to my eyes. "Harder!" he cried again.

After the exam, I lay on the table looking up at the ceiling. My legs had turned to throbbing slabs of meat, and I didn't think I could even shift them on the table. My brain felt like an overripe peach, swollen, bruised, and delicate. I worked on smoothing the catches in my breath before they could turn into sobs. *Odd,* I thought, *I don't really feel upset. I don't really feel anything.* The tears seemed to condense directly from the exhaustion that throbbed through my body. I focused on my lungs expanding, contracting, expanding, trying to crowd out any internal speculation about what the neurologist would say.

The doctor proclaimed, "Your strength is within the normal range. There's nothing neurologically wrong with you."

I couldn't make sense of what I was hearing. That was obviously impossible.

"You have chronic fatigue syndrome," he said.

Fatigue? I thought. Sure, I'd been tired for years, and I'd wondered if chronic fatigue syndrome might explain it. But *this* wasn't fatigue. I couldn't fucking walk! And wait—the neurologist hadn't even done any fancy tests. He'd only pushed on my legs.

I struggled to speak—I knew what I wanted to ask, but the words scampered away from me like a flurry of mice. I finally mumbled something about further testing.

"Well, yes, I could order an MRI, or maybe an electromyogram," he said, "but I already know the results will be normal."

Treatments? I asked. Nothing he knew of. Other doctors? No, he knew no one to suggest.

I tried to kick my brain into gear. If only I could think, find the thing to say that would penetrate, clear up the confusion. If only I weren't too sick to show him how sick I was.

Finally I asked, "What would you do if it were your wife who was sick like this? Your daughter?"

He shrugged. His round face was blank as the moon.

William and I drove home quietly. I narrowed my consciousness, smaller, smaller, examining the glove box in front of me, fingering the seat belt. I couldn't wonder what was going to happen, couldn't absorb the spectacular uselessness of that neurologist, couldn't contemplate what it all meant. I allowed in just one thought: *Get home, rest.*

LATER, I SAT ON WILLIAM'S BED with its glorious view of the Golden Gate Bridge and Googled "chronic fatigue syndrome." I read the definition aloud to him. Patients with chronic fatigue syndrome—abbreviated CFS—had severe, lasting fatigue not alleviated by rest, along with at least four of eight other symptoms. I went down the list: yes to unrefreshing sleep, muscle pain, increased symptoms after exertion, and concentration problems; no to sore throat, tender lymph nodes, joint pain, and increased headaches. So I guessed I qualified—but my most obvious symptom, near paralysis, wasn't anywhere on the list. Also, "concentration problems" didn't seem like it included becoming nearly unable to speak. Nor did the list include the way my face would swell until I could barely open my eyes.

When I read that many patients are housebound or bedbound for decades and that severe cases of CFS are as bad as full-blown AIDS, congestive heart failure, or late-stage cancer, I couldn't bring myself to read that part aloud. William would have to find that out on his own.

I learned that about three-quarters of patients are women and wondered if unconscious sexism might have explained the neurologist's casualness in tossing me into the CFS pail. The cause was unknown, but the most common understanding was that some event, such as a viral infection or toxic exposure, threw the immune system into chaos, kicking off all the other symptoms. I came across a 1990 *Newsweek* cover article on CFS calling the illness the "yuppie flu." I also read a CFS joke: A doctor diagnoses a patient with CFS. "The good news is that it's not going to kill you," he says. "The bad news is that it's not going to kill you." *Ba dum dum,* I thought. *Hilarious.*

William and I talked strategy, avoiding any longer-term questions. Obviously, we agreed, I hadn't found the right doctor. If chronic fatigue syndrome really explained what was going on with me—doubtful, but possible—I needed a chronic fatigue syndrome specialist. Google revealed one in the area, but only one. *What is the deal with this illness?* I wondered. *Is it really so rare that a single specialist suffices for the entire San Francisco Bay area?* But I'd read that a million Americans had the disease, so that didn't make sense. *Whatever,* I thought. *One is better than none.*

And this doc, an independent practitioner named Michael Rosenbaum, had even written a book on the illness, years earlier. I was unnerved, though, by his Web site's mention that he also specialized in anti-aging. *Would you like your medicine with a side of hocus-pocus?*

With no better options, a week later William and I were sitting in Rosenbaum's waiting room, looking at a framed poster hawking an anti-cellulite treatment, showing the smooth hip of a supine young woman. We giggled at a flyer nearby advertising acai berry juice, which Rosenbaum sold in wine bottles for $35. The brochure rhapsodized about the mysteries of the Amazon jungle where the berries grow, pointing out that darker fruits contain more healthful antioxidants and that acai berries are so dark that "they reflect no light!" When the doctor called us in, I couldn't help but notice the wattles on his neck and his thin, aged skin, neither of which were apparent in his Web site photograph. An anti-aging expert, huh?

But when we started discussing my situation, Rosenbaum seemed surprisingly sane and knowledgeable, citing studies and explaining the physiology underlying my illness. I mentioned that I wrote for *Science News,* and I got the impression that Rosenbaum was trying to impress me, perhaps hoping I'd write about him.

He explained that I had suffered an immune system freak-out called a "cytokine storm." The ordinarily innocuous vaccination I'd gotten for our Peru trip had triggered an exaggerated response from my disordered immune system, he said, and it was the flood of immune molecules that had crippled me.

He recommended supplement after supplement, citing studies showing how this one helped rebalance the immune system, that one supported the cells' tiny power plants called mitochondria that provide energy, and this other one healed broken metabolic pathways. Rosenbaum didn't have an overarching theory to explain the illness, but he seemed to have a reasonably promising bag of tricks.

I walked out with a sackful of supplements and orders for a thousand tests. As I paid up, the office attendant earnestly testified that drinking Rosenbaum's acai berry juice had been the best thing she'd ever done for her health. I passed.

The tests later showed a hodgepodge of findings, none terribly alarming. A couple of viruses my body had long ago beaten down were mildly reactivated. My iron stores and vitamin B_6 and B_{12} levels were all a tad low. My body didn't seem to be metabolizing carbohydrates well. My gut had more *clostridium* bacteria and yeast than Rosenbaum liked. He refined his supplement list and said it was good news: I should be better in no time.

I started taking dozens of pills every day, more pills in a week than I'd taken over my entire life. Each time I parceled out a handful of candy-colored pills, I hesitated before gulping them down—supplements had always struck me as an efficient way of parting the gullible from their money. Few had received any kind of testing, and although I was somewhat reassured by Rosenbaum's references to studies, I would have had to analyze the studies myself to have confidence in their quality—which felt like way too much work, being so sick.

And I thought it unlikely that the research would be very impressive. I thought about how difficult it was, for example, to determine whether postmenopausal hormone therapy increased or decreased the risk of cancer—and serious scientific firepower was devoted to that, with giant, expensive studies over many years. That kind of money wasn't available to test supplements, so the few studies that existed were tiny and unreliable. With little way of determining what worked and what didn't, and lots of plausible stories one could invent about why one compound or another *might* be useful, I figured that most supplements were bound to be useless. Some might even hurt.

And emotionally, for me, supplements were the worst of all worlds: My mother would certainly have rejected them on the grounds that they were medicine, and mainstream doctors would generally have rejected them on the grounds that they were quackery. Having this be the most promising path available to me made me want to weep. I felt no better when I found the same supplements being sold on the Internet for far less than what Rosenbaum had charged me.

But hey, they might work, I reminded myself. *His stories about them sounded good.* In any case, I felt like I had to try something, and at the moment, this was the only thing I knew to try. I bought a tackle box for the pills—perhaps if I could organize them tidily in a box, I could also fit them tidily in my mind.

I was talking with Chris, my therapist, twice a week during this period, sitting in my car a couple of blocks away because it was the only place I could get privacy from William. Chris knew a lot about chronic fatigue syndrome, since his wife was suffering from the illness. They had become convinced that her problems were caused by an exposure to mold and heavy metals, and they'd spent hundreds of thousands of dollars on treatment for her and upended their lives. She was still quite sick, though.

I listened to his stories about their experience, feeling both interest and skepticism. It didn't sound to me like all that money had accomplished much, and although they were certain they were on the right track, I was unconvinced. In any case, I didn't have that kind of money to spend.

Chris recommended that I check out the Web site of a doctor in England. I dutifully did so and was immediately creeped out. She claimed, for example, to have a cure for autism. *That's got to be total BS,* I thought. *If she really had a cure for autism, people would be all over her and I would have heard of her.* Plus, I didn't think "cure" was the right model for autism in the first place, and anyway, why would an autism expert have anything to offer someone with CFS? So I ignored her. *Hey,* I figured, *Chris can continue to be helpful to me psychologically even if he likes stupid doctors, right?*

But the next session, Chris asked me what I thought of her. Uncomfortably, I explained my dubious reaction, citing her autism claims in particular. Chris said that her alleged cure involved some kind of psychological something, so of course people would resist it. *It did?* I thought. *Guess I didn't read that far.* But Chris barreled on, claiming that the fact that I hadn't embraced her approach was proof that I too was resisting something.

I was outraged. My therapist, to whom I was paying good money and who was my only source of support outside of William, was hounding me because I didn't believe in his crazy doctor! I wanted to fire him on the spot—but then I'd have even less support, exactly when I needed it the most. I tried discussing my outrage with him, and he saw my response as further evidence of my resistance. I seethed, but I concluded that talking to him about this was not a good use of my very limited energy or money. I needed him, so I simply steered our conversations away from such topics and toward the areas where I found him helpful.

With no better ideas about what to do, I rested. Sometimes I could walk, other times I could only stagger or crawl. When I felt my best, I worked on stories for *Science News,* managing to carry a reasonable portion of my load. At a moment when I was feeling strong, I went to the grocery store, hoping to pitch in and ease the burden on William—after all, I still had no idea what I'd do if he decided my illness was too much for him. I relished being out of William's bedroom and in the world, admiring Berkeley Bowl's fifteen types of tomatoes and dizzying display of squashes. *I'm getting better!*

But as I lifted the grocery bags into the car, I heard myself groan with the effort, and driving home, my leg shook when I shifted gears. Halfway through dinner, I could no longer lift my arms. William had to help me to bed. I awoke in the night needing to pee, but I got stuck after a couple of steps and couldn't move. I had to ask William to get me a makeshift bedpan—especially horrifying because I knew of his disgust at bodily fluids—and help me back to bed.

But the experience proved useful, because it made me realize that exertion was the key to my ups and downs. I began a program of aggressive rest, and gradually, my strength became more reliable.

This program paid off: Over the following months, I was able to incrementally reduce the restriction on my activities, achieving a carefully regulated but semi-normal life. I exercised, gently, and I learned that the first moment the thought "I'm a little tired" wafted through my mind, I had to stop immediately. If I continued for even five more minutes, I paid for it the next day with pain and paralysis.

William never announced that he could handle it after all, but day by day, he kept showing up. And we were able to find pleasures within my limitations, discussing a movie or walking a few blocks to a café even though we couldn't go hiking. Indeed, a new sweetness was blossoming between us.

Even with my increasing robustness, I at times found myself mysteriously stuck in bed for days, paralyzed, hoping rest would again restore me. The worst was "brain fog," when thinking made my brain throb and feel like it was swelling against the back of my eyeballs. I was barely able to form words and completely unable to do my work. My brain came to feel like an object separate from me, to be managed, coddled, nursed. Or, even more disturbingly, it wasn't separate from me: When it dissolved, I dissolved.

When my internship ended, a regular job or another internship were clearly beyond me. So I started freelancing, ramping up my workload as my health improved. I often worked from bed or sprawled on the carpet. I watched my deadlines carefully, aiming to give myself a comfortable margin in case I got too sick to work. I tapered off the supplements, annoyed and impoverished by the hundreds of dollars they cost every month, and I found that almost none of them seemed to be making a difference.

After immense deliberation, William and I even took our trip to Peru together. I found two stories to report while we were there, and the reporting was a highlight of the trip. One story was about an ancient, primitive astronomical observatory that archaeologists had recently discovered in a 4,000-year-old village, and the scientists gave me and William a private tour. The second was about macaw research in the Amazon, and while we were in the jungle reporting it, a macaw flew into the dining room, stole food off William's plate, and turned to look at me, its beak lining up perfectly below William's own beaklike nose as he grinned and I giggled.

The trip included some minor disasters—when we visited Machu Picchu, the walk up to the town site left me so exhausted I collapsed on the grass and slept—but still, it felt tremendously exotic and expansive: *I'm an international correspondent!* I had barely even considered traveling internationally before, and I felt like William was literally opening the world to me.

After we got back, I kept looking for a doctor who wasn't a quack, or a semi-quack, or a know-nothing. I'd given up on Rosenbaum after concluding that his supplements were almost certainly useless. Still unconvinced that CFS really explained my symptoms, I went to a neurologist at the University of California, San Francisco, who specialized in gait disorders. To guarantee that I could display my own special disordered gait for the doctor, I went for a long bike ride in the Berkeley hills a few hours beforehand, abandoning all restraint, reveling in the joy of pushing my muscles. I got home, bounded upstairs, and danced a jig in front of William. Then, within a couple of hours, I crumpled like a week-old flower. I had successfully crippled myself.

This time, we were savvy enough to ask for a wheelchair to get me into the doctor's office. The doctor then watched me stagger down the hallway. My gait, he said, didn't match any he'd seen before—it wasn't the MS teeter or the Parkinson's shuffle. Instead, he declared that it might be "conversion disorder." That is, it was psychosomatic.

"Fine, then what do I do about it?" I snapped. The doctor had nothing to say and shifted uncomfortably in his chair.

After we left, I felt as though I'd barely escaped with my life. I'd read stories of CFS patients who had gotten locked in psych wards, kept from contact with friends and family so that doctors could dredge out their "false illness beliefs." I wasn't inherently offended by the notion that my psyche could be contributing to my illness—my mother had drummed into me the idea that my patterns of thought could have a profound impact on my body. What angered me was that, coming from this doctor, the idea was so useless. It only added a dollop of blame to the news that the doctor had nothing to offer.

The next stop was a CFS doc who hadn't turned up in my earlier search, one with the stamp of the UC San Francisco teaching hospital. But the doctor turned out to be in the "integrative medicine" department— which, I soon realized, meant that he was integrating standard medicine with the not-so-standard kind. He listened so attentively and warmly that I couldn't help but like him. But ultimately, he recommended almost all the same supplements as Rosenbaum—and added that he'd take a "shamanic journey" after our appointment to see what else he could recommend. He never got back to me, and I felt cheated. If he wasn't going to have anything new that was scientifically grounded to offer me, hey, I at least wanted my damn shamanic journey! Oddly, I felt less uncomfortable with that absurdly unscientific notion than I did with supplements. I knew precisely nothing about shamanic journeys, so who was I to say it was bunk? At least it didn't *claim* to be scientific—and who knows, he might have been able to tell me something thought-provoking.

I dug into the CFS research literature myself, and I quickly realized why the doctors were so useless. The research offered nothing solid to go on. Some researchers focused on "latent infections"—viruses that lots of people get and recover from, but that apparently got fired up again in CFS patients. Rosenbaum's tests had indicated I had some, but then, healthy people sometimes had those too. Other CFS researchers believed that some unknown virus or retrovirus must be actively infecting patients. A reasonable enough theory, I thought, for the patients whose condition had started with a sudden flulike illness, but mine had been a gradual decline with no apparent infection.

I read about a bizarre panoply of other abnormalities, vague types of immune dysfunction and strange cardiac irregularities and gut problems and nervous system issues, but none of these anomalies had the cut-and-dry quality I expected of medical science. Either the abnormalities had no clear treatments, or they might not even *be* abnormalities, or the proposed treatments were untested and suspicious-sounding.

As far as I could tell, saying that I had chronic fatigue syndrome meant little more than that I was tired and sick and no one knew why. I was on my own.

CHAPTER 4

THE SPLIT BETWEEN THE WORLDS

It was a hard thing for me to absorb: Doctors weren't going to help.

It wasn't just that there was no magic pill to fix me. Plenty of other illnesses couldn't be fixed with magic pills—but at least they had legitimate specialists who would try to help. Chronic fatigue syndrome, it seemed, didn't count as a "real" illness. The problem was less that people explicitly asserted that CFS was psychosomatic—my friends never said that, and only that one doctor I saw had discussed the possibility—and more that it lacked all the trappings of legitimacy, with proper doctors and blood tests and researchers and conferences and solid information on Web sites. If you told people you had cancer or multiple sclerosis or lupus, you got lots of sympathy. If you said you had chronic fatigue syndrome, you often heard, "Oh yeah, I'm tired all the time too."

I tried to avoid the name, saying something vague, like "Well, doctors haven't really figured out what's going on with me. Seems to be some strange neurological something." I might add, "Some have called it chronic fatigue syndrome, but that doesn't really mean anything." After all, it wasn't at all clear that whatever was broken in my body was also broken in the bodies of other CFS sufferers. The only thing calling my illness "chronic fatigue syndrome" seemed to add was a stain of stigma, as if the name provided a window into my soul and displayed some moral failing within me.

I focused on learning to manage my illness, living richly in spite of it, and looking for ways to make myself feel better on my own.

I read online patient boards, hoping to learn something useful from my fellow patients, but I was put off by all the ridiculous treatments people discussed seriously: A woman wore magnets in her underwear to balance her hormones; a man was shining a red light up his nose; someone even contemplated drinking cow urine. Even worse was the endless, frightening misery. *These people aren't like me. This won't be my future.*

Even the hopeful stories, when people reported that plausible-sounding treatments were making a difference for them, put me off. None of these treatments seemed to work consistently across patients, nor did I see patients recovering and resuming their lives, only feeling a bit better for a while. That's pretty much what I would have expected to see if none of the treatments were really doing anything and the improvements were random upswings that patients attributed to whatever treatment they happened to be trying at the moment.

Even with that intellectual skepticism, I felt the emotional pull of these stories: *Maybe that would work, maybe, maybe!* In some ways, this frightened me much more than the ridiculous treatments, because I could imagine following that hopeful tug and then gradually getting sucked into one of the cliques that formed around a particular theory or treatment, sucking in all available evidence and interpreting it in support of their theory, repeating unproven claims so often they began to feel like facts.

So I shut my computer and analyzed my experiences for myself. I scoured my activities, my diet, my environment, coming up with endless theories about what might have caused the downturn. For a couple of weeks, cutting out gluten seemed to help—hurrah! But then I got worse again. Still, I thought, maybe the downturn was caused by something else and cutting out gluten really was helping—you never know. I tried gorging on bread and didn't have any problem immediately afterward or the next day, but I felt lousy the day after that—could I have had a delayed reaction? Or maybe the problem wasn't gluten, it was milk, or sugar, or nightshades, or all of the above, or something else entirely.

I kept up the dietary experimentation, but I had lots of nondietary ideas too. Maybe, I thought, I needed to rest absolutely as much as possible, or to build up really gradually, or to just get over myself and stop worrying so much about overdoing it. Maybe I wasn't getting enough vitamin D—or maybe my new vitamin D regimen was causing me problems. Lying in bed after one crash, I pondered how I walked home in the cold just before I crashed—could that have caused it? But I'd also been upset that day about a story I'd written that had gotten killed, and I'd gone to a concert that turned out to be really loud and over-stimulating, so maybe it was one of those things.

But the truth was, I couldn't find any compelling patterns that predicted when I was strong and when I was bedbound. I felt as though my illness might as well have been controlled by the Greek gods, creatures more irrational and capricious than the human mind can comprehend.

Friends constantly mentioned their ideas about things I should try: green smoothies! a paleo diet! this supplement, that supplement! quacky-sounding doctor number one or number two or number three!

One friend suggested a doctor he knew who, he said, had cured every single person with CFS who had gone to her. *Yeah, right,* I thought. But my friend persisted, and I could see how it hurt him to believe my stubbornness alone was keeping me sick. So I capitulated. His doctor recommended various supplements I hadn't tried that seemed fairly harmless, so I took them for a few months. In the end, they had no apparent effect.

My friend soon pushed his next cure-all on me, but this time, I firmly told him I wasn't interested. He clucked his tongue at me. "You're pretty stuck," he said. "Mainstream doctors have nothing to offer, and you're closed to alternatives, so I guess you're just going to stay sick."

I sputtered. I tried to explain that running off after every quack treatment my friends pushed on me just made me feel desperate and hopeless. The reality was that nobody knew what to do about this fucking disease—if they did, I would have heard about it by then. I figured that my life would be richest—and I'd also be more likely to get better—if I accepted that reality and dealt with it, rather than running from it and imagining that the next random treatment some friend recommended was going to magically cure me.

And anyway, I didn't feel stuck, I told him. I felt like the way forward lay in cultivating a curiosity about my illness, simultaneously enjoying my life as it was while scrutinizing my experience to find ways to make things better. Also, although I certainly wasn't a Christian Scientist as my mother was, her religion had fueled the belief in me that diligent attention to one's internal feelings and attitudes was the best place to start in solving a problem, allowing one to act more powerfully in the world and sometimes opening the door to change in ways you couldn't predict.

My friend frowned. "Okay, okay," he said. "It's your life."

FORTUNATELY, my life was mostly pretty rich. Occasionally, I was strong enough that William and I could bike around Angel Island or walk down to Stinson Beach; sometimes I was stuck in bed; and most of the time, I was in-between, carefully regulating how active I was so that I could do the things I most cared about.

I still worried that my illness felt like an imposition to William, but our day-to-day life was undeniably sweet. We moved out of his two rooms in a shared house and into a proper apartment together. We both worked from home, and we'd check in throughout the day, bringing one another little snacks or consulting about some work puzzle. He composed music, and I'd hear the strains of his guitar coming from his office. We went to lectures by leading lefties that he admired and that I usually found uncomfortably radical, and we'd gently argue about them afterward. And my career was growing nicely—I'd gotten hired to write a weekly math column for *Science News*, and I was having success in placing stories in other science magazines as well.

But the illness also intruded, even frighteningly sometimes. Walking home from a café one day, I found myself limping a bit, then limping a lot, then barely able to move either leg. Finally I stood motionless on the sidewalk, as stuck as a mouse in a glue trap.

I only had four blocks to go, but it might as well have been 400 miles. William was gone for the day, so I couldn't call him for rescue. *Fuckety fuck fuck fuck.*

A fellow I'd seen before was out cleaning his car and looked up, hearing my groans as I struggled to walk. Horror flashed across his face as relief flashed across mine: *I'll bet I can talk this guy into giving me a ride. He doesn't look like a rapist.*

He quickly agreed to give me a ride home and helped me into his ancient Rabbit. The backseat was filled with car batteries—he'd converted it into an electric car. I got him talking about this, deflecting the obvious questions he might otherwise ask.

Finally he said, "Uh, you okay?"

"Yeah, well, this just comes on sometimes. They don't really know why." I avoided those toxic words "chronic fatigue syndrome," not wanting to lose his sympathy.

When we got to my house, I couldn't bring myself to ask my rescuer for help up the stairs to our second-story apartment, so I thanked him from outside. Once I closed the door, I sat on my butt and lifted myself with my arms, stair by stair. Then my arms failed, so I turned on my belly and slithered, bellowing like a woman in childbirth with each wriggle, finally flopping, spent, at the top.

This, I thought as I panted, with my face mashed into the carpet, *this blows. This really blows.*

I DISCOVERED my most effective management tool through serendipity, when William and I visited a hot springs resort in the Sierras. As always, I'd imagined that I'd catch an upswing and be able to tramp through the snow under the great dark pine trees, but in fact, short walks were the best I could manage, and my paralysis came on several times. We hung out at the hot springs and in the body-temperature pool next to it, where I listlessly floated on my back in the womblike embrace of the warm water. I looked at the trees towering above me, imagining the energy flowing through them into the sky, their sap traveling a hundred feet up through their sturdy trunks despite the freezing cold. Every tree felt like an unattainable miracle of verticality and life force.

After paddling around for a bit, I prepared myself to stagger back to the locker room—but when I got out, the problem had disappeared. *Thanks for the break, Greek gods,* I thought.

The next time I was paralyzed, I floated in the warm pool again, and again, I was able to walk. A third time too. *Hmm . . .*

I didn't have a warm pool handy at home, but I thought that maybe the warmth wasn't essential to the magic—after all, a warm bath had never helped. So when we returned home, I decided to try going swimming during the middle of an episode. I staggered and groaned my way to the pool using a walker, dragging my legs forward with my hands, feeling ridiculous as the Speedo-clad athletes gave me startled looks. I should have used a wheelchair, but that required a level of acceptance of the illness I resisted.

When I reached the pool, I collapsed into the water. The weightlessness in the water felt reassuringly good, though as I looked at the impossibly faraway end of the pool, I thought, *This might be the stupidest thing I've ever tried.* I reminded myself that I didn't have to swim that whole distance. I put my goggles on, pushed feebly off the wall, and pulled my arms in a slow breaststroke.

After just a few strokes, a wave passed over me, as if a current traveled from my brain down through my body and filled me with the power I'd been missing. *Holy shit!* My kicks began propelling me forward, and my arms moved fluidly. I reveled in the delight of being able to move freely, forcing myself to stop after five laps to make sure I didn't overdo it.

Then I lifted myself from the water with ease, folded up my walker, and walked smoothly away. As soon as I got back to my phone in my locker, I called William, giddy: "It cured me!"

This turned out to be a reliable miracle. The front desk workers and lifeguards no longer looked alarmed when I lurched past them, groaning. Once, I stopped in the hot tub first and chatted with a garrulous gentleman who had watched me stagger over. I explained to him that once I swam I'd be fine, but he barely noticed my words, continuing his flirtatious banter without a hitch until I grunted my way to the pool. When he saw me get out of the pool a few minutes later, walking flawlessly and carrying my folded-up walker, he hollered, "Look at her! Did you see her before? She couldn't walk, and now she's cured! She's a mermaid!"

The mysterious swim cure generally lasted the rest of the day, but while it could stop a paralysis episode, it couldn't prevent one. That meant that I had to keep staggering to the pool while semi-paralyzed, and getting to the pool in that state was the hardest physical task I'd ever done.

I looked for a medical explanation for what swimming might be doing to my body—*it's got to be an important clue about what's wrong with me*—but I never found anything, and doctors I asked were stumped.

I made an observation that led me to come up with my own theory:

When I was having trouble walking, I found it oddly easier to move if someone pushed against my leg, providing resistance—I thought that might explain that first neurologist's claim that my strength was normal, even as I lay unable to shift my legs on his table. Perhaps, then, I thought, the uniform resistance of the water somehow helped reset my brain's ability to communicate with my legs. That would also explain why a bath had never helped: There wasn't enough water to provide much resistance.

But the swimming effect was so bizarre that I also wondered if I wasn't just crazy. Could that gait disorder specialist have been right about conversion disorder after all?

WHILE I NEVER BELIEVED that my illness could truly be all in my head, my childhood grounding in Christian Science made it natural to view my illness in a psychological and spiritual context and to hope that working on that level could support my healing. So despite my irritation with my therapist about the quack doctor he'd so aggressively pushed on me, I threw myself into our work together.

We started by discussing the most basic emotional fact of my childhood: I grew up believing that I had been brought into this world to save my mother.

As a child, I could have articulated neither that duty nor what threatened her, but my responsibility was as apparent to me as my dirty blond hair or skinny, coltish legs. Something wasn't right with the person I was most devoted to in all the world. Throughout my childhood, my mother didn't have friends, or a job, or a husband. She'd been alone since she'd left her husband six months after I was born, taking me and my two siblings with her; my father, with whom she'd had an affair during her marriage, had chosen to stay with his wife and five other children. My mother relied, somewhat precariously, on family money to pay her bills. She spent hours every day sitting on her bed playing solitaire. She sometimes careened into towering, inexplicable rages. When I was seven, she sent my older brother and sister away to live elsewhere, leaving just me and her in the house together.

As far as I could see, I was the person to fix whatever undefinable thing seemed to be ailing her. Certainly, no one else seemed to be volunteering for the job. How to accomplish this wasn't so obvious, though.

I quickly realized that people in the outside world weren't likely to help, because I couldn't talk about it with them at all. One morning when I was seven, I arrived at school in tears. A beautiful fifth-grader—royalty!—named Lupe wrapped her arm around me. As we walked down the open-air walkway of our San Diego school, Lupe asked me with maternal gentleness what was wrong. I snuffled that my mom was mad at me, and she asked me why.

I was astounded. She thought that question would be answerable? I realized she expected me to say something like "I forgot my lunch and we had go back home to get it" or "I was slow putting my shoes on." It wasn't anything like that. My mother was mad at me because—well, I barely knew myself. Because she had a headache and that meant my "thought was wrong," or something like that, something I knew would sound ridiculous to this good-hearted girl. Lupe's kind face and the sweet weight of her arm around me, I realized, existed in a different realm from my challenges with my mother.

So I had to figure it out on my own, just as I would many years later with chronic fatigue syndrome. The two experiences had very much the same quality for me, lying outside language, outside acceptability, outside any structure in which I could expect to receive help or even understanding. I spent time with Chris talking about the strategies I had used as a kid for dealing with my mother, because I recognized that I would naturally be inclined, for better or worse, to think about my illness in similar ways.

As a child, I had instinctively figured that the place to start on my overwhelming task was to deeply, sympathetically understand my mother's view of the world. Though she'd formally left the Christian Science church after the scandal broke about my extramarital conception, her religious beliefs hadn't shifted. For her, the physical world of chairs and stomachaches and paychecks was an illusion: True reality was purely spiritual. Thus the way to achieve what you want in the physical world was to work on this deeper, underlying, *real* plane, to refine yourself spiritually.

That meant, for example, that to solve her money problems, she shouldn't go out and look for a job—she should work on her own thought, creating a more perfect understanding of the abundance that was available to her and coming to more fully know that God provided all that she needed. That internal, spiritual work would produce results in the material world, and the practical solution to her problem, she trusted, would emerge. And it was my job to talk with her as she rooted about in her mind like in a toy box, looking for the rotten belief that was hiding out in there like a long-forgotten ham sandwich.

Talking with my mother and trying to figure out how to perform my savior's mission absorbed my full intellectual and emotional capacities. My mother had me memorize the "Scientific Statement of Being," the tersest summation of the Christian Science religion, read at every Sunday church service. It started out, "There is no life, truth, intelligence nor substance in matter. All is infinite Mind and its infinite manifestation . . ." The words themselves were tricky—what exactly did "manifestation" mean? But it was even harder to relate them to, say, the problem of filling my mother's bank account. She and I spent hours sitting on her bed, discussing passages from Christian Science texts and considering how they might shed light on her fraught relationships with her siblings, or her aggravation at the paper boy's repeated failure to throw the paper over the gate, or what she should do with her life.

If I had a friend over to play, my mother would frequently call me away, wanting me to talk with her about what she was feeling or to "fix my thought." I would sit on her bed with her, pushing away images of my friend, surrounded by the model horses we had just put into elaborate families. I knew it was essential to suppress my frustration and annoyance—telling my mother she was wrong or unreasonable never worked. It also didn't work to try too desperately to make her happy. The only thing that seemed to help was full, empathetic attunement, accepting anything she said as truth, allowing my body and soul to resonate with her like an antenna. I had to trust that even though I couldn't solve her problem directly, my presence and love could help open a path forward, one that could both lead to the freedom to play peacefully with my friend and even, perhaps, eventually, to a resolution of my mother's problems.

All these years later, I was listening to my body the way I had once listened to my mother. Carefully managing my activity levels was a practical tool, but it was also a sort of spiritual one, a way of attuning myself to my body's needs and abilities. Just as I had not allowed myself to be irritated with my mom as a kid, I didn't let my attitude toward my illness harden into frustration or allow myself to view my body as broken or misbehaving. On a level so deep it was nearly beyond articulation, I believed that being fully present to the experience of this illness, loving myself and my body in spite of it all, would somehow open a path forward, one that I hoped would lead to health, or at least to a détente that would allow me to live my life with the illness peacefully.

I could imagine that effort being effective on a variety of levels: It might simply help me waste less energy on anxiety and fear; it might directly heal my body, calming my nervous and immune systems; it might work in some deeper, more mysterious way that I didn't understand. And even if my efforts didn't impact my illness at all and my notion of some cosmic connection between the inner and outer worlds was bunk, this perspective still made my life richer and deeper. For example, regardless of whether my cyst as a teenager was truly connected to my relationship with my mom, exploring the possibility had helped me draw a needed boundary with her and cast the experience as a meaningful and valuable one rather than as random suffering.

And as a child, I certainly believed the approach I took to dealing with my mother paid off enormously. The benefit of managing my absurd responsibility for my mother well was that she then treated me with a deep respect for my integrity and autonomy—and I rarely received that from the outside world.

I knew my mother could look crazy to others and even to me, but the outside world often seemed at least as crazy. I was a child who was born old, and the expectations and constraints the world placed on me because of my age felt like a violation of my basic dignity. Even at four years old, I was outraged when I was forced to take a nap at a new preschool. I was perceived as simply throwing a tantrum—*I am not tired! I don't take naps in the afternoon!*—but for me, not being able to control my body in such a fundamental way felt like a deep intrusion.

As I grew older, the limitations the external world placed on me only felt more outrageous and out of step with my capacities. One day in fifth grade, for example, a girl made faces at me every time the teacher looked away. The other students in the class, who had themselves often been tormented by this girl in the past, discreetly looked away. I ignored her, but her smirks only grew more extreme: She stuck her tongue out, rolled her eyes into the back of her head, and stretched her mouth wide with her fingers.

My outrage mounted—not just at this ridiculous girl, but at my passive classmates, at the unaware teacher, at my own hot cheeks, at the stupidity of the whole situation. What was I doing, participating in this farce? I didn't belong here, listening to a lecture on stuff I already knew, while an 11-year-old exerted a petty power over me.

My aggravation was also fueled by something I couldn't have articulated: To my mind, school was about helping me acquire the tools I needed for my mammoth task of saving my mother. It certainly wasn't about performing for a teacher and politely enduring the tyranny of other children. I felt as though my chest were growing with my rage, that I was far too big to fit in these little chairs in this little school full of little people wasting their time on little tasks.

I felt myself rise and walk out of the classroom. I seemed to be floating above my body, my heart pounding distantly. I watched myself turn right toward the lighted red exit sign and heard the double doors clang as I pushed through.

I blinked in astonishment as the bright sunlight and traffic noise hit me. *What am I going to do now?*

The sensible thing would be to go back in, pretending that I'd suddenly had to go to the bathroom—but I knew I wasn't going to do that. *Hmm . . .* Home was a 20-minute drive away, since this was a special program for gifted students that occurred at only a few schools around San Diego. I didn't have a dime for a pay phone to call my mom.

I walked to a strip mall a few blocks away and asked to use the phone in a small, friendly looking drugstore. I spun a story to explain my presence in the middle of the school day—I was a homeschooler, I extemporized, and my mom was supposed to pick me up but she hadn't, so I needed to call home. The cashier told me I could use the phone in the back, but then she kept delaying and asking me strange questions about my family, and I couldn't figure out why. My chest reignited with rage at my own powerlessness. *What kind of messed-up world is this, that just because I'm a kid I can't even make a phone call?* Later, my mother told me that the clerk had called Child Protective Services and was trying to keep me there until they arrived.

When the clerk's back was turned, I slipped out and ran. Once out of sight, I settled in for a long, hot walk home: Would it take two hours? Three? The traffic whizzed past me as I walked under a billboard with a giant XXX hovering above two enormous, bikini-clad breasts, twin poster children for one of many strip joints that peppered this Navy-dominated area of town.

A car pulled up next to me. "Hey, good-looking, want a ride?" It was my mother, leaning over to open the door for me, her smile easy and teasing. "I figured I'd find you!" she said. Her dark, wavy hair fell on either side of her face, a familiar white streak of hair rising elegantly from her forehead.

The air-conditioning caressed my sweaty face as I slid into the car. My mom leaned over and kissed me and then reached for my hand, her olive-skinned fingers with their long, painted nails wrapping around my pinker, stubby-nailed hand.

The school had called her in a panic, she told me as she pulled back into traffic, but she hadn't been worried. She knew I had a head on my shoulders and could take care of myself. She didn't ask me what had happened, waiting until I offered the tale on my own. I breathed in deeply, feeling each rib separating, making more space.

That was the thing about my mom—she never squished me the way the outside world did. My childhood dramas weren't piddly affairs, to be discussed in that high, altered voice reserved for kids. They were part of a much bigger struggle, even a planetary struggle, so that my decisions were as significant as hers, or my teacher's, or those of the president of the United States. My fifth-grade tormentor might have been a cosmic cousin of Leonid Brezhnev, her grimaces an expression of the same malign force that led Brezhnev to invade Afghanistan. And my ability to maneuver around her stupidity might, in its own small way, affect the balance of the world, resisting that malevolent force wherever it occurred, even helping democracy outmaneuver communism. My mother's perspective almost made the culturally enforced puniness of life as a child bearable.

So I felt as though I were a dual citizen of two universes, or perhaps only a visitor in each. My mother's world felt more generous, psychologically bigger, with more possibilities, but it came with preposterous responsibilities and could veer into simple craziness. The outer world felt more grounded and comprehensible, and I *had* to participate in it to connect to others—but it also chained me into a child's role that I felt violated my integrity, and it rigorously enforced a narrow conventionality. So I performed a kind of mental juggling act, holding my mother's world in my mind privately as I moved through my day at school. When one of these worlds felt foreign and uncomfortable, I took comfort in the other.

As an adult, these childhood experiences made the insanity of the outside world's view of my illness feel entirely natural to me. I was used to such violation. I was used to conventional views being at odds with the most obvious truths about my life. And I was used to dealing with that craziness by taking solace in the world I lived in with my mother, a world based on the faith that deep attunement was a tool that could find unseen paths around seemingly insurmountable obstacles.

And my childhood experiences had taught me that, at least sometimes, working on that level could indeed be remarkably effective. When I was 15, I managed to—well, perhaps not save my mother, but certainly to help change her life.

A couple years earlier, I'd told my mother I was fed up with school and wanted to quit. I'd just come home after a semester at a fancy East Coast boarding school that was supposed to be the "best high school in the country," but I'd hated it, feeling that it had only provided small, high hoops to jump through, when I wasn't interested in performing at all. "Okay," she'd said, "but I'm out of ideas. You have to figure out what to do next."

I ended up taking correspondence courses for a while, enrolling at the University of California, San Diego, when I was 14, and then making my way to St. John's College in Santa Fe a year later. At St. John's, I found an intellectual home for myself for the first time. The college had a Great Books program, so I was reading and discussing Plato, Shakespeare, Kant, Euclid, Newton, and more. Grappling together with the profound questions in these books at last felt like a challenge that could expand my soul. I couldn't have spelled out the connections between that and my work with my mother, but intuitively, it felt relevant. If I was acting as an antenna resonating both with my mother and the world at large and thus providing a link between them, it felt as though my experiences at St. John's were lengthening that antenna, making it more powerful and sensitive.

Just a month after I arrived, I persuaded my mom to join me. She became a graduate student there while I was an undergraduate.

After she moved to Santa Fe, her playing cards, soft as fabric from all those games of solitaire, sat unused in their boxes. Rather than discussing Christian Science books, we discussed books from the college. She bought a house—far more affordable in Santa Fe than in San Diego—and renovated it beautifully. I would come home to find her chatting with friends on the patio or heading out for a tennis date. She threw dinner parties and displayed a knack for getting people to share their most vulnerable, budding ideas and feelings.

I felt vast satisfaction, watching my mother live a relatively normal life. My task wasn't yet fully accomplished—for one thing, she still didn't have a way to earn a living, and she was running out of money. But her frightening rages had vanished, and I no longer felt like I had to straddle a vast gulf between her and the rest of the world. All those hours I had spent entering her perspective, empathizing with her, looking for threads connecting her to the outer world, seemed to be paying off.

As an adult, I no longer believed that one person could save another (much less that a child could save a parent), but those experiences nevertheless gave me a kind of stabilizing faith with my illness. I didn't imagine that some great old man in the sky had sickened me to teach me some lesson, and that once I'd passed the test I would graduate back to health. But I did believe that my illness was opening a window onto an aspect of the world I would never have experienced or appreciated otherwise, and that was something I could open myself to, embrace, experience deeply, allow to change me. I believed that being sick could be an experience worth having. I believed I could function most powerfully with the illness by opening myself to it as fully as possible, just as I had with my mother.

Most of all, I believed that the world was a vastly more complicated place than our little human minds could grasp, and that just because I didn't have a rational plan I could spell out that started where I was and ended up in health, that didn't mean I couldn't get there.

CHAPTER 5

THE GREAT COLLAPSE

My efforts to manage my illness and fashion a satisfying life for myself with William in Berkeley paid off. By carefully limiting my activities, using bizarre tricks like the swim cure, and expanding my conception of the tolerable, I was able to reduce my illness to little more than a really big nuisance. I could do my work as a freelancer, travel, exercise as I was capable, go to talks and movies with William—albeit with some inconvenient interruptions during bad days or bad weeks. I felt as though I were walking around carrying a hundred pound weight. It slowed me down, but hey! I was strong, I was capable, I could handle it!

The illness was more than a nuisance, though, when it came to long-term planning. I had wanted children all my life, and William wasn't sure. He worried that there wouldn't be enough to go around—enough money, enough time, enough energy, enough love—and my illness sharpened the edges of those worries considerably.

I brought up "the kid question" from time to time, and William mostly avoided it. Our relationship felt like it balanced on top of a jagged rock, and either we would figure out how to shore it up or all would come tumbling down. My therapist, Chris, told me that William's continuing ambivalence almost certainly meant that he didn't really want kids and at most would capitulate to my desires. William denied that, and I chose to believe him. *We love each other,* I thought, *so surely we'll find our way.* But to all appearances, we were well and thoroughly stuck.

In the spring of 2009, when we'd been together for three years and during a period when my health wasn't too bad, we took a trip to South Africa. Africa had felt like the land of fable to me since I'd been a child and read books like *Born Free* and *A Story like the Wind* and *The Flame Trees of Thika*. We had to plan around my limitations—I couldn't, say, go on significant hikes, or do a bike trip—but to be able to go at all was intoxicating. Also, William and I both felt in some inchoate way that the trip would get us through our stuckness about the kid question, though neither of us could articulate how this might happen.

South Africa brought my fantasies to life. On a safari, our bodies vibrated with the roar of a lion just yards away from us; we scuttled back into the Land Cruiser when a huge bull elephant flapped his ears and stamped his feet at us; and we guarded our lunches from glaring baboons. We each flew in a tiny microlight plane—essentially two lawn chairs with wings and a propeller—high over a crystalline bay on the Indian Ocean, then swooped down just feet above hippopotamuses dozing with their heads resting on one another's backs in a lake. We each suppressed our shock when we talked with an Afrikaner farmer who lamented the end of apartheid, arguing that the country had disintegrated after that. We took an easy bike tour around a township and talked with a black woman running a daycare center who continued to care for the children even when the parents couldn't pay. William and I enjoyed one another tremendously, and throughout the trip, my body held up so well I hardly seemed sick at all.

After we returned from the trip, my health improved, spectacularly. Within a month, I was running again. Running! After so many years of not being able to push myself during exercise, every run was a thrill, a small miracle.

Months went by, I ran faster and harder, and the illness quickly began to seem like a nightmare from long ago. I figured my health problems had just faded away, as I'd always hoped and expected they would. I didn't have a very compelling explanation for what had happened to me or why I'd gotten better. But of course, one can always generate ideas: I figured I'd set the stage for healing through my aggressive rest, through my care with exercise when I felt stronger, through my careful organization of my life so that I never had to do more than my body could handle, through my healthy diet. Plus, I thought it was important that during the periods when I was doing badly, I'd stayed calm and had confidence in my body's ability to bounce back. I couldn't point to any great psychological or spiritual revelation that might have contributed, but still, I figured that it couldn't have hurt that I'd viewed the illness as an experience worth having, rather than just a big fucking drag.

In any case, my joy at my recovery made the reasons for it seem like a trivial matter. Also, my experience with Geoff had taught me not to expect straightforward explanations even for major experiences in my life. I still couldn't say why Geoff had collapsed as he did, or how I could make sense of it in my life, or what I'd learned from it all. But I felt myself slowly, slowly digesting those events and allowing them to change me. In a similar way, I imagined that even though I couldn't make much sense of my illness yet, over years, it would rework me and come to have a meaning I couldn't yet see.

I was also struck by how different the experience felt to me than it would have if I'd had a clear, unambiguous, scientifically ratified explanation for what had happened. The upside was that the experience had an openness, a fertility about it—I felt more room to create my own meaning. It felt potentially, if not actually, profound. If I'd had, say, an especially bad bout of mononucleosis, I imagined that the simple, mechanistic explanation would have felt so complete and compelling that it would have left room for little else, and the experience might have felt banal.

The downside was that my mysterious recovery reinforced the scent of illegitimacy about the illness, even in my own mind. That dichotomy struck me as peculiar: Clearly, *something* had been going wrong inside my body, and medicine's failure to understand what that something was didn't change the fundamental reality. But without a known explanation, the illness felt a bit like Schrodinger's cat: neither dead nor alive, neither physical nor psychological, and yet rich with possibility.

Unlike a cat that truly can't be simultaneously dead and alive, it seemed to me that my illness had to be both psychospiritual and physiological. We experience the world on both of these levels, and they are so interwoven that even conceptually, we can't truly separate them. Take the simple example of pain: The intensity of neural firing correlates only loosely with a person's subjective experience of pain, and that subjective experience is strongly impacted by our interpretation of what we're feeling. If we believe we're being damaged, it hurts a lot more than if we believe the pain is harmless. It's all woven together.

But I was far more concerned with moving forward with my life than engaging with that endless puzzle. With my health so much better, the kid problem felt more pressing, and I had more energy to tackle it. The conviction William and I had shared that the trip would break the jam seemed to be nothing more than a fantasy. I finally did something I'd been resisting for ages: I gave William an ultimatum. Agree to a kid by my 37th birthday in a few months, I said, or I'm leaving.

A month or so before my birthday, he said yes.

Finally, the family I've been trying to create since my mother died! At long, long last, my life seemed to be falling into place, the blockages I'd been stuck on dissolving.

William wanted to wait a few months before conceiving, and in the meantime, we bought a lovely cottage together in Berkeley, with room for a baby and with stairs that we figured were no longer a problem for me. When we moved, I hauled furniture and boxes all day without a second thought. I shipped the glass Christmas ornaments my mother and I had collected together from storage at my house in Santa Fe to our new home. I felt a huge contentment, standing healthy and strong with my beloved partner, seeing my own sparkling Christmas tree in our own comfortable house. The next time we brought the ornaments out, I figured, we'd have a baby in our arms or in my belly.

BUT WILLIAM STILL WASN'T quite ready for us to get pregnant. We decided to get a puppy first, as a test run on our ability to coparent—though, since I was far more interested in the puppy (and the baby) than he was, I accepted that more of the work would fall on me. I found a 10-week-old, brown, floppy-eared puppy on a rescue organization's Web site. When I met her and picked her up, she melted against me and snuggled her nose into my neck. We named her Frances, after the badger in the children's book *Bread and Jam for Frances.*

I was astonished by what a miracle this puppy was: her sweet breath, her soft little body, her growth every day, her instant connection to us. I knew my reaction was absurdly intense given that she was a perfectly ordinary puppy, but her ordinariness only increased the miracle: *Imagine! We live in a world filled with puppies!*

I also thought, *Man, if I'm this over the moon about a puppy, imagine how I'll be with a baby.*

The coparenting experiment, however, was a spectacular failure. Anytime Frances peed in the house, William became convinced that she would never get house-trained and that it was my fault for not watching her closely enough. He wanted her never to bark under any circumstances, and god forbid she chew anything she wasn't supposed to. Raising a puppy with William proved far more difficult than raising a puppy by myself, and I quailed to imagine what raising a child with him would be like. Chris's view that William fundamentally didn't want to have children—and even more, that he wasn't cut out for the task—became hard to deny.

I found this almost impossible to take in. Just a few months before, I thought my family was finally coming together. But when William fumed if Frances cried at night and equally fumed if she snored when sleeping beside us, I felt like the last thing I wanted to do was have a baby with this guy.

I tried to dismiss the problems as adjustment, and I focused on maintaining my own emotional equilibrium as William, I hoped, found his way back to his. I also tried to look at the bigger picture: We'd been together for four generally happy years. Despite his fear that he couldn't handle it, he'd stuck by me through my illness. And I loved our life together. I loved our house, I loved walking up to downtown Berkeley together for dinner at our favorite Indian or Mexican or Nepali restaurants, I loved the parties we threw that felt like a ratification of our life together, I loved watching how William's mind worked as we discussed a movie or a lecture. I simply enjoyed his company. Although I couldn't regard his behavior with Frances as anything but ridiculous, I hoped he'd find his way through it and become a reasonable partner again. *No need to freak out, Julie. It'll be okay.*

LATER THAT SPRING, in 2010, I went for my usual run and found that it didn't feel so good. I stopped a bit early and dragged the rest of the day.

The next run, I could do even less, and within a week, I couldn't run at all anymore.

My recovery, apparently, was only a remission. And it was over.

Some days, I couldn't think clearly enough to work. Occasionally, I even had trouble walking again. It seemed that I had once more displeased the Greek gods.

And then at the beginning of the summer William told me he'd changed his mind about getting pregnant. No kid, he said—not then, not ever. "It'd be hard enough if you were fully healthy," he said. "Even if you get better again, I'll always know you could get worse at any moment, and I could be stuck taking care of the kid and you both. I'm just not up for that."

I gasped for air, as if the wind had been knocked out of me. Even though I'd been having severe doubts of my own, I was so angry that leaving William didn't feel like sufficient punishment: I wanted to scratch his eyes out. I desperately wished I had never met him. Even if I left William right then, finding a new partner and building the relationship to the point where we were ready to have a kid would take years, and I was already 37. *I may have lost my children.*

One night, William held me while I sobbed so hard that I burst capillaries around my eyes, leaving a constellation of purple spots the next day. William remarked in the morning that he was sorry I was in so much pain, but the good side was that he finally understood how deeply having a child mattered to me—though that didn't change his mind or anything. His remark only made me want to kick him in the balls. *You didn't understand that years ago, you fucking asshole?*

Still, I couldn't bring myself to leave William. He wanted to stay together, and he continued to bring himself to the relationship with vulnerability and commitment. The idea of frantically looking for some new man to father my children made me feel ill. And the idea of being alone, again, overwhelmed and depressed me. I imagined myself returning to Santa Fe, starting over again—but this time, starting over when sick and possibly too old to have a kid. And even if I met someone else and built a new relationship, a prospect that sounded far more exhausting than exciting, who was to say it wouldn't just fall apart too?

Over the next few months, I limped along in a haze. I slowly developed a plan of sorts. I'd always figured that if I neared the end of my child-bearing years without a partner, I'd have a child on my own. My mother had raised me by herself, and while I had been aware of my father's absence, I had felt loved beyond measure. That alone, I felt, had given me the foundation I needed. Plus, I'd watched my sister raise a fabulous daughter by herself.

Of course, I hadn't counted on being sick while being a single mom. Still, I was confident that I could continue managing my illness as I'd done for years—why wouldn't I be able to do so with a kid too? Heck, I'd built a house by myself with a sick husband while my body was falling apart!

So in the fall of 2010, I decided to get pregnant using donor sperm. I told William, and although he and I both knew that our relationship almost certainly wouldn't survive that, we stayed together in the meantime. I didn't have the heart to wrench myself away from him, and he seemed to be hoping that I wouldn't be able to get pregnant and the problem would thus go away. The situation felt awful to me, awful almost beyond imagining, but I couldn't come up with a better solution.

I did my research. In a few months, I would start trying to get pregnant.

In December, Frances and I went for a hike in Santa Fe. William and I had been spending much more time in Santa Fe—he had offered that as a concession, hoping it might make our life together more satisfying for me. My house was rented out, but any time we wanted we could stay in the pair of travel trailers I'd brought onto the land while building. Frances and I stayed a couple of extra weeks after William had returned to Berkeley. My health had improved, not back to a full remission but enough that I could do a gentle four-mile hike like this one.

I soaked up the land greedily. We hiked along the stream, past the oak tree with branches that stretched horizontally into an arbor across the trail. I breathed in the always-cool air at the "Anasazi icebox," where a huge, damp, north-facing rock acted as a natural refrigerator. Then we turned right into a side canyon almost no one ever went in, up to the saddle where I'd discovered an error in the contour lines on the official federal topographic map, and down along a hidden arroyo with a trickle of water running under the ice. Frances streaked past, dodging around me at the last possible moment before barreling down the trail. I delighted in the joy she took in her strong, sleek, nine-month-old body, tearing up and down the trail with none of my ever-present caution.

I had begun the bizarre process of choosing a "donor" for my child—*do I want the blond guitarist business major, or the Italian-American who loves bicycling?*—and was planning to start donor insemination soon after I got back to Berkeley. I fantasized about someday coming here with a baby on my back. In my daydream, it was summertime, and I'd stop in this little cottonwood grove and my baby would crawl in the long grasses.

And then I realized: I was getting tired. *It's time to stop, right now.*

I sat down on a rock. I knew I'd pay for every additional step I took, even though similar hikes hadn't been causing me problems lately. But stopping wasn't an option: I was still a mile deep into the wilderness. Frances ran back to me, smacked a kiss on my cheek, and ran off again. I wished I could ride on her strong back, or suck some of her ample energy off her.

I rested until the cold rock hurt my butt, and then I started walking slowly. Another rest, another gentle walk. The walking stretches got shorter, slower, harder. *Please, god, don't let me get paralyzed out here.* When I made it across my bridge and then into my trailers, I rested my head against the fake wood paneling inside and sobbed.

The next day, I couldn't walk, couldn't think. My bones hurt, my eyes swelled, just moving my lips was hard work. *Don't freak out,* I thought. *It'll just be a couple of bad days, and then you'll be okay. Time to rest.*

But I didn't get better. I delayed my return trip by a few days, but I still could barely walk. Finally, I hired a couple of local boys to help me pack, and I drove back to Berkeley. Fortunately, even when I was quite sick, I could almost always manage to drive.

After I got back, day after day, I could barely get out of bed. The image often arose unbidden of a giant shovel scooping me up and tossing my ragdoll body on the compost pile. The idea of getting pregnant was now ridiculous.

Frances spent hours cuddled up next to me, a tight brown ball of warmth and comfort. Then her puppy energy would take over: She'd tear around the house, full of flapping ears and pig grunts, her claws leaving scratches on the linoleum floor as she spun out on the turns. Since I was too weak to take her for walks, we instead went to the dog park—but then I didn't have the strength to chase after her when she refused to go home, deafly cavorting with her buddies. I'd have to ask others for help luring her in. When I was strongest, I'd walk slowly, slowly two blocks to a café and try to work, but I often found that when I got up to go home I couldn't walk anymore and had to call William for a ride.

I fought off panic as the nonfunctional days piled up, my work undone, with no idea when or if I would improve. I sent apologetic e-mails to the editor of my math column at *Science News*, promising that I'd get him something next week—and then, well, *next* week. Because many of my symptoms were so intangible, I even doubted myself. *Maybe I'm coddling myself, being lazy*, I thought. *If I just tried harder, I could get something done.* I'd use the tricks that had gotten me through procrastination in the past, telling myself things like "Write the next paragraph and then you can have a piece of chocolate" or "Cut the fucking crap and get to work!" But none of those tricks seemed to work much anymore. I thought my inability to work was a direct product of my illness—but how do you ever know?

Then I'd have a day where I couldn't turn over in bed and could barely lift my head, and I'd stop the obsessive self-questioning. Or, rather, I'd turn it around and wonder why, when I felt a smidgen better, I couldn't seem to remember just how sick I really was.

It was clear: I needed help. The only source for that seemed to be the doctors I'd given up on. On the online patient boards, occasionally someone mentioned one faraway specialist or another who seemed to be genuinely scientifically minded, levelheaded, competent. But most of them had waiting lists of six months to two years. Other specialists chose the patients they were most interested in, and the rest waited forever.

But one physician, a Florida immunologist named Nancy Klimas, had a clinic that was relatively new, private, and didn't accept insurance—and thus had a shorter waiting list.

I read everything I could about Klimas and watched videos of her on the Internet. I read that in the 1980s, she'd been a young immunologist captivated by the puzzle of AIDS, both decoding it in the laboratory and treating its victims. But other patients had come to her as well, patients who didn't have AIDS but were profoundly exhausted, brain-fogged, and in pain and who found that if they exercised, they paid for it later. Klimas tried to turn them away—she didn't know anything about this strange disease, if it even *was* a disease—but they begged her, convinced that something was wrong with their immune systems. She relented and tested their blood, and she found such a consistent pattern of immune abnormalities that she knew they were sick with some real disease. And these patients had no doctors to treat them.

So Klimas became their doctor, treating them alongside her HIV/AIDS patients. She became one of the most respected and committed researchers and clinicians for chronic fatigue syndrome in the world, dividing her time between treating patients, research, and advising governmental committees about the disease. Two years earlier, she'd told the *New York Times*, "My HIV patients for the most part are hale and hearty thanks to three decades of intense and excellent research and billions of dollars invested. Many of my CFS patients, on the other hand, are terribly ill and unable to work or participate in the care of their families. I split my clinical time between the two illnesses, and I can tell you if I had to choose between the two illnesses in 2009, I would rather have HIV."

When I called Klimas's office, I got the first available appointment, in March, less than two months away. *Not bad,* I thought. *Now I just have to get through until then.* In the meantime, I tried to ask myself as few questions as possible, avoiding thoughts about whether I'd get better, about what meaning I could create out of this experience for myself, about whether William and I would stay together, about whether somehow I'd manage to have the child I so longed for.

Day by day, breath by breath, bathroom trip by bathroom trip, I got through.

ONE MORNING as I was counting down the days until my appointment, I was reading the *New York Times* on my phone—sitting up to use my computer was far too hard—and came upon the headline "Psychotherapy Eases Chronic Fatigue Syndrome, Study Finds."

Psychotherapy? Are they saying this is a mental problem?

Reading further, I learned that the study claimed that both psycho-therapy and a gradual increase in exercise could make CFS patients feel significantly better. The article continued:

> While this may sound like good news, the findings—published Thursday in the *Lancet*—are certain to displease many patients and to intensify a fierce, long-running debate about what causes the illness and how to treat it . . .
>
> The new study . . . is expected to lend ammunition to those who think the disease is primarily psychological or related to stress.

The article noted that the type of psychotherapy the researchers used, a particular form of cognitive behavioral therapy (CBT), aimed to change the psychological factors "assumed to be responsible for perpetuation of the participant's symptoms and disability."

I felt the heat rise to my face. *Oh my god, what will my editors think?* I'd been juggling deadlines, trying to tell my editors enough so they'd cut me some slack but not so much to alarm them. I imagined them reading the article and figuring: *Ah! Julie's not getting me that story because she's fucked in the head! Too lazy to get out of bed and exercise. Science has proven it.*

I groaned. I'd worked with Chris for seven years during my illness, and while he'd helped keep me from losing my mind as my body deterio-rated, he couldn't stop me from losing my health. I'd finally quit work-ing with him when my health was good and William agreed to have a baby, so I felt like my life was going well (*snerk!*).

As for exercise, my very first strategy when I'd started getting sick was to swallow my pride, start with only slow, short runs, and gradually build up. It hadn't worked, though I'd tried it again and again. *If this study is right, shouldn't I be cured by now?*

At the same time . . . jeez, the *Lancet*. That was about as good a medical journal as there was. Plus the study, nicknamed the PACE trial, was enormous by the standards of chronic fatigue syndrome: 641 sub-jects, $8 million. *Could there somehow be something to this?*

The study was everywhere: CNN, NPR, the BBC, Reuters. Some articles were far more effusive than the *New York Times* had been: "Got ME? Just Get Out and Exercise, Say Scientists," declared the *Independent*, using the acronym for the international name of the disease, myalgic encephalomyelitis (which I'd only recently learned). "ME Sufferers 'Better Pushing Their Limits,'" proclaimed the *Times of London*. Many reported that the study showed that 30 percent of patients who received cognitive behavioral therapy or gradually increased exercise had a full recovery. *Recovery!*

The *New York Times* article was the only one that expressed reservations about the study. Although it presented the trial at face value, it pointed out that researchers defined chronic fatigue syndrome in varying ways, and that the PACE trial had used a broad definition that could include patients who were depressed and didn't have CFS at all. And the article added, "At least one survey has found that exercise therapy can significantly worsen many patients' symptoms."

Um, yeah, I thought, remembering my unfortunate hike a couple of months before that was no greater than other hikes I'd been doing at the time. And I knew that at government clinics in the United Kingdom, cognitive behavioral therapy and exercise were pretty much the only treatments offered to patients. I'd heard of many patients who went from moderately ill to bedbound under that regime and who complained that they were browbeaten into accepting that they weren't really physically ill. Patients were sometimes threatened with loss of disability payments if they refused these treatments, or even thrown into psychiatric hospitals against their will.

And the study completely contradicted what I'd learned through hard experience: I had to stop as soon as I felt the slightest bit tired. It didn't matter if I'd swum for 10 minutes without difficulty the day before—if I felt tired after five, it was stop or else. Steadily increasing my exercise regardless of my symptoms was a surefire path to disaster, and every patient I'd spoken with had learned a similar lesson.

I fiddled with my phone to get to an online patient forum, feeling annoyed at the tiny screen but far too exhausted to sit up to use my computer. I found patients who had zoomed past my befuddlement straight into fury. "I'm losing it right now," wrote one patient. "This obscene bullshit is just killing me."

The background on the study only made it worse: The theory driving the PACE trial was that something happened to CFS patients initially—perhaps a bad bug, a pregnancy, or maybe even just being a workaholic—and they got out of shape. Then, when they tried to exercise again, they found that it didn't feel like it used to. Rather than working gradually and consistently to get back in shape, these patients either didn't try to exercise at all or they pushed their bodies too hard, bringing on fatigue and pain. Either way, they became convinced that they had a dread disease, so they grew afraid of exercise, focused excessively on their symptoms, and, as a result, remained unfit. Along with that came more fatigue and other symptoms, perpetuating a vicious spiral.

The solution, the team said, was simple: CFS patients just had to exercise. They needed some guidance to help them start slowly and build up gradually so that they didn't overdo it, because then they'd get scared silly when they got sore and tired. And perhaps patients needed some therapeutic help to get through their fear about it, to focus less on their symptoms, and to overcome any associated depression. The PACE trial, the researchers claimed, had proven that they were right.

It wasn't just in the United Kingdom that researchers were pursuing psychological explanations for the disease: I'd been ignoring a steady stream of similar but less well-publicized research in the United States. Just a few months before, for example, a study by the Centers for Disease Control and Prevention (CDC) claimed that 29 percent of CFS patients had a personality disorder, compared with just seven percent of the general population. It was important for doctors to understand this, the paper concluded, because "this might be associated with being noncompliant with treatment suggestions, displaying unhealthy behavioral strategies and lacking a stable social environment."

When I read about that study, I thought, *Fuck you! Let's give* you *a horrendous illness, deny you decent medical care and disability payments, have your friends and family tell you you're crazy, and then see how your mental health fares!* Comparing CFS patients with healthy folks was absurd—they should have been comparing them with other chronically ill patients. And indeed, a 2003 study in the *Journal of Psychosomatic Research* compared CFS patients with those with multiple sclerosis and found equal rates of neuroticism and depression (which isn't the same as a personality disorder, but still . . .).

As absurd as they were, these US psychiatric studies were small and obscure. I found them irritating, especially because they were a dreadful waste of money—but hey, there's plenty of lousy research on all topics. At least they didn't get published in top medical journals or garner world-wide headlines.

But the PACE trial did.

I felt sick. I'd heard so many stories from other patients about their friends and families not believing they were really ill, and I'd always felt lucky that had never been a problem for me. I wasn't immune to the cor-rosive effect of the skepticism focused on my illness—I could hear even in my own head a sense that my illness didn't quite measure up. But I'd never been told that I just needed to exercise and stop obsessing about my symp-toms. It was painful to hear from anyone, but from the *New York Times*? *The Lancet*? It felt like science itself—my refuge from craziness and irra-tionality and stupidity—had turned on me. And my science-writer col-leagues were cheering them along.

I put my phone down again and decided to put the whole thing out of my head. My priority at that moment had to be taking care of myself, not worrying about some dumb study. And, after all, I knew perfectly well that occasionally science goes wrong—though this flub was more dra-matic than I was used to. Regardless, I just needed to get through the days until I saw Klimas. Through her, I hoped, I'd find some good science to help me.

CHAPTER 6

THE MIRACLE

As William and I flew to see Klimas in Miami, I was exhausted by the effort of keeping myself upright in my seat. I was also exhausted, I realized, from the effort of dealing with my own terror. For all these years, I'd kept my life and dreams going in spite of being sick, but my best efforts weren't enough to accomplish that anymore. Now it wasn't just my future children that were at risk—it was my ability to have a meaningful life of any kind. I wasn't merely looking for some small incremental improvement, or the simple reassurance of having a doctor behind me. I was looking for a miracle, plain and simple.

And deep in my gut, I didn't believe I was going to get my miracle. CFS patients as sick as I was rarely improved dramatically, as far as I could tell. New, relatively mild cases often spontaneously resolved. But by this point, more than a decade had passed since the day I'd struggled to walk up the path to my house and first thought that perhaps I was sick.

Part of the reason I was so frightened was that my previous efforts at miracle generation hadn't worked out so well. Late in my sophomore year at St. John's, while my mother was a graduate student, she came down with what seemed to be a flu. After nine days, she wasn't feeling better, and she confessed to me that she hadn't pooped that whole time. I persuaded her to go to the nurse at the college, and the nurse sent her to the hospital. That night, my mother was on the operating table, and the next day, we learned that colon cancer had spread through her abdomen.

My mother was serene: She believed that God would save her and that this miraculous cure would prove that she'd lived her life right. I didn't believe that. Instead, I believed that *I* would save her—that had always been my job, after all. I had faith that I'd find the way forward, just as I had in the past.

I started working on the external level, insisting that she do chemotherapy. She agreed, but only for my sake, and as soon as she found a crack in my resolve to force her, she stopped. Within months, blood tests indicated the cancer was growing wildly. I couldn't summon the will to fight with her about it further, and it was probably too late for chemo to beat the cancer anyway.

So I started thinking on an internal, psychological level. My mother's illness felt oddly unsurprising to me, like it flowed naturally out of how stuck she was. Despite all the changes in her life since she'd moved to Santa Fe, I knew the prospect of running out of money terrified her. She had an immense internal power but few external skills, and help wanted ads rarely called for such a combination. She wasn't willing to mess around in some puny job—she wanted to be her full, grand self, right away. Neither of us had great ideas about how to make that happen, and she was running out of time.

Cancer provided a way out of that mess—but not one I was very happy about. Her complacent expectation that God would rescue her felt to me like a willingness to leave her problems, and me, behind.

Figure it out! Get a job! Do something! I wanted to yell at her—except that the notion of yelling at her was so preposterous that I forced the urge down nearly before I was even aware of it. I just couldn't help but believe that if she'd find the courage to truly face her situation and come up with a solution, maybe her body would manage to fight the cancer too.

I didn't talk much about my theory, knowing it might sound to others like the kind of magical thinking a distraught 18-year-old could easily take solace in. But then I read a book that backed me up: *Cancer As a Turning Point* by the psychotherapist Larry LeShan. LeShan argued that while thoughts and feelings neither cause nor cure cancer, they do strongly affect the immune system. As a result, working on a psychological level could help marshal the body's own self-healing abilities. He backed these assertions up with reports of dozens of studies along with his 35 years of experience both as a researcher and a clinician.

LeShan reported the stories of patients he'd worked with who had turned their lives around and beaten their cancer in the process, or at least given themselves extra time. Each of these stories was reported with a combination of deep compassion and scientific authority.* LeShan fingered stuckness and hopelessness as immune system killers—my mother's exact responses to her need to make a living.

I crammed the book into my mother's hands, demanding she read it. I felt as though I might have found both the key to saving her life and the link I had been longing for between my mother's world and the outer world of science. It gave a plausible physiological mechanism for how living one's life well and attuning oneself to the currents of life could help one's body function better.

And hey, I figured, even if I was wrong and there was no connection between my mother's stuckness and her cancer, surely finding a sustainable and satisfying way for her to live was a good idea regardless.

My mother read the book and seemed generally agreeable, if less lit up by it than I was. Full of the uncracked conviction of an 18-year-old, I contacted LeShan through his publisher, determined to fly with my mother to work with him. But LeShan told me that he was old, he was tired. He didn't treat patients anymore—sorry. I should find a local therapist. Good luck!

I hung up the phone and dug the heels of my hands into my eyeballs. A few minutes later, I called him back. I recited a story to him from his own book: Many years earlier, he'd considered quitting his practice to spend more time with his kids. His daughter had told him he couldn't quit: "Your patients need you." I echoed her: "My mother and I need you."

"Okay, okay," he grumbled. "Come to New York. We'll do a few sessions."

The next step was to convince my mother to go, but I knew I could do that. We flew to New York, stayed in a hotel that was shabbier than any I'd ever seen, and walked to LeShan's elegant, book-filled apartment. He was right—he was old and tired, reclining in a La-Z-Boy

---

* At least, it sounded scientifically authoritative to me at the time. Since then, I've become skeptical of much of the science around mind-body medicine. The links may exist, but proving them scientifically requires enormous care, and so far, little work has been done that meets that standard.

through the sessions, his skin sallow and drawn.

And he was no match for my mother. She was there only to please me anyway. The truth, I gradually realized, was that she wasn't interested— God was on the way.

I didn't give up. My mother and I went to a local therapist (together, because she wouldn't go on her own and I hoped that I could somehow make the sessions useful to her). We went to a workshop in Phoenix where we were told to beat on phone books with batons made of garden hose and scream about our troubles.

I realized that I wasn't going to find anyone who could reach my mom. I was on my own. The only tool I had was the one I'd used since childhood: my ability to stay connected with my mother.

She had started growing weaker, her once-athletic arms and legs shriveling as her belly grew firm and bumpy with her tumor. Her eyes looked too big for her face. One day she got impatient with my attempts to start our ancient gas lawn mower and grabbed the string herself, only to find that she could barely move it at all. She started puking green-brown bile many times a day, and soon we had to upgrade from the one-quart Pyrex measuring cup to a two-quart model.

Still, my mother insisted that she was going to live. She started adding this, though: "If there's no hope, I want to take the pills and die." When she made no effort to procure such pills, I went to the library and checked out a book called *Final Exit*.

I went into her room one morning and found my mother confused. "Can Tom fly?" she asked, an absent, awestruck expression on her face. I told her I was quite sure Tom, a college friend of hers I'd met a few times, couldn't fly. She looked so disappointed that I almost felt guilty.

Frantic, I called the doctor and got the soonest appointment. When it was time to leave, my mother was sitting at the kitchen table in her underwear with a T-shirt stretched taut over her belly. Her head was down, her ordinarily gorgeous salt-and-pepper hair hanging slack over her face, and when she looked up after I called "Ma," her eyes were empty. I couldn't see how I could get her to the doctor. I'd have to go alone.

I told her I was leaving and that she needed to go back to bed. She said she didn't want to, her voice filled with the petulant finality of a toddler. "Okay," I said, "but then you have to wait until I'm back." Her head made a motion vaguely like a nod. I tried again, my voice urgent and clipped: "You have to stay right there until I get back. You can't walk on your own. You might fall. Do you understand?" She nodded a bit more distinctly.

I left, not knowing what else to do.

I told the doctor about my mother's muddleheadedness and asked what could be done. "Nothing," he said. "She's dying, and people often get delirious when they're dying. You should call hospice."

I rushed home and found my mother still at the kitchen table. *Thank god, thank god, thank god.*

I sat on the window seat next to her and tried to figure out what on earth I was supposed to do now. She looked up and said, with surprising clarity, that I seemed upset. *She seems like she's here at the moment.*

I took a deep breath. "The doctor says that you're dying, and that's why you've been confused." I paused, studying her face to see if she was going to reject that, but I saw nothing. "Do you want to take the pills?" I kept my voice even, neutral, as if asking your mother if she wants to kill herself were no different than asking if she'd like some lunch.

She smirked at me. "You can't get rid of me that easily, girlie," she said.

Tears bit at my eyes and I looked down. *It's a joke,* I told myself. *It's just a joke.*

"I'm going to live," she added, and then her head dropped back down.

I spent the next day in a frenzy. My whole life I'd accepted and worked with my mother's beliefs, no matter how odd they might sound to outsiders. But one couldn't glance at her without seeing the death upon her, with her swollen belly and shriveled limbs and cheekbones protruding like she was a concentration camp victim. I didn't believe that a miracle would just happen without our doing something to create it, and my mother was obviously not capable of participating in that.

So what was I going to do? Did I believe she was going to live or not?

And then I felt like a miracle did occur—not one that made the cancer melt away, but a miracle nonetheless. A kind of grace entered me. If my mother still believed that she could live, then she could live, goddammit. If she needed me to look at her great swollen cancer belly and be convinced she would survive, that was exactly what I was going to do. I was going to measure her belly every day, and it was going to shrink. I felt complete clarity. I wasn't in denial about how sick she was, or how unlikely it was that she'd live. But I was somehow able to hold those contradictions all at once, to look directly at the illness and stare it down, to believe that she'd live in spite of it all. My days felt altered, heightened, as though all the mass had been drained out of the world and replaced with light.

And then, of course, my mother died.

When her breath slowed, the death rattle drawing out longer and longer until it stopped, I thought, *Do I believe this? Now do I accept she's dead? Is this enough to make me stop believing in my miracle?* And then I fled the room.

FLYING TO MIAMI two decades later to see Klimas, my psyche couldn't reach toward a miracle. I'd come to believe, in a deep, preconscious way, that the world unfolded in a different pattern. I felt like this terrible thing, this illness, had been given to me, and when such things arrive, you can't return them. The dreadful gift is yours, and the way forward is not to beg God to take it back but to stop pushing it away and get to know it, embrace it, confront it, reach absolution.

I took that kind of observation about the nature of the hidden world underlying physical reality seriously. But at the same time, rationally, I didn't see any reason that I couldn't get my miracle. Some patients had great results from anti-virals, and a lymphoma drug had recently brought full remissions for a few patients. A number of patients had pursued a new theory that CFS was caused by a retrovirus known as XMRV by taking AIDS drugs (since HIV is also a retrovirus). Some reported that they had benefited, even though the research on the XMRV theory was becoming embroiled in controversy. Even if I didn't get some dramatic recovery, I might at least find a small-scale miracle, something that would pick me up off the floor and allow me to return to my simple hundred-pound handicap.

So sitting on the airplane, I narrowed my focus, chanting with each breath: Small miracle. Small miracle. Small miracle.

WHEN I STAGGERED, SEMI-PARALYZED, into Klimas's office and saw the same sturdy, unflappable face that I'd seen in her pictures on the Internet, I felt like a fan girl meeting a rock star. But being crippled also left me feeling raw, exposed, as though my skin had been stripped off along with my nerve sheaths.

Klimas smiled and said wryly, "Your legs aren't working too well for you there! We should be able to get you feeling better." I nearly cried.

Klimas laid out her understanding of what this disease was, her voice warm and practical and smart. First of all, she said, she was confident that CFS is not psychosomatic. The abnormalities she'd seen in patients' blood work were far too consistent for that.

Her quick-and-dirty explanation for the illness was that it boiled down to neuroinflammation. That was what was screwing up my legs, she said. The international name for chronic fatigue syndrome, myalgic encephalomyelitis, fit with this explanation: "Myalgic" means pain, "encephalo-" means the brain, "-myel-" means the spinal cord, and "-itis" means inflammation. Because the name chronic fatigue syndrome is so misleading, Klimas and others often called the disease ME/CFS, as a way of sneaking the less familiar international name into the American consciousness.*

---

* At the time of writing this book, there is no good name for this illness. "Chronic fatigue syndrome" is horrendous—trivializing, inaccurate, and overly broad—but "myalgic encephalomyelitis" has its own drawbacks.

I know of no scientists who use the term "myalgic encephalomyelitis" on its own. They point out that we have only a small amount of scientific evidence to support the idea that patients' brains and spinal cords are inflamed (though it sure felt like it to me!). We don't know at this point if all patients have neuroinflammation, and we certainly don't know if neuroinflammation is at the root of the diverse array of symptoms that plague patients.

From a patient perspective, however, "myalgic encephalomyelitis" has a lot going for it. Those who are seriously affected pretty much all have both pain and neurological symptoms that seem related to inflammation. The scientific evidence for neuroinflammation has grown over the last few years—and of course, with so little research funding, it's hardly surprising that more evidence doesn't yet exist. The name has a deeper pedigree than "chronic fatigue syndrome": It was coined in 1956, and the World Health Organization continues to list it. And, of course, "myalgic encephalomyelitis" has a serious tone that is appropriate for the seriousness of the condition. The patient community has increasingly embraced the name ME. Many consider ME to be distinct from CFS, reserving the term ME for more severe forms of the illness.

The National Academy of Medicine suggested the name "systemic exertion intolerance disease" in its 2015 report on the illness, but that name has received little support.

For myself, I found the scientific objections to the name ME too compelling to ignore. I've stuck with ME/CFS as a compromise solution, especially because federal agencies are using that term and it's one my journalism editors would accept. There's no question that it's a klunky compromise. It's especially problematic for those working to distinguish ME from CFS.

The name issue is intimately connected to the issue of definition. Just what illness are we naming here? Both ME and CFS have multiple competing definitions, each of which captures a different patient population. Most likely, none of the definitions carves nature at its joints, capturing a precise set of patients who share a common root physiological problem. Very broad definitions of chronic fatigue syndrome, such as the Oxford definition which requires only six months of disabling fatigue as the primary symptom, certainly don't.

I don't think we'll find a name or a definition that the community as a whole will embrace until high-quality science reveals the underlying mechanisms of the disease.

Klimas said that she found it useful to explain the disease as neuro-inflammation because people can grasp the idea quickly and understand that the disease is real and serious. But, she said, the reality of ME/CFS is so much more: It also involves immune dysregulation and autonomic problems and out-of-whack hormones and screwed-up sleep and on and on and on, the menagerie of abnormalities that I'd found overwhelming and confusing.

The menagerie came together, in her mind, as a problem of "homeostasis." Ordinarily, she explained, the body regulates itself to maintain a state of health. If your core temperature gets a little low, for example, the body fires up the engines to get back to 98.6 degrees. Similar mechanisms regulate blood pH and glucose levels and oxygen levels and all the other levels, adjusting the internal physiology to maintain health. But in ME/CFS patients, the body had gotten pushed into a different mode, and the state the body worked to return to wasn't a healthy one.

ME/CFS patients, for example, tend to have low levels of cortisol, a hormone that fires up the body, increasing energy, immune function, and memory. Klimas said she found that when she gave patients regular supplemental hydrocortisone, she could initially get their cortisol levels up to normal. But after a while, she'd have to increase the dose again and again. The body responded to the supplementation by reducing its own production, as if it were regulating itself to maintain a lower set point. Her theory was that many complicated feedback loops stabilized the body in a very suboptimal state.

Klimas described health and illness as two valleys with a mountain between them. If you push a ball from the floor of either valley up the side of the mountain a bit and then let go, it will roll back to the bottom of the same valley. Klimas's job, for patients like me, was to push the ball from the valley of ME/CFS all the way up and over the mountain, so it would roll down into the valley of health. There, my body would naturally maintain that healthy state.

Klimas's approach was to identify as many different ways my body was out of whack as she could, and then to simultaneously nudge all of them in the right direction. Not only would that make me feel better in the moment, it might get me over the mountain.

I asked her about the notion that chronic fatigue syndrome is a "trashcan diagnosis," a wastebasket doctors throw unrelated patients into when they don't know what to do with them. Is it really a single disease?

"First, I have to say that that depends on how you define it," she said. Neither scientists nor clinicians had settled on a single definition of the disease, which was a huge problem, especially for research. Different studies were analyzing different types of patients while describing them all as having "chronic fatigue syndrome." Some of the definitions of the disease were so broad—for example, including all patients with six months of otherwise unexplained fatigue with no other symptoms required—that yes, patients could have entirely unrelated ailments. Many such patients, for example, were suffering from primary depression.

But she didn't find *her* patients hard to recognize. The problems they had were quite similar: fatigue, difficulties standing for long, cognitive and neurological problems, sleep issues, flulike symptoms—and most of all, an inability to tolerate exercise. Furthermore, when she took up her researcher's role and looked at patients' immune markers and gene expression and other biological signals, she found that they looked similar too.

But, she said, even among her patients, there are different doors into the disease, and as a result there are different doors out as well. Some patients, she theorized, got pushed over the mountain into the valley of ME/CFS because they got a particularly terrible virus; others had messed-up hormones; others had gotten too much exposure to some environmental toxin; most had a combination of those and other nasty shoves. Each patient therefore requires a slightly different combination of counter-pushes to get them back into the valley of health.

So does that make it one disease or many? She preferred to think of it as one, but with overlapping subgroups.

In any event, Klimas said, the first step to getting me functional was to do loads of tests. She'd test my blood for immune abnormalities, particularly looking at the functioning of my natural killer cells, the immune system's appointed assassins for cancer and other baddies. She'd also check the levels of tiny immune regulators called cytokines. (My ears pricked up at the word "cytokine," remembering the explanation offered by Rosenbaum, the very first ME/CFS doctor I'd seen, that I had suffered a "cytokine storm" after the vaccine. Klimas said yes, that's likely what had happened, creating neuroinflammation.) She'd check various hormone levels and look for old viruses that may have seized their chance to reactivate when my immune system started malfunctioning. She'd order an MRI of my brain. She recommended aggressive cancer screening, because low natural-killer-cell functioning leaves ME/CFS patients vulnerable to cancer.

And right in her office, Klimas would test me for a problem called orthostatic intolerance—essentially, low physical tolerance for being upright. "But I already know you have it," she said, laughing. "Look at you!" She gestured at my nearly horizontal position, slumping down with my feet propped up on another chair. When most ME/CFS patients are vertical, she explained, their blood pressure drops and their heart rate climbs—that's why I'd instinctively stayed as horizontal as I could. The problem, she said, is that ME/CFS patients typically have about a liter less blood than people who are healthy, and as a result, there isn't enough available for the body to get it all the way to the brain when the patient is standing.

I was doubtful. Even before I'd gotten sick, I'd tended to get dizzy when I first stood up, but it hadn't gotten worse with the illness, nor did I notice my heart racing. Klimas explained that low blood pressure doesn't necessarily manifest as dizziness. It can manifest as generally feeling like crap—and I certainly did often feel like crap when standing up.

To formally test me for orthostatic intolerance, Klimas's assistant strapped me tightly to a table and attached electrodes and a blood pressure cuff to my body. After the assistant monitored me for a few minutes, she tilted the table until it was nearly vertical.

Although I was strapped tightly enough that standing was effortless, after four minutes, I didn't feel so well. After six minutes, the assistant said my blood pressure had dropped from a perfectly normal 119/78 to 88/60. Soon thereafter, a wave of heat, light-headedness, and nausea passed over me, and I begged her to stop the test. "Wait!" she said. "I'm just about to take another reading!" She put me down moments before I would have puked or passed out. At eight minutes, she told me, my blood pressure was way below normal at 80/52 and my pulse was 140.

Klimas's assistant parked me in a massage chair in the waiting room and hooked me up to a liter of saline to increase my blood volume before she retested me. The massage chairs were the only luxurious things in the office. As I sank into one gratefully, it felt as basic and essential as the IV bag hanger next to me.

While the IV dripped, I chatted with a young man who, despite his bulging muscles and strapping appearance, had been sick with ME/CFS for three years. I felt stupidly surprised to see such an apparently vital man suffering from this illness—ironic given the number of times people had told me that I looked great even as I strained under the effort of holding a conversation. The young man told me that working full-time from home was all he could do, and he was afraid even that might soon be beyond him. His first stop had been at the prestigious Cleveland Clinic, he said, where he'd been told his problem was psychological.

When Klimas's assistant came back for me and had me repeat the tilt-table test, I was able to finish the full 30-minute protocol, though by the end, my heart rate was somewhat elevated. So Klimas prescribed a beta-blocker to keep my heart from racing, and in lieu of IV fluids, she recommended something simpler: Gatorade. The electrolytes and water, she said, would increase my blood volume and help with the problem.

I was oddly buoyed by failing the tilt-table test so dramatically. It wasn't just that it suggested a treatment. My relief was more basic: Finally, a doctor had found something clearly, dramatically wrong with me. But my reaction struck me as peculiar. Wasn't it already obvious that something was clearly, dramatically wrong when I, for example, couldn't turn over in bed? This, however, was an accepted test, one that generated objective numbers and had nothing to do with my effort or lack thereof. It felt *real*.

KLIMAS AND I TALKED again after the tilt-table test, and I asked her in a small voice whether it was practical to have a child while dealing with this illness. My chest felt tight enough to crush my heart.

"Yes!" she cried. "Do it! Don't delay!"

Oh my god, I thought. *I can have a kid!* But almost immediately, horror mixed into my exultation: *How will William and I deal with that answer together?*

Klimas reported that most of her patients felt great during pregnancy.

One had kept herself pregnant almost all the time because it was the only way she felt good, ending up with seven kids (a less-than-excellent strategy, I thought, for coping with illness). Klimas's theory was that her pregnant patients felt better because pregnancy increases blood volume, helping their bodies maintain their blood pressure when they stood. Three months after birth, though, blood volume drops again and women can end up feeling terrible. Klimas assured me, though, that she would watch carefully for that and treat it before it became a problem. Studies showed no significant risks to the child, she reported, but I should get started right away: Women with ME/CFS tend to go through menopause early.

"But will I be well enough to take care of a baby?" I asked, forcing my tongue to form the words.

"Oh yeah!" she said. "You're going to get better. The only thing is that you'll have to make sure you get your sleep, which of course can be a challenge with a newborn. You'll just need a supportive partner," she said, beaming at William.

Uh-oh, I thought.

EVEN BEFORE WE GOT the remaining test results, Klimas had other treatments that she hoped would help. She prescribed an immune modulator to convince my immune system that my body wasn't under constant attack. She recommended a rather mysterious drug called naltrexone because she had discovered that tiny doses of it sometimes makes ME/CFS patients feel better—even though the drug's primary use, at higher dosages, is to block opioids in the brain, thereby making recreational drugs less satisfying and helping addicts kick the habit. She also recommended various research-backed supplements, and as she described them, I flashed back to my meeting with Rosenbaum: This one will help the mitochondria, that one will regulate my immune system, this other one will calm inflammation.

Sleep, she said, is a huge issue in this disease, but to figure out how to improve my sleep, she needed more information. So she recommended I start using a device to monitor my sleep, and on a follow-up appointment, she'd analyze that data to make recommendations.

She also discussed how to exercise safely. Of course, she said, avoiding overdoing it was key. She told me to wear a heart monitor all the time and set it to beep when my heart rate got too high. She also said I'd likely do better if I exercised in a horizontal position, making it easier for my cardiovascular system to pump blood up to my head. And she recommended five minutes of exercise alternating with five minutes of rest, giving my body recovery time as I went. I told her about my miracle swim cure, and although she was enthusiastic about swimming as a good, horizontal exercise, she was as flummoxed as everyone else about why it was so restorative for me.

None of the ideas I'd come in with passed muster for her, though. She didn't recommend anti-virals unless my test results showed that my viral levels were very high, because the drugs, she said, are expensive and hard on patients. As I figured, the recent ambiguous results on XMRV had convinced her to discourage patients from trying antiretroviral drugs. And the lymphoma drug that I'd heard about was still highly experimental and needed more study before she could recommend it.

Toward the end of my seven hours in her office, Klimas flopped in one of the massage chairs next to me. She had just returned from presenting at an ME/CFS conference in England, and the jet lag was making her chattily punchy. She described how challenging it was to run her clinic. She could help only a tiny percentage of the patients who needed her, but to expand, she'd need to take insurance, and to take insurance, she'd need to double her staff, and to double her staff, she'd have to spend more time on management rather than seeing patients. She was also frustrated that she hadn't been able to train more young doctors in the field. There was so little research funding that ambitious young researchers were stymied and turned to other diseases.

I asked her how her patients did—was she really able to help them? "Yes," she said, and then paused and looked thoughtful. "I don't think any of my patients are just stuck." She warned me not to judge my prospects for recovery by what I read on the online patient forum, pointing out that when patients get better, they go live their lives and don't hang out on the forum anymore.

I felt a surge of hope—but also of skepticism. Maybe a warning like the one she gave me about the forum applied to her: Perhaps she never saw her patients who got stuck, because they gave up and no longer made the long trek to see her. But I pushed that out of my mind.

As I left her office, I felt weak with both fatigue and relief. At last, I had found a true authority with a genuinely scientific understanding of my illness and a great deal of caring for her patients. Her very existence felt like a balm for my soul. In a way, she wasn't doing anything so amazing—she was simply being a good doctor. But with an illness so misunderstood, being a good doctor felt like a noble and brave thing.

William and I were planning to fly out late the next day, and before that, we planned to go to the Everglades. But in the morning, I was unable to even sit upright for long. We had to check out of our hotel room, so we sat in the car, feeling rather forlorn and homeless as I lolled lifelessly in the seat.

Then William suggested we go to Klimas's office so I could rest in one of her lovely massage chair recliners—*brilliant*. The office manager welcomed us and got me a Gatorade, and once the revolting neon-red fluid slid down my throat, presto! I felt the life come back into me. I drank a second one and was able to walk a bit. I could hardly believe it.

Half an hour later, we decided to go to the Everglades after all. When we asked at the gate if they had a wheelchair we could use, the attendant asked if I was permanently disabled. I hesitated and then said yes. She gave me a Golden Eagle pass that brought free entry into any national park, for the rest of my life. William and I grinned at each other.

William pushed me in their wheelchair along a canal, dodging the sunbathing alligators lolling across the path. Great rivers of grass blew in the wind. A green-black cormorant swam through the clear water like a feathered fish, lazily pecking at the algae on the streambed. I leaned my head back to kiss William.

I had gotten my miracle after all. And lo, it was Gatorade.

CHAPTER 7

ALONE

The morning after we returned from Florida, I woke up barely able to move, groaning as I staggered to the bathroom. *Gatorade time!* But Gatorade wasn't in our normal supplies, so I asked William to go get some.

"I have work to do," he said. "It's only two blocks. Get it yourself. You can't expect me to take care of you all the time the way I did on the trip."

I gasped. It was true that he'd been wonderful in Florida, supportive and present, figuring everything out with me. I knew how hard my illness was on him, and I'd thought that perhaps our connectedness on the trip showed we'd gotten over a hump together. *Well, thanks for clearing that up,* I snorted to myself.

I caught myself before I snapped at him, my aggravation wilting into weary futility. I knew that William would get the Gatorade for me when I insisted—he knew as well as I did that it was all but impossible for me to. But as he walked to the store to get it, he wouldn't be suffused with his love for me, nor would he pat himself on the back for being such a great boyfriend. When he returned, my genuine appreciation would be salted with irritation, and William would feel deprived. And then my next need would feel even more onerous to him.

As clear as our pattern of resentment was to both of us, neither of us knew how to get out of it. So we reenacted it, just as I'd imagined. He got the Gatorade and then went back to work as I sucked down my glowing urine-colored elixir, the few feet between us a frozen crevasse.

I remembered William once telling me that he thought the illness was harder on him than on me. I'd raged to myself, *Just which one of us is paralyzed here?* But the irony was that in a way, he was right. The intensity of my illness crushed him and made his life feel narrowed, reduced. He felt constantly aware that my illness might suck the happiness from our lives, no matter what we did. On top of that, I didn't, in his eyes, sufficiently appreciate his sacrifice and devotion in staying with me despite that.

But I didn't want staying with me to be an act of sacrifice and devotion. I believed we could live richly in spite of the illness—or at least, I was hell-bent on doing so. To me, living with the illness felt like learning to fence with one arm tied behind my back, and then with my legs tied together too. Sufficient skill, I was convinced, could overcome the handicap. That belief provided the lubrication that let the agony slide past and made the illness bearable.

I stopped my cogitations when I realized that the Gatorade miracle had worked again: *I can walk!* I decided to take advantage of my reclaimed ability to go to my usual café two blocks away and work on a report I was months behind on.

I walked slowly, slowly, feeling as though all that Gatorade I'd just sucked down might spill out my ears. As I settled in at my old table next to a window, I soaked up the chatter of other humans, the smell of the yeast and flour, the feeling of sitting up in a hard wooden chair. I pulled out my computer and, blessedly, worked.

After a couple of hours, though, my thoughts grew slow and stupid and I had the familiar feeling that my brain was swelling against the back of my eyeballs. I packed up my computer and went to stand up—and found that I couldn't. And I didn't have any Gatorade.

Fuck. I'll be damned if I'm going to call William right now.

The most important electrolyte, I knew, was sodium, so I unscrewed a salt shaker and poured a small mountain of salt into my hand. I slugged it down with a full glass of water and then sat, stuporous, for 10 minutes. I felt my brain start to clear, and I braced myself on the chair and table and tried getting up again: Voilà! I was able to walk home without making a spectacle of myself. I felt a giddy delight: I had mastered one more fencing move. *Ha!*

By the time I got home, though, I was exhausted and went back to bed. *Well, two hours of work are a lot better than no hours of work,* I thought.

In the weeks following the appointment, I found that I was no longer stuck in bed nearly all the time, as I'd been before the trip to see Klimas, but my abilities were still constrained and unpredictable. I took my six-year-old nephew to a museum for an hour and ended up in bed and in pain for the next two days. I rallied for an interview on NPR's *All Things Considered* about the prize a mathematician won for discovering, among other things, that there are 28 different kinds of spheres in seven dimensions. While I thought I sounded reasonably coherent and even lively on air, I could barely say my name or get back to my car once the interview was over. Gatorade could be counted on to raise me from the lowest points, but it didn't provide reliable function overall.

The endless self-focus of illness, the consuming minutiae of judging and predicting and managing my physical state, aggravated and bored me. And when I was stuck in bed, I was consumed by uncertainty about what kind of life was open to me now. Most of all, I obsessed about whether I'd be able to have a child. Klimas's encouragement was all well and good, but it was predicated on having a "supportive partner." Not only was William unwilling, he was incapable.

The "kid question" felt like a dark force glowering in the corner. William was caring for me far more than he ever had before, while knowing that our future together seemed damned whatever happened: If I got better, I'd leave him to have a kid; if I didn't, my illness would continue to limit our lives. My heart broke, for myself but almost more for William. I remembered how my own hope for a future with Geoff had slowly suffocated under his illness, and how hard it had been to continue to care for him once that hope was snuffed.

I knew the idea of having a child while I was this sick was insane, with or without William. But it seemed even more insane to not have a child. My children felt present to me, like they already existed. I loved them; I felt as though I almost knew them. To not manage to bring them into the world seemed like an unforgivable failure. I also imagined living a kind of half-life if I remained childless, like a huge part of me would never be expressed. If this damned illness deprived me of my children, I'd never forgive it. And I knew I couldn't forgive William either, no matter how much sympathy I had for his concerns.

As I spent hour after hour lying in bed, looking at William's back as he worked at his computer, I began fantasizing of my own home and land in Santa Fe, of my stream and my ponderosa trees, a quiet place I could be alone to think my own thoughts. *I can't do this anymore,* I thought. *I can't be this sick, be unable to have a child, and have my illness drag my partner down too. I've got to get out.* Of course, if I went home, I'd be all alone, far from town, with no one to help me—but the cost of William's help was too high, and I didn't have anyone else to turn to.

I told William I needed to go home, and he agreed that I should go to Santa Fe for the summer. He talked of my return to Berkeley in the fall, but I knew I wouldn't be coming back.

Pulling out of our driveway in my packed Subaru a few weeks later with William waving good-bye, I felt as though I were ripping my heart right out of my chest. William and I had intertwined so deeply that leaving him felt like an act of violence—but also like a grasp at life. As I drove away, my lungs seemed to have forgotten how to breathe, and sounds I didn't recognize came from my chest as I labored to pull in air.

I tried to take comfort in a dream I'd had the night before: I'd been too sick to walk and had to cross a river in flood. Somehow, I had not only managed to get across, I'd carried a half-drowned deer to safety with me.

I couldn't help but hope, yet again, that changing my life would change my health. Surely, I thought, escaping the tightening noose our relationship had turned into and returning to the land I so loved would make me feel at least a little bit better. How could it not?

I PICKED UP my friend Sheila, who had volunteered to help me move back home. She was a fine art photographer and had never been to the Southwest before, so I got the joy of seeing the familiar desert landscape we were crossing through Sheila's eyes. She goggled out the window at the mesas and cacti and occasionally hollered that we needed to stop so she could take a picture. Except for my occasional inability to get up out of the car or sustain a conversation, the drive felt like two girlfriends on an ordinary road trip.

When we turned east toward the mountains just north of Santa Fe, I felt my chest expand. The road began to rise and fall through the foothills before dwindling to a single lane and turning into my narrow, oak-filled valley, a riot of bright-green leaves. We turned across the bridge I'd built, strong enough to hold a concrete truck, and drove under my own great ponderosas. We got out of the car, and I sucked in a great lungful of butterscotch-scented air. Sheila was spinning around slowly. "I can see why you wanted to come back here," she said.

My house was rented out, but the pair of old travel trailers I had lived in while building the house were empty, and they were to be my home again. I saw their ugly tin-can sides and knew that by any objective standard they were crappy, but I'd come to love them over the decade I'd owned them. I'd installed hardwood floors, supplied the kitchen/bathroom trailer with water from a rainwater purification system I'd developed myself, fixed their leaks, replaced the appliances one by one as they'd broken. Their many windows looked out toward the stream, and the breeze blew through them on hot days. The kitchen was tiny but efficient, everything within a step, and I even loved the minuscule bathtub I could just fold myself into.

We discovered that uninvited mousy tenants had set up housekeeping while I was gone, decorating the place with their droppings. Sheila dauntlessly donned a mask, banned me from the trailer until she was done (lest hantavirus do in my compromised immune system), evicted the mice, and cleaned up their turds. I couldn't have brought myself to ask her to do such an unpleasant job if she hadn't volunteered. When she was done, I pulled a panel off the wall to uncover the spot where the pipes entered the trailers, and I stuffed steel wool around the gaps, hoping to prevent new squatters from taking over the place.

Over the next week, Sheila unloaded the car, followed my instructions about unpacking, and helped me cook a huge mass of food that I froze in individual containers, insurance in case I was too sick to cook for myself.

I was determined to show Sheila the spots up the stream I so loved— the oak tree arbor, the rock-cooled "Anasazi icebox," and most of all, the 20-foot waterfall that sprayed its grotto with mist. But each time we went up the trail, I had to turn around within a quarter mile.

The day before Sheila left, though, I woke up feeling good, and I sent us on an expedition to one of the most beautiful places on earth, a wonderland of sculpted, eroding white cliffs an hour away. I walked for five minutes, lay down for five minutes, and then walked again, following the advice Klimas had given me to exercise safely. Sheila matched my slow pace by pausing to take photographs, and Frances looped back from time to time before sprinting off to check out another crevice. I felt as though I were expanding, untwisting, growing into the landscape. *Thank god I'm home.*

I drove Sheila to the train station for her trip home and told her what a hero she'd been. She tilted her head and shrugged her shoulders. "I'm glad I could help, kiddo," she said. "But it's not adequate. It's just not adequate." She hugged me, her body thin and long against me.

My only plan was to hope that I improved—but in fact, I mostly felt like crap after she left, worse than in Berkeley. Sometimes my groans were so loud as I pulled myself up the stairs into the trailer with the bathroom that the tenant in my house ran out to help. I got a pee bucket to put next to the bed and hoped that at least I'd be able to use that. But sometimes I was too weak to even roll out of bed to use it.

Probably just the exertion of moving, I figured. *It'll get better.* I opened the bedroom door so I could look from my bed out through the ponderosas at the stream and listen to the birds' chatter and the burble of the stream. Frances would find a stick, toss it in the air, and chase it down, over and over, or she'd run after a squirrel and dance at the bottom of the tree while the squirrel lectured her on her bad behavior from its safe perch. In the evenings, she curled up in bed with me, warmth and energy thrumming into me from her strong, solid body.

I reminded myself that it had only been a couple of months since I'd seen Klimas, and her treatments hadn't taken full effect yet. A couple of weeks before leaving Berkeley, I'd had a phone consultation with her to get my test results, and she reported signs of reactivated viruses everywhere: My blood teemed with antibodies to Epstein-Barr, cytomegalovirus, *Mycoplasma pneumoniae*, and varicella. The immune messengers called cytokines indicated lots of inflammation, and one cytokine in particular, INF-gamma, was extremely high. "That's your natural antiviral," Klimas said. "You're cranking! That's more evidence that there are viruses, and, hey, your body is trying to deal with them! For a lot of people with ME/CFS, their bodies are too worn out to do that. That's pretty cool."

But my immune cells were dying off faster than they should, an indication that my immune system was starting to wear down, and my natural killer cells barely functioned. Still, Klimas said that many of her patients' natural killer cells were even weaker than mine, and at my level, prospects for improvement were good. To her, all of that meant we were on the right track. The immune modulators I was on should help out my immune system. Stay the course!

But that meant I had no new treatments to pin my hopes on—I just had to give the current treatments more time. *Be patient,* I told myself, and I found the admonition more effective than it had been in Berkeley.

FROM TIME TO TIME, I considered what I'd do if I didn't get better. It was a question I could only look at out of the corner of my eye, in quick glimpses.

I didn't feel like I had any family I could turn to. My mother had estranged herself from almost all of her family—and me along with her. One of my aunts had reached out to me just after my mother died, sending me a kind note and a box of pecans from her orchard. Given my mother's rejection of her family, the box of pecans felt dangerous to me, like betrayal and enmeshment lay hidden inside the ruddy shells. I cracked a pecan open and found it rotten. I laughed, threw the box away, and didn't respond. Years later, when I had managed to separate my sense of myself from my mother more, I reached out to my aunt and even went to visit, and she was extremely kind. But still, we barely knew each other. I certainly didn't feel like I could throw myself on her mercy.

My sister Robin and I kept in touch regularly, and I felt her love. We'd grown up together until I was seven, when my mother sent her and my brother Ty to live elsewhere. I'd seen Ty only twice since then, but Robin moved back nearby when I was 11 and she was 19. She really felt like my sister, but our mother had stood between us when she was alive. I was my mother's golden girl, while Robin tried and tried to make her happy and only rarely received her approval. I was always amazed and impressed that Robin didn't resent me for my unearned, blessed status. After our mother died, Robin and I had slowly grown our relationship, but the web of connections between us certainly wasn't strong enough to bear the weight of her supporting me through long-term disability.

I'd never known my father, and he had died a few months before my mother did. I had always known that he had five other children, though growing up, I hadn't even known their names. I'd finally tracked them down eight years earlier, a few years after Geoff and I had split up. It had occurred to me to ask Robin for their names—she had played with them as a kid—and she provided those she remembered (some of which turned out to be wrong).

Armed with the names, I sat at my desk in my office, with its little octagonal window that looked out on the ponderosas and made me feel like I was in a tree house, and used the newly popular search engine Google to look for traces of them on the Internet. I managed to track down a phone number for my half brother Wes in Austin, and that evening, I called him up. He wasn't there, so I left a message. As I spoke, I thought fast: *What should I say? Does he know I exist? Will he even believe me?* I settled on the vague statement that I was a family member trying to get in touch.

A few hours later, I got a call from a very stunned Wes: He'd asked his maternal uncle who I might be and heard for the first time that his dad had had an affair with my mother in the years after Wes's youngest sister, Tricia, had been born, and yes, there had been a child. Wes had never suspected it. Although his parents had separated a few months before his—our—dad died, Wes had seen their long marriage as a mostly happy one.

We exchanged some basic information, and I felt a tentative warmth from him trying to reach its way through his shock—though he took pains to mention that his dad's estate had no money in it, a possibility that had never occurred to me.

Some months later, after more phone calls and e-mails, I visited him and his sisters in Austin. I knocked on the door of a giant tract house and a tall, blond-haired man opened it. "I'm not quite sure what to do here," Wes said, "but I guess I should give you a hug." And he wrapped me up.

Wes sat me down at his kitchen table and pulled out the photo albums. For the first time, I saw a picture of my father, taken not long before he died: a graying man with a high, round belly and heavy-browed, deep-set, squinty eyes. My eyes, only gray. When Tricia came into the room, her eyebrows flew up: Our eyes were mirror images of one another, like his but dark. "I guess you *are* my father's daughter!" she said.

They began telling me stories, stories of my father, coming from these people I'd just met. Someone mentioned his favorite brownies, with caramel in the middle—I knew those brownies! My mother had made them, and it had been my job to unwrap the Kraft caramels, cellophane crinkling and a deep golden sweetness seeping from between my teeth as I chewed and worked. Another sibling dug out a letter my father had written to her son with an outline of his hand: "Someday," he had written, "your hand will be this big." Barely breathing, I held my hand against it. Mine was much smaller.

For the next two days, I was swept into the hubbub of a big family so unlike my own, which had been mostly just me and my mom, until it was mostly just me. And at the end of the weekend, the whirlwind tossed me back out to my ordinary existence.

Lying alone in my trailers these years later, I thought of my half siblings sometimes and wondered what it would be like if one of them got terribly ill. Would the others swoop in to help? Probably, but they'd grown up together, and they still barely knew me. We'd had occasional contact since then, but building those relationships would require continuing effort over years, effort I couldn't make at the moment. In the meantime, I was on my own.

ONE EVENING, a science-writer friend, Christie, was visiting Santa Fe, so a group of us got together for dinner. I pushed myself to go despite feeling poorly. One friend talked about his progress in his book about cancer, another described reporting her *New York Times* story about Navajos resisting a uranium mine. I mentioned a story I'd written for my *Science News* column about the mathematics of beer bubbles, but forming words took so much effort that I quickly quieted.

I caught snippets of their accounts of future projects and goals and frustrations, but I couldn't stay tuned in long enough to follow what they said. My friends seemed to be floating away from me on this great river of conversation and stories and success, while I was drowning in the shallows. I wondered when I'd next work on a story I deeply cared about. I watched their faces, trying to catch when to nod or laugh.

I noticed myself sagging lower and lower in the chair, head propped on hand, and I finally thought, *Ah! Low blood pressure! Must have salt!* I surreptitiously poured some into my hand under the table, tossed it down my throat when my friends were distracted, and slugged some water down.

It helped some, but I could still feel my energy sinking, sinking, sinking. I tried again: salt under table, toss in mouth, water. The Gatorade miracle seemed to be fading, and I wondered if perhaps my kidneys had gotten more efficient at disposing of the extra electrolytes. The conversation continued to drift past me, and I decided it was time to give up. I made my apologies and left.

As I walked away, my left leg started to drag, and I staggered down the stairs, supporting myself against the wall and pushing my leg down with my hands, step by step. *Just a block and a half to the car,* I thought. *You can do it, Julie.* But my steps were getting shorter, the grunts I couldn't suppress louder. I had to cross a road, and though I had barely noticed the slope in roads for drainage when I was healthy, that grade now felt like a mountain. I got across the road only to face the intimidating slope of a sidewalk cut. My steps diminished to a couple of inches apiece, an inch, and finally, nothing. I was stuck.

I leaned against a building and caught my breath. My heart rate monitor was beeping stridently, warning I had exceeded safe limits. I took a deep breath and considered my options. *I guess I need some help.* I called one of my friends but got no answer. I started looking for the next phone number.

A very young woman in a restaurant uniform came out, face earnest, carrying a chair from the restaurant. She urged me to sit down, asked me how she could help, volunteered to drive me home, told me she didn't mind if she got fired for disappearing from her job as a bus girl. Her intensity and kindness overwhelmed me. My eyes sprang tears, which belied what I wanted to say: *This is normal for me, no big deal really. I just need to get one more block back to my car and then I'll be fine, and my friends can help. No need for concern.*

I stammered out, "Look, the gray hair of the man there, up on the balcony, he's one of my friends, right there!" I persuaded her to let me call Christie, but then I struggled to find the right number. My brain felt like it was short-circuiting and might set on fire as the nice young woman kept talking. My phone started calling Christie's number, but it had automatically chosen her work number. I stabbed at the phone to make it stop, it kept ringing, the bus girl was telling me how she'd do anything I needed, how she knew what it was like, how she just had to do something when someone was hurting. I finally managed to make the phone hang up.

Just before I asked the young woman to go upstairs to get one of my friends, my phone rang. Apparently Christie's work number *was* her cell phone number. Yes, absolutely, she said, she'd come help.

The young woman told me that her mother was sick, and that's how she knew what it was like. She started crying, and I gave her a hug from the chair, thinking back on my own terror when my mother was dying. The girl was so tiny I felt as though my arms could wrap around her twice. When Christie arrived, the girl and I were both teary-eyed, in an embrace.

Christie helped me up from the chair, and I saw the shock and fear on her face when I couldn't stand up straight and could barely move. The only reassurance I could offer was through specific instructions: Push forward on my lower back, no, a little harder, yes, that's it. In the hubbub, I barely gave the young woman a good-bye, absorbed by the effort of moving my legs. I swore later that I'd go back and thank her, but I never did.

After I'd made it home, settled back in bed, and curled up around Frances, I thought, *Well, you chose it, Julie. You chose to be alone, and this is part of that reality. Better get used to it.*

PART 2

SOLITARY

CHAPTER 8

RAGE

During the long days I was stuck in bed after I returned to Santa Fe, I started dipping into the online patient forum from time to time. I didn't find it nearly so off-putting as I had previously: Having disintegrated so thoroughly myself, I now found their suffering familiar rather than frightening.

I dug around, looking for an idea that could make me feel better, but I still found the treatments I read about patients pursuing uncomfortably unscientific. I mostly found myself drawn to threads about the PACE trial. That was the study from the previous February that had so puzzled and upset me, the one that had claimed that psychotherapy and gradually increasing exercise could effectively treat or even cure ME/CFS.

I had tried to put the trial out of my mind in the previous months, hoping it would fall into obscurity just as other, similar scientific studies had. But on the forum, I read about how the study had worldwide influence: Web sites for the CDC, the Mayo Clinic, UpToDate, and Kaiser, for example, all highlighted cognitive behavioral therapy (CBT) and graded exercise therapy as the only proven treatments for ME/CFS.

As absurd as that seemed to me, I was startled by the intensity of the fury the study inspired on the forum. It seemed that for many patients, the trial had acquired the wickedness of Mordor, a locus of evil and hate focused on them. *I can't believe these scientists are villains in a Tolkien novel.*

The anger grew especially intense on any mention of the trial's principal architect, a fellow named Simon Wessely. On the patient forum, his name often came attached to some condemning adjective: "evil," "warped," "morally bankrupt." *A wee bit over the top, maybe?*

Then I read some of his articles and speeches. He didn't quite say that ME/CFS was all in our heads, but he came very, very close. He said that ME/CFS and psychiatric disorders had pretty much the same causes, with the main difference being that ME/CFS patients had "a powerful lobby group that dislikes any association with psychiatry." ME/CFS patients turn to doctors for "validation," he said, and "once that is granted, the patient may assume the privileges of the sick role: sympathy, time off work, benefits, etc." Patients look for physiological explanations for their illness, such as a virus, he said, because "it preserves self-esteem." And doctors should be wary: "It is important to avoid anything that suggests that disability is permanent, progressive, or unchanging. Benefits can often make patients worse."

My heart pounded as I read.

At the same time, if directly asked, he vigorously denied that ME/CFS was "all in your head." No, no, he said: It's in your brain. Just like mental illnesses are.

I found all this puzzling: Depression is a mental illness because its primary symptoms are, well, *mental,* even if those symptoms are rooted in physiological abnormalities in the brain and body. If ME/CFS had physical causes and physical manifestations, what possible sense did it make to argue that it was essentially psychological?

When I beat through the clouds of obfuscation, Wessely's positions on ME/CFS seemed to boil down to these: Patients need to realize that their continuing symptoms are a manifestation of their own psychology and poor levels of fitness, so they have the power to change them. The more they believe that they have a physical illness, the less likely they are to recover. Their path to wellness is to get over their fear of exercise, quit seeing problems as catastrophes, stop focusing on their symptoms, and give up the search for physiological treatments.

So while doctors should be empathetic, they should refuse to get dragged into a counterproductive search for physiological problems. Instead, they should steer patients toward CBT and graded exercise, since both will train them to ignore their symptoms and get active. Sadly, Wessely admitted, those treatments might not cure everyone, but they were the best medical science had to offer. And one shouldn't expect better treatments anytime soon—since ME/CFS is a brain problem, we'll have to wait until we've cracked the functioning of the brain for that.

Every last one of those statements struck me as wrong, offensive, and damaging.

I found it even more galling to read Wessely evade criticism with misleading descriptions of his own position. For example, in a 2002 article in the *Guardian* about a "war" between ME/CFS patients and his psychiatric camp, Wessely said, "Oh, it's years since anyone has denied there is a biological basis to CFS. That's just tilting at windmills. We have been most active in looking at the biological basis of CFS." I knew from his writings, though, that the only "biological basis" for ME/CFS Wessely believed in lay in the brain—that is, he considered ME/CFS a *real* mental illness, just like depression or schizophrenia.

But the *Guardian* writer ended his piece declaring the differences between the two camps scant. He wrote, "All the combatants have said how hurt and upset they've been by enemy action. Wessely himself recently issued a call for some sort of peace. So what are they all waiting for?"

I, for one, wasn't ready to make peace with Wessely's view of the illness. And Wessely's philosophy was at the heart the PACE trial. The rage of the patients on the forum no longer seemed so peculiar.

BUT ALL THAT ONLY made me more puzzled about the trial itself. Given how ludicrous the PACE researchers' theory was, shouldn't the trial have crashed and burned? Or—I forced myself to admit this possibility—did their success show that they were on to something? Perhaps their theory was bunk but their treatments worthwhile. After all, science is supposed to get solid answers, even if the scientists happen to be assholes.

The only way to find out was to dig into the science. On a day I was feeling especially clearheaded, I started reading the *Lancet* study. I also dug deeper into the hundreds of posts on the forum dissecting the study's science. To my surprise, I was dazzled by the quality of the analysis: This was a community of serious citizen-scientists unleashing their full geekitude upon this study. And geeks were my people.

The first problem the forum geeks pointed out was pretty amazing: It wasn't clear that the patients in the trial even had chronic fatigue syndrome! Participants were only required to have six months of disabling fatigue as a primary symptom—the very definition Klimas had criticized as overly broad. None of the other symptoms ordinarily required for an ME/CFS diagnosis, including brain fog, pain, blood pressure regulation problems, or sleep problems, were necessary—not even problems after exercise, which most experts considered the hallmark of the illness. And while patients with many fatiguing illnesses were excluded, it was okay to have major depression, even though that alone could explain the fatigue, and depression was well known to respond to exercise and CBT.

But that was just the beginning of the problems. The forum geeks pointed out that suspiciously, the only sign that CBT and exercise had helped patients was that the patients said they felt a bit better. Objectively, though, they hadn't improved at all: They hadn't gotten back to work, hadn't gotten off welfare, hadn't gotten more fit. Even the patients who exercised for a year did no better on a fitness test, and while they were able to walk slightly faster than at the beginning, they would still have lost a race with a patient in heart failure, severe multiple sclerosis, or chronic obstructive pulmonary disorder.

Even more suspiciously, the researchers then pooh-poohed their own objective measures as flawed or irrelevant. It was the subjective self-assessments, they said, that really meant something. After all, they pointed out, how else can you tell how tired people are, other than asking them? *Okay,* I thought, *but shouldn't the researchers acknowledge that the lack of objective improvement is disappointing, to say the least?*

Furthermore, when I looked at how much better participants said they felt, it struck me as fairly pathetic. Patients started out feeling pretty terrible: They rated their own physical function at less than 40 on a 100-point scale that any moderately healthy person would ace. At the end of the trial, CBT and exercise improved their scores by fewer than 10 points. So a typical patient reported that he still couldn't vacuum his house, climb more than one flight of stairs, or walk more than a few blocks—but he struggled a little less carrying in his groceries and, maybe, could just manage a single flight of stairs when he'd had to rest in the middle before. If I'd put a full year of effort into therapy, I think I would have felt pretty disappointed.

And even these slight improvements were suspect. I imagined myself as a participant in the trial: I come in and I'm asked to rate my symptoms. Then, for a year, I'm told that to get better, I have to pay less attention to my symptoms. Then I'm asked to rate my symptoms again. Won't I feel a lot of pressure to say I feel a bit better, in order to do as I'm told, please my therapist, and convince myself I haven't wasted a year of effort?

The irony, the geeks on the forum pointed out, was that the researchers' modest results in fact offered compelling evidence *against* the theory that it was psychological problems and deconditioning that kept ME/CFS patients sick. After all, the researchers had given patients the best treatments they could to address those problems, and it had barely helped. CBT and exercise did no more for ME/CFS than for illnesses like lupus, multiple sclerosis, and fatigue from cancer treatment, all of which are known to be primarily biological in origin.

But one of the PACE researchers in a press conference described patients getting "back to normal." Many news reports said that about 30 percent of participants had recovered and that 60 percent had improved. *Recovered! Normal! Sixty percent improved! How could that be, when the results are so puny?*

My new friends the forum geeks had the answer for me: The researchers had changed their definitions of "recovery" and "improvement" after the trial began—weakening them so dramatically that patients deemed "recovered" at the end of the trial could be both more fatigued and less functional than when they began treatment.

They could get worse and be called recovered?

Originally, patients had to assess their own physical function at 85 or higher, among other requirements, to qualify as "recovered." That was perhaps slightly low, given that fully healthy people would ace the test with 100—but hey, I would have been thrilled to score an 85, so it was plausible enough.

After the trial began, though, the researchers lowered the threshold for recovery to 60—which, shockingly, was worse than that of 92 percent of the working population and typical of an 80-year-old. But not only that, it was worse than the threshold of 65 for entry into the trial—which the researchers characterized as "significant disability."

Similarly, patients could say they were more fatigued than when they entered the trial and still qualify as "recovered."

At this point, I got downright furious. The PACE team's changes in the definition of recovery—a definition colleagues of theirs touted as "strict" in an accompanying commentary—were absurd, and I couldn't see how anyone could have failed to recognize that. *This isn't just sloppy science. This borders on research misconduct.*

The forum geeks pointed out that the researchers had strong motivation to claim a positive result: Some of them had worked as consultants for private disability insurance companies, earning money advising them that CBT and exercise would get patients back to work and that companies should deny payments to patients who hadn't done these treatments—a fact they failed to disclose to participants in the trial. Plus, these researchers had invested their careers in this. They'd look terrible if the treatments failed.

Even though I had never had CBT or graded exercise pushed on me, I felt personally affected by the trial. *No wonder this disease is so alienating!* Wessely had first developed his theory nearly 25 years earlier, and his ideas had spread into US researchers' and physicians' ideas about the illness. These were the people who had helped turn chronic fatigue syndrome into a mark of shame.

I sometimes felt as though I were stewing helplessly in bile. I longed to expel my adrenaline-fueled fury with a rock-kicking, branch-breaking hike up a steep hill. Instead, I lifted a five-pound weight a few times, as much exercise as I could safely do. *Fucking ironic,* I thought as I set the weight down again, rage still pounding through my bloodstream.

I grew even more furious as I watched what happened to the forum geeks when they tried to bring these problems to light. They wrote blogs; they contacted the press; they successfully submitted carefully argued letters and commentaries to the *Lancet* and elsewhere. They even published papers in peer-reviewed journals. The PACE researchers dismissed all the criticisms with spurious responses, explaining, for example, that they chose their extremely broad definition of chronic fatigue syndrome— so broad that it likely captured people who were depressed and didn't have ME/CFS at all—"to make sure our findings applied to the greatest number of patients." I laughed when I read this. Why not include cancer patients too? Or stroke patients, or cardiac patients? Then you could apply your findings to even more people! The researchers certainly never offered any justification for their claim that patients could simultaneously be "significantly disabled" and "recovered."

And the PACE researchers didn't stop there. They and their defenders painted critics as unhinged crusaders who were impeding progress for the estimated 30 million ME/CFS patients around the world. The editor of the *Lancet,* Richard Horton, for example, went on the attack against the study's critics, calling them "a fairly small, but highly organized, very vocal and very damaging group of individuals who have, I would say, actually hijacked this agenda and distorted the debate so that it actually harms the overwhelming majority of patients."

When the forum geeks filed Freedom of Information requests to obtain various portions of the raw data from the trial, the researchers denied the great majority of the requests, some on the grounds that they were "vexatious" and qualified as harassment.

And the press joined in the pile-on. They wrote credulous stories about how ME/CFS patients had sent death threats to researchers—a claim that was never substantiated.* Wessely led the charge with these accusations: Because of the death threats, he said, he'd had to have panic buttons installed in his home and office and have his mail x-rayed. No journalist described seeing these purported death threats or confirming the allegations with the police, but in article after article, Wessely painted his critics as lunatics who had stepped beyond the bounds of reason or legality. He said he'd quit ME/CFS research to study health in the military, and "I now go to Iraq and Afghanistan, where I feel a lot safer." I couldn't help but laugh when I read that, weighing the image of a desperate, enraged patient in his sick bed tapping out hateful e-mails against that of a desperate, enraged Iraqi insurgent with an IED.

Maybe Wessely did in fact fear for his safety, and if so, I was sorry for him. But those threats sure seemed like a handy way for him to smear all

---

* Indeed, in a court hearing in 2016, one of the researchers admitted that neither they nor any PACE trial participants had ever received a threat of any kind, though one researcher was heckled at a talk.

those who disagreed with him and deflect attention from the scientific criticisms of his work. Routinely, these articles lumped together critics of PACE with the purported crazies. An article in the *BMJ* about the death threats quoted one of the PACE researchers as saying: "The paradox is that the campaigners want more research into ME/CFS, but if they don't like the science they campaign to stop it. They want more research but only research they agree with."

The death threat meme certainly served them well. I once contacted a journalist who wrote a credulous story about PACE, and he remarked privately, "To be honest, not knowing much about the study at the time [I wrote the article], it was easy to side against the people who threatened the researchers with physical violence."*

For me, the press coverage was perhaps what hurt most. My colleagues were writing stories that belittled me and my fellow patients and dismissed the serious scientific errors that had allowed the PACE researchers to have such influence. And when I talked about the trial to my science-writer friends, I feared I could hear the taint of crazy in my voice. The severity of the problems I complained of sounded so unlikely. After all, it was the *Lancet*!

Another journalist I contacted about his uncritical story about PACE wrote back:

> You, and the commenters, seem to see fatal flaws in the whole business; what has stopped it being investigated further, overturned, formally disputed, written off altogether in the annals of medicine? It's as partisan a debate as I can fathom, but sound scientific consensus should normally weigh in here . . .

Yes, it should! I thought. *But so far, it's not. And it only will if folks like you act as watchdogs and make it happen!* I wrote back to him with more information, but he had moved on to his next story and wasn't interested in digging further.

---

* The death threat meme also served Wessely quite well personally. In 2012, he was awarded the John Maddox Prize, for promoting "sound science and evidence on a matter of public interest" and "the way he has dealt bravely with intimidation and harassment when speaking about his work and that of colleagues." He was also knighted in 2013.

I contemplated pitching a story about the PACE trial myself: "Dear Editor, I want to write a story about the biggest treatment trial in the history of chronic fatigue syndrome, published in the *Lancet,* led by some of the most reputable psychiatrists in Britain, which has influenced public health recommendations around the world and has received nearly no public criticism by the scientific establishment. But I, Julie Rehmeyer, can tell you it's a crock of shit. Oh, and by the way, I'm a patient, I'm personally offended by this work, and I might be too sick to finish the story." *Hmm. Not a very compelling pitch.*

I felt betrayed by the institutions of science and journalism both. I took breaks as I researched, looking out my bedroom door at the sheltering ponderosas, listening in on the stream's eternal conversation with itself, working to remind myself that I was here, now, in this body, that this rage and powerlessness didn't encompass the entire world.

Still, my grief built into desperation as I read about the toll the PACE trial was taking on patients. Parents of children with ME/CFS in the United Kingdom were frequently accused of keeping their children sick through their "false illness beliefs," especially if the parents resisted CBT or exercise for their children. Authorities sometimes threatened to remove such children from their families and place them in foster homes or psychiatric wards. PACE didn't study children, but it strongly influenced attitudes and beliefs about the illness, persuading many that the only problem ME/CFS patients faced was their own belief that they were ill.

The stories of such children broke my heart. I read about Ean Proctor, a 12-year-old British boy with severe ME who had been confined to a wheelchair and couldn't speak. In 1988, Wessely diagnosed Proctor as having a psychiatric illness and recommended him for "wardship." Social workers, accompanied by police, then forced Proctor into a psychiatric unit and kept his parents from visiting him. Proctor reported that he received "treatments" such as being put face down in a pool of water, in order to force him to swim. Too weak to do so, he said, he had to be rescued. After a court battle lasting five months, he went home and slowly recovered. Proctor's parents managed to get a commission appointed to investigate their charges of professional misconduct, but the commission defended the medical personnel and instead accused Proctor's parents of mistreating him.

This case was one of the worst I heard of, but it was far from unique.

In England and elsewhere in Europe, authorities continued to threaten to take children with ME/CFS from their families. The Tymes Trust, an organization that supports families of children with ME/CFS, reported that over 10 years, more than 140 families had turned to the organization for help after their children with ME/CFS were threatened with removal. All of these families succeeded in keeping their children, but sometimes only after a major fight.

Adults weren't free from risk either. One patient, Sophia Mirza, was so ill, according to her mother, that she couldn't tolerate any light or sound or touch, was unable to speak, and was in severe pain. Her doctor repeatedly and forcefully recommended an ME clinic that practiced graded exercise therapy. Mirza refused, and under her mother's care, she gradually improved a bit. In 2003, when Mirza was 29 or 30, police smashed in her door and took her to a locked mental hospital, where, she said, she received nearly no nursing care. Two weeks later, after a tribunal, Mirza was released, but she was far sicker than she had ever been. Over the next couple of years, she deteriorated further, becoming entirely unable to eat or to move. In November 2005, she died. An autopsy found extreme neuroinflammation in her spinal cord and kidney failure. Mirza became the first person officially ruled to have died from ME.*

Reading about Mirza, I found my little trailer starting to feel like a coffin. What if I got worse? What if my paralysis episodes started lasting long enough that I wasn't able to wait until I could use my pee bucket? What if I couldn't get my own food? Mirza's mother took care of her for years—I had no one to do that for me.

As it was, my house tenant sometimes helped me get up the stairs to the other trailer when he heard my groans. Another neighbor shopped for my groceries when I asked her to, and if she found my bedroom door closed, she let herself into the kitchen, put the cold stuff straight into the fridge, and disappeared silently. I hired a housekeeper to clean for me and to help me cook.

---

* At the time of publication of this book, these abuses of patients continue. In February 2013, a 24-year-old patient, Karina Hansen, was taken from her home in Denmark, forcibly admitted to a psychiatric hospital, and allowed very little contact with her family. A court-appointed guardian—the chief of police in her area at the time of her removal—made all decisions about her care. When her father visited her in the spring of 2016, she was no longer able to speak, stand, or even apparently recognize him. She was finally released in October 2016 and returned to her family's care.

But I didn't have any other help, and I had no idea how to get more if I needed it. What would I do if I couldn't take care of myself? I couldn't even think of whom I might call, what steps I might take.

About the only thing I could picture was becoming so poor that I qualified for Medicaid and could go to a government-funded nursing home. *Could that really happen to me?*

I was also slowly losing hope that Klimas's treatments were going to help. In a follow-up appointment that fall, six months after my first one, she made a few adjustments to my medications, but she didn't seem to have much else to offer. She confirmed my guess that my kidneys had become more efficient at expelling electrolytes and that was why the Gatorade treatment wasn't doing much anymore. There was one treatment, Ampligen, that worked miracles for a few patients, but it wasn't FDA approved, cost $25,000 per year, and was only administered in a few places around the country—and even then, it didn't always work. The lymphoma drug that had brought remissions to a few patients was highly experimental, difficult to get, and extremely expensive.

Eventually, perhaps, science would find a treatment. But PACE showed me that science could be a force for evil as well as for good. And with research being funded at $5 million a year by the National Institutes of Health—only enough to fund a handful or two of small studies—"eventually" looked like it might be a very long time away.

For years, I'd been sustained by an unshakable, ungrounded optimism that I'd recover. I'd been convinced that I'd find my way back to health using some combination of the attunement I'd cultivated to deal with my mother, the intuition and analytical skills I'd used to do mathematics, and a kind of receptivity and openness to whatever my life would bring, along with whatever medical treatments I managed to find.

But lying in my trailer with my body nearly paralyzed, my brain swollen, and my mind numb from researching PACE, that optimism was looking not just irrational but silly, even self-centered. Plenty of people spent their lives with horrible illnesses they never recovered from—why not me? What made me think I had some special quality that would magically protect me from such suffering?

This—or worse—might well be my life forever.

CHAPTER 9

A LIFE, LIMITED

Oddly, despite the fright and fury I felt from researching the PACE trial and my dwindling hope that coming home would help my body, life didn't feel so bad. I felt overwhelmingly grateful to be back on my land. I also felt a sweetness in being by myself.

That sweetness astonished me. I'd found aloneness terrifying for years, ever since my mom died. I remembered not having anyone to spend Thanksgiving with one year during graduate school and feeling like eating dinner alone might erase my very existence from the earth. But now, I felt a plenitude in the silence that seemed to reach to the space between my cells. Even when I was in so much pain that I had to breathe through it moment by moment, I felt as though the great expanse of the entire Rio Grande Valley had penetrated my body and created room that had never been there before. I was still bound, but I wasn't pinched.

Life became simple: When I couldn't turn over in bed, I didn't. When I could work or run errands, I did. My only choices were to worry or not to worry, and when I put it to myself that way, the choice became easy. So I set the rage and the fear aside and sank into the immediate moment I occupied.

My connection to the world seemed to be growing more remote, as if the very ground off my property were turning to mist. I found that my mother often felt very close, as if by pulling away from the outer world, I was pulling closer to her.

I also felt much as I had back in my math days when I was stumped on a problem and had set it aside, leaving my subconscious to keep nibbling at it as I absently ordered a latte or walked down Mass Ave to class. Then I'd notice a whisper of an idea tugging at my mind, an approach or possibility I hadn't considered, appearing as if by magic. I rarely felt like Archimedes leaping from his bathtub to run naked through the streets of Syracuse yelling "Eureka!" It was more like some subconscious part of me was trapped in a locked room in a hidden world, inspecting the cracks in the walls and prying at the doors, and it had just discovered the slight jiggle of a loose window. Then I'd return to actively working on the problem, seeing if I could use that slight looseness to break the lock.

Lying in my trailer, out of ideas about what to do, I felt as though I were waiting for that little jiggle. In the meantime, I was mostly just staying out of the way, letting my subconscious prowl around that hidden locked room as I listened to my stream and cuddled with my dog.

My experiences in mathematics were part of what reassured me then, allowing me to occupy the formless moment I was in without terror. Math had convinced me that the hidden worlds I'd occupied as a child with my mother weren't mere insanity. As I saw it, math was the immaterial structure that underlies the world, the thing that invisibly drives the pattern and meaning in all that we experience.

Just as my mother saw that you could solve problems in the outer world by working on the spiritual level, so I saw as a teenager that you could solve problems in, say, physics by working on the mathematical level. A few scribbles on a page, a bit of pure thought, and you could predict the precise force needed to apply to a lever to lift a weight—no experiments necessary. In fact, any physical measurement seemed only a messy approximation to the true, beautiful mathematical law. Math was the pure reality, material the crude imitation. Math was mysticism incarnate.

When my mother died, I had turned to mathematics as a haven, a foreign land that I hoped would accept me as an immigrant. I felt at that moment like the sole survivor of a catastrophe that had wiped out not just my mom but my entire culture, as if I were an ancient Indian who was the only remaining speaker of my native language. The language of mathematics had just enough similarities that I could imagine myself making a home in that new world.

I couldn't specialize in math at St. John's, because its all-required curriculum didn't allow for majors. So I transferred to Wellesley College. When I arrived, I found myself in a peculiar position: I had just spent two and a half years at St. John's reading and analyzing texts by mathematicians in the thick of their art—but the content of those texts was ancient and foundational. So while I'd developed a lot of mathematical sophistication, from a modern perspective, I hardly knew any math.

I had an extraordinary stroke of good fortune: A Wellesley professor, Leonard Miller, volunteered to meet with me individually to help me get up to speed. For our first meeting, Lenny asked me to prove some apparently simple things, including that $0 + 0 = 0$, using building blocks called "axioms" that I could assume were true. One such axiom, for example, was, "if $x = y$, then $y = x$."

I solved most of the problems he gave me, but the statement about zero stumped me. I was embarrassed to confess my failure.

Lenny's cheeks bunched into apples as he said, "I don't immediately know how to prove it either. I've never worked with this particular axiomatic system. But I know that I'll be able to figure it out, because I'm a mathematician, so I've learned how to do this kind of thing. Keep at it, and you'll get there too."

His kindness brought tears to my eyes. I was astonished to hear math presented as a simple skill you develop rather than a test of your intellect. And he reassured me that I might indeed be able to make a life for myself in mathematics.

Ultimately, Lenny had me prove a big portion of undergraduate mathematics for myself. Rather than having me crunch my way through calculus problems, Lenny would give me one of the critical theorems in calculus to prove, and then he'd patiently encourage me, with occasional hints, as I figured it out for myself.

I felt, quite literally, like I was building an entire universe from scratch, one that underlay and connected with the physical world we live in. It made me think of the long hours I'd spent sitting on my mother's bed talking with her, feeling my way toward the invisible threads of meaning I believed underlay the world, deep within its inherent structure. I didn't think that God had squirreled away messages for us to find like cleverly hidden Easter eggs, but I did think that great beams and columns were inherent in the architecture of the universe, and that listening empathetically to my mother, no matter how crazy her words seemed, was a way of perceiving that invisible architecture. Perhaps, I'd believed, this would reveal alternate pathways to travel through to impact the world—and even, maybe, to solve my mother's problems.

Mathematics felt like a non-woo-woo version of this exact thing.

Sitting down with a problem set, I often found that the problems weren't just hard—they seemed to have no connection to anything I'd ever learned in my life. I had to fight panic to be able to even start thinking about them. I'd eventually manage to come up with one dumb little idea, then another, nothing that seemed the slightest bit profound or adequate. But eventually I'd manage to set the problem in this great superstructure of mathematics, and it would unfold, its roots sinking deep into the soil of math and its branches reaching toward heaven. The solution would then emerge naturally, like a swelling fruit.

In the end, I would write up my proof with strict logic connecting each step, but logic played a secondary role in discovering it. Intuition was my guide for discovery, and becoming a mathematician was all about training that intuition, working examples, seeing patterns, developing a feeling for how ideas connected. I felt like I was learning to navigate an invisible city, first finding my way around using landmarks and only later codifying that knowledge into a formalized map.

The process of doing mathematics reworked my brain, teaching me a new way of thinking. I was entering a kind of priesthood, removed from ordinary reality, living in the realm of the spirits—just as my mother most valued. And just as in childhood, I couldn't describe anything about what I was learning to those who weren't initiated. When I was a graduate student at MIT, I could tell people that my master's thesis was about homotopy colimits, but if they weren't already mathematicians, I couldn't tell them what a homotopy colimit was.

Graduate school, however, pulverized me. My professors seemed . . . not human. I could find no point of connection. My male colleagues seemed to fit in far better than I did. And the thing I most valued about myself mathematically—my ability and determination to understand mathematics deeply, from the ground up, grasping its interconnections and deep structure—seemed to be viewed only as slowness and boneheadedness.

Two years into graduate school, Geoff and I spent a summer in Santa Fe. We wanted to snatch a bit of happiness to power ourselves through the gloom of grad school. I'd been telling Geoff stories about Santa Fe for years, describing it as a Shangri-La with wildly colored rocks, enormous blue skies, and green chile to make your eyes water. At the end of the summer, we could barely make ourselves go back to Boston, and we promised ourselves that if we were just as miserable after another semester, we'd hop in our car and drive back to Santa Fe. We figured it was a kind of noble lie—*surely we won't really abandon graduate school*—but a few months later, we took leaves of absences, packed the car, and barreled back down the highway.

I hoped I'd find some less agonizing way of doing math and finish grad school, but I couldn't figure out how. Then we bought the land, and I started teaching at St. John's, and research mathematics gradually faded away.

Fifteen years later, lying in my trailers on my land feeling my connections to the outside world grow less reliable with my illness, this mystical-maternal-mathematical universe grew more dominant. The complete uselessness of doctors had closed off the direct, medical, logical, accepted, well-understood paths to healing my body. Science gave me no brightly lit highway to speed down. But I still felt promise in these other, deeper, harder-to-express levels.

I could use the tools I had developed over the course of my life, the intuition and attunement, listening deeply to my body and my experience, paying attention to logic but not relying on it exclusively or even primarily. Those tools had brought me significant (if not ultimate) success in changing my mother's life, despite the overwhelming impediment of being a child with little power in the world. They had gotten me into the elite level of mathematics. I believed I could also use them to find my way out of this horrid disease.

LYING IN BED for hour after hour, I discovered, had a major downside, peaceful as I was feeling: It's terribly boring. But during that summer, I found a project I could work on even from bed—to train Frances as a service dog.

I'd first come up with the idea before I left William, but it seemed so implausible I could barely bring myself to mention it to him. My idea was that she could carry a small, foldable scooter—basically a skateboard with a handle and a brake—in a backpack, and when I couldn't walk, she could pull me on it. The idea made me laugh: ludicrous but clever, thoroughly Julie-ish. Just contemplating it made me feel like me. Plus, if I was going to stay this sick, maybe it really could make life more manageable.

I couldn't find a scooter for sale like I had imagined, though I figured that I could have one custom-built if necessary. But it occurred to me that even without a scooter, just wrapping Frances's leash around my waist and having her pull me might be enough—she could play the same role as Christie's hand, pushing on my lower back to help me move.

So I did some research about training a service dog. Formal service-dog training schools generally started with specially bred, eight-week-old puppies, whereas Frances was an 18-month-old mutt. But I found a community of people training their own service dogs—and I even found a trainer who worked over Skype. I also found an elaborately detailed set of instructions for training all the basic behaviors a working dog needs to know, such as how to behave in public.

So I jumped in and started training her. About a month later, I seized a day I was feeling good and took her into town in her "service dog in training" vest. That day, I just walked her into a café, gave her treats every couple of steps, gave her a few simple commands, and walked out. Then we celebrated her fabulous success with a play-dance outside.

Later, we started working on one of the big challenges: She had to ignore every crumb on the floor in a café, even when I wasn't paying attention. We'd already worked extensively on "leave it," starting by my holding my fist out to her, a piece of cheese inside. Her first response had been to nuzzle at my fist, trying to get at the cheese. When nuzzling didn't work, she paused, trying to think of a new strategy. As soon as she left my hand alone, I clicked a little noisemaker called a clicker (to tell her the precise moment that she did something right), opened my hand, said "take it," and let her eat the treat. We built up in tiny steps from there—

she had to wait longer before getting the treat, I offered the treat in an open hand and made her wait for permission, I put the treat on the floor, etc.—until she was able to step back from a wriggling lizard or a tossed-aside Kentucky Fried Chicken bone, eager to get her bit of cheese.

Now I just had to make "leave it" her default behavior when we were out in public. I began by setting a crumb near her wordlessly, looking her in the eye and placing the crumb very deliberately. That clued her in that something was up with that crumb, so even though I didn't say "leave it," she hesitated before hoovering it—click, treat! I built up until I could toss any tasty morsel her way without a word and she wouldn't make a move toward it. Eventually, when she walked up to a crumb, she'd look at it, turn toward me (and the treat bag), and lick her lips.

Much harder than crumbs for Frances were people. Frances *loved* people, and cafés were filled with them, their hands crying out for a friendly lick, their crotches alluringly close to her snout. Plus, she knew that if she wiggled at them hard enough, she could probably seduce them into petting and cooing over her. I started working on this in a more controlled setting, hiring a 10-year-old neighbor, Ida, to be my assistant. Learning to greet Ida calmly, I figured, would help Frances learn to stay controlled and look to me for direction when she encountered strangers in public.

The mornings my body was up for it, Ida would appear at the end of the driveway, her black bangs framing her shyly smiling eyes. I would sit on the deck with Frances in a sit-stay next to me, and as Ida approached, Frances would try desperately to keep her butt on the ground as it wriggled back and forth against her will. Often, she would lose the fight and leap up to squirm toward Ida. Ida would immediately turn around and walk away, I'd call Frances back into her sit-stay, and we'd try again. The second time, Frances would manage a bit longer, and eventually, Ida would reach her, sit down, and giggle as Frances covered her face with kisses. We repeated this each session, and the first morning that Frances succeeded on the very first try, she exploded into full-speed laps around the ponderosas, every leap of her body radiating delight and pride.

I was particularly eager to train Frances to go to the pool with me. I continued to rely on my miracle antiparalysis swim cure, but getting to the pool was a Herculean feat. Sometimes I was too weak to go, and I simply had to lie in bed and wait to hit an upswing that would make the trek possible. Once I arrived, I would call the front desk at the pool and they would meet me at my car with a wheelchair. I'd put on my swimsuit before going, so that I could just pull my clothes off and slither off the chair into the pool. I planned to train Frances to pull me to the car at home and then from the car to the pool.

The trick to training her, always, was to create a ladder of easily learnable steps that would lead her to the behavior I wanted. The first time we went to the pool, Frances's eyes about bugged out of her head, apparently unsure what these strange critters in the water were. So I kept it very simple: I asked her to sit, lie down, give me five, anything I could think of to give her something to focus on as she regained her composure. Then we walked once around the pool as she examined the swimmers.

The next time we went, I put her in a down-stay by the pool. At home, she could stay for several minutes, but since this environment was so unfamiliar to her, I started from scratch. I stepped back a foot, returned, gave her a treat. Then two feet, treat; then five feet, then ten feet, etc. Over seven training sessions in the course of a month, we built from there until she could hold her stay while I swam a full lap.

The two of us were very popular with the lifeguards, and on the days I was feeling too lousy for training and left her behind, they asked after her as they watched me stagger and groan my way into the pool.

The service-dog trainer I found over Skype helped us work on specific service skills, such as retrieving objects and, most importantly, pulling. I got a special harness designed for pulling, and I had Ida walk in front of us facing backward, encouraging Frances forward with treats, while I provided slight resistance on the leash from behind. Frances was suspicious: I'd drilled into her that she always had to keep the leash loose. But once she understood, she was thrilled.

Over time, Ida gave fewer treats, and then she walked beside me for short periods. Then we started working on niceties, like teaching Frances the commands for right and left and stop. Often, the session with Ida and Frances was my only time out of bed for the day.

Training became one of Frances's very favorite activities. In public, she knew when she was on duty, and a veil of concentration fell over her as she looked to me for direction. At home, she often came over to me with an alert expression, sat very straight in front of me, and looked right into my eyes. Her meaning was clear: "Let's train!" Training ended up substituting for taking her for walks, the mental challenge burning her energy almost as much as physical exercise (though the neighbor dog who visited for wrestling sessions helped too).

The most important thing was to always make sure that I was asking no more of her than she could do—but I didn't always judge that correctly. One day, I asked my friend George to meet me and Frances at a mall, to help us practice polite greetings in public. Frances and I arrived first, to give her some time to get used to the mall, and when George showed up, he sat down some distance from us.

Frances lost her cool upon sighting him, tugging at the leash and wiggling, her meaning clear: "There's George! Mom, it's George! We have to go say hi, right now! Come on, Mom!"

Unable to get her attention, I led her far enough away that she could calm down a bit and gave her rapid-fire cues to focus on: sit, down, sit, high-five, touch, down. Then I tried walking back toward George, rewarding her very frequently for staying at my side.

But Frances had calmed down only slightly. Convinced George was in a group of folks walking past, she tugged on the leash to follow them. When the group disappeared, she looked around wildly for George. Then she sat down, threw her snout into the air, and did something I had never seen or heard her do before: She yodeled. Not a bark, not quite a howl, but I knew precisely what it meant: "George! I'm over here, George! Where *aaaaaaare* you?" I had to laugh, though my cheeks also burned at this complete breakdown of service-dog behavior.

I spent so much time training her that I occasionally felt guilty, wondering if that time would be better spent on my work, or on doing something to get myself better (not that I knew what that might be). The image of a skeptical William easily came to mind.

But working with Frances fit my abilities at that time perfectly. She needed short bursts of training, which were all I could manage. When I was too ill to leave home for a week, her training in public could pause without harm. I could think up new strategies even when I couldn't move. And my fascination with the project made my brain function better.

Plus, working with Frances was the single most satisfying thing in my life. It connected me to myself, gave me something to think about other than my dismal health, provided an outlet for my maternal energies, and gave me hope that I could continue to respond to this illness creatively, even if I never managed to get better. Every time I felt her soft, wet tongue licking a piece of cheese from my fingers, I felt grateful to her.

Training her also felt downright profound, like the process was reworking my brain and my fundamental relationship to the world. The most basic tenet of the dog-training approach I was learning was that the process always had to be fun for the dog. When I'd trained dogs in the past, the word "no!" had always been a fundamental training tool, but I almost never said that to Frances. It was my job to set situations up for Frances so that she'd naturally do what I wanted her to do. I could see the impact this had on her, the deep trust she had for the world, her basic expectation that the world was a wonderful place filled with games and treats and joy and love.

Was it possible that all of life could flow out of easy play? Could I approach my own life that way? Could I train my brain the way I was training Frances's? Could I, like her, come to feel that the world was a wonderful, gentle place and that challenges were games to be enjoyed that always ended in a treat?

I wasn't sure what the answers were to those questions, but I did feel the gratitude that I felt working with Frances suffusing my life. Despite my fear about the future, the immediate present had a lot to offer. Even when I was too weak to move—often—I could take comfort in a peculiar feeling of *rightness* about my life, right there, in bed, in my trailers, on my land, with my dog. I could fling the door open and look out from my bed toward the stream, I could catch wafts of butterscotch scent from the ponderosas, I could listen to the chatter of the birds.

When I thought of everything I wished I could be doing—the stories I longed to write, the hikes I longed to take, the people I longed to be with, the children I longed to have—I grieved. But I found that I could control how hard I pressed against those griefs, allowing them to wash in and out like the tide without drawing too much of my concern or energy.

All my life, an ambition had driven me, a feeling that I needed to accomplish things, to find my place in the world, to make use of all the gifts I'd been given. But those goals and dreams were currently so impossible that their prick had dulled. And I was astonished to find that a gentle gratitude lay underneath, all the time, like a drum beat, like my own heartbeat.

I could look at my house that I could no longer afford to live in, occupied by a renter, and feel the agonies of years earlier. When Geoff was at his sickest and I was struggling to finish the house, I commented to my therapist that I felt like I could no longer hear God's voice. I didn't imagine that some great old man in the sky had ceased whispering in my ear, but I did feel like the attunement I had spent my life developing had somehow led me to a dead end, like I could no longer feel my way forward along the invisible thread I had been following, hand over hand.

Gradually, over the decade since we'd split up, I'd started to realize that throughout Geoff's illness I'd heard God's voice perfectly well—I just hadn't liked what it had said. What it said to me was, "Suffer." It said, "Hurt without understanding. Be broken. Let all of this pain pour through you, and let it change you."

These years of illness had allowed that message to seep between the cracks in my psyche and make a kind of sense I couldn't grasp back then. So much of the pain I experienced then was a result of outrage. I insisted that my suffering had to make sense, that I must be able to control it, that it must be an outcome of a mistake I'd made and would vanish once I corrected it. My rage grew out of my conviction that I had power in the situation, a belief that looked pretty silly now that I no longer had the ability to even lift my head. At this point, suffering felt like just one more experience to be attuned to, as valuable and welcome as joy or silliness or excitement, if far less fun. And I found that when I stopped resisting my suffering, I had more room for other things, like my pleasure at training Frances or at listening to the stream.

This acceptance that had grown within me gave me a source of comfort and strength in dealing with this stupid, formless, misunderstood illness. I had an invisible cord to follow, and I was willing to continue through whatever bog it threaded through. Just as I had survived both my mother's illness and Geoff's illness and was beginning to see how they had opened me and made me bigger, I would survive this illness, I would survive the breakdown of science, I would survive the hypocrisy and prejudice. And in the process, I'd become more fully who I was.

CHAPTER 10

THE CIRCUS

In November, I received an e-mail from an editor at the online publication *Slate*, asking if I wanted to write a story for them. The theory that the retrovirus XMRV caused ME/CFS had recently been debunked. That wasn't so shocking, but what happened next was: Judy Mikovits, the researcher who had made the claim, got fired—and then she was arrested for stealing her own laboratory notebooks and was at that moment sitting in a California jail cell. The editor wanted a piece explaining what the hell was going on.

I'd been groaning as I watched the situation degenerate into farce. XMRV had finally gotten serious, mainstream scientists to pay attention to ME/CFS, but now the whole thing was becoming a circus that only deepened the impression that some contagious craziness was seeping out of the pores of ME/CFS patients and tainting anyone who touched them.

To my eyes, though, the current absurdity looked like a natural and not terribly surprising outcome of the nasty politics and history of the disease, which I'd been learning about in the last months. I'd finally read Hillary Johnson's *Osler's Web,* which describes the disease's history between the mid-80s and the mid-90s. It changed my understanding of what I was grappling with and transformed how I saw the XMRV story.

So I took the *Slate* assignment eagerly, just hoping that my body would hold up long enough for me to get the story written.

The roots of the XMRV circus, to my mind, went back to at least 1985, when the Centers for Disease Control and Prevention began to investigate a mysterious outbreak of a peculiar illness around Incline Village, Nevada, near Lake Tahoe. A pair of doctors, Paul Cheney and Dan Peterson, had seen about 150 cases of what they believed could be a new disease.

Osler's Web described how, along with nearly unimaginable, crushing fatigue, the patients experienced an astonishing array of other odd and debilitating symptoms: They got dizzy, they broke out in rashes, their guts didn't work, their hair fell out, light hurt them, their hearts pounded, their vision blurred, they couldn't think straight, they had seizures. Some were too ill to walk or even to speak. Despite the severity of the illness, standard lab work on the patients was mostly unremarkable.

But when the CDC investigators arrived in Incline Village, they quickly became skeptical. The illness looked nothing like ordinary contagious diseases. Plus, their investigation quickly got stymied on a practical problem. The first step in probing any apparent epidemic was to develop a working definition, a set of symptoms common to everyone who had the illness. Investigators could then use this to determine who their patients were. Ordinarily, that step was easy. But in this case, the patients' symptoms were all over the place: While they all had extreme fatigue, one might have rashes, a sore throat, and swollen lymph nodes, while another was throwing up and having seizures. Some of the patients didn't even look all that sick.

Also, the investigators were trained to be suspicious of purported epidemics. Clusters of illness often happen purely by chance. The classic analogy to explain that is to imagine firing a shotgun at a wall from a distance. Inevitably, there will be a few tight groups of buckshot appearing at random in the constellation of holes, even though there's nothing special about those spots on the wall. Similarly, one expects to find that from time to time, lots of people will get sick in a particular area, just by chance. Enormous resources can be wasted chasing after apparent contagions that simply don't exist.

So after a cursory investigation, the investigators concluded that the only epidemic in Tahoe was an epidemic of diagnosis, not disease. The doctors, they decided, had simply "worked themselves into a frenzy," Hillary Johnson reported in her book.

Eventually, Peterson and Cheney managed to dig up some objective abnormalities in their patients by using less-common tests: Patients had white speckles on MRI brain scans indicating lesions, their immune systems were altered in ways that had never been seen before, and they lost as many as 40 IQ points, almost entirely in nonverbal skills. To the doctors, this was incontrovertible evidence that these patients were truly sick.

The CDC was unimpressed, though, because none of these abnormalities were consistent across all patients.

Then the illness failed to vanish as the investigators expected—it was popping up in Los Angeles and San Francisco; in rural Yerington, Nevada; around Boston; in Ottawa, Canada; and elsewhere. (I found this puzzling as I read about it in Johnson's book. *What is the deal with epidemics of ME/CFS? I've never heard of one recently. Do they not happen anymore? Or is no one paying attention?*) The doctors treating these patients didn't need objective tests to persuade them the disease was real. Dr. Byron Hyde in Ottawa, for example, told Johnson that the disease was "simple to diagnose—there is no disease even vaguely like it."

One might imagine that at this point, the CDC would start taking the illness seriously, since it wasn't politely going away as a good illusory epidemic should. But in fact, this is the point where things really started going wrong. The agency's dubiousness had already crystallized. When the CDC received a deluge of frightened phone calls from the public after the press started writing about the illness, it only increased the belief that the whole thing was a manufactured hysteria. Frustration about the protean nature of the symptoms rapidly curdled into downright contempt.

Johnson reported that around this time, the main CDC investigator of the mysterious disease posted a letter on his door, making fun of an imagined patient. "I would like a list of recommended treatments . . . in descending order of trendiness, including acyclovir, gamma globulin, WXYZ-2, 3DOG . . . alternating sensory deprivation and walking on hot coals, purified fruit-bat guano injections, and bed rest." The letter concluded, "Please inform me about how to get social security and workman's compensation benefits for the above diseases. I have had them for over forty years now, and I am only twenty-nine years old."

Under pressure from the public, the CDC developed a case definition for the illness. The symptoms they required, fatigue plus a selection of such things as sore throat, swollen lymph nodes, muscle pain, and weakness, were sufficiently common that no one knew how many patients were being captured that didn't have the same disease at all. But the widely varying symptoms among patients made it difficult to come up with something more precise.

The disease probably wasn't new. Doctors connected it to "myalgic encephalomyelitis," a term coined in 1956 to explain a similar-sounding disease that occurred in clusters: in a Los Angeles hospital in 1934; in Iceland in 1948; in Adelaide, Australia, in 1949; in the Royal Free Hospital in London in 1955; and more. Symptoms varied, but they generally included extreme exhaustion, tender lymph nodes, sore throat, pain, and neurological problems suggestive of encephalomyelitis, the inflammation of the brain and spinal cord.

The CDC knew about these similar illnesses, but the investigators nonetheless chose a new name: "chronic fatigue syndrome."

The illness was cropping up in the United Kingdom as well, equally confounding and frustrating British doctors and researchers. Simon Wessely began publishing papers on ME/CFS in 1988, and reading one, I felt like I was reading PACE's ancient ancestor, the Lucy of psychiatric ME/CFS studies. He argued that patients simply got out of shape after having come down with a virus, and they needed help getting over their fear and getting more active.

The National Institutes of Health, which funds and leads most of the nation's health research, had its own contribution to the problem as well. At that point, the pattern that is nearly universal with poorly understood diseases began playing out: ME/CFS was declared to be psychosomatic.

Peterson contacted Stephen Straus, a leading researcher at the NIH, and asked him to examine some of his Nevada patients at the NIH hospital. Peterson selected several patients with abnormal brain scans, immune system abnormalities, dramatic weakness, pain, and cognitive dysfunction. Straus sent each one home with the declaration that they were suffering only from psychiatric problems, Johnson reported.

Then, in 1989, Straus published a study claiming that most ME/CFS patients were mentally ill. Newspapers nationwide picked up the press release, with headlines such as this one in the *Washington Post*: "Chronic Fatigue Linked to Psychiatric Troubles." None of the stories noted that the study consisted of only 28 patients. Nor did they point out that out of the 21 patients who "had been or were currently affected by psychiatric illness," only 10 had such problems before getting ME/CFS, and of those, eight suffered from simple phobias, such as a fear of heights. The stories didn't comment on the lack of a control group or the prevalence of depression and other mental problems in all chronic illness (one study put it at 70 percent in AIDS patients). In most news stories, the only source quoted was Straus himself, who became the most commonly quoted expert on ME/CFS for many years to come and who became a lasting advocate for the psychiatric view. The reporters certainly didn't talk to Cheney, who told Johnson, "Straus's article is an absolute *lie*. . . . There is a very conscious attempt to misrepresent the data."

Straus's study was the first example of a species of science that thrived for decades, culminating in the PACE trial. Even if these studies had been good—and they weren't, suffering from the same kinds of flaws as Straus's study—I was struck by how astoundingly *unhelpful* this psychiatric approach was. It sure as hell wasn't going to help me get better—though perhaps it would reassure healthy people that the disease was nothing to worry about. And it had certainly done a fine job of discouraging doctors from taking the disease seriously.

On top of that, the CDC made a hash of the physiological research by developing and pushing a definition of the disease that was absurdly broad, capturing 2.5 percent of the American population. It quadrupled the number of patients from the definition in widest use at the time. That happened just as doctors and researchers were pushing in the opposite direction, trying to narrow the definition to avoid capturing patients who really had major depression, for example. Under this new, broad CDC definition, 38 percent of people diagnosed with clinical depression qualified as having ME/CFS. Expanding the pool of patients in this way made it harder to find physiological abnormalities and easier to find psychological ones, and it made it impossible to compare studies using different definitions.

Along with guiding research into ME/CFS in psychiatric directions, the federal agencies starved it for money. In the 1990s, Congress gave the CDC money specifically for ME/CFS research, but the CDC used that money for other purposes and then lied to Congress to cover it up. *Osler's Web* revealed this misuse of funds, leading to an investigation by the General Accounting Office.

The NIH joined the starvation game. For years, the NIH had been spending around $5 million a year on ME/CFS research, when the illness was estimated to affect a million Americans—five bucks a patient. *I could root around in my couch cushions and find more than that,* I thought. *No wonder we know so little about this damn illness.* By comparison, multiple sclerosis, which is similarly devastating, was getting nearly $300 per patient in research funding each year.

Reading about ME/CFS history in *Osler's Web* made me feel a little bit like a victim of Hurricane Katrina—a natural disaster had walloped us patients, followed by a highly unnatural one. The societal structures I had assumed were there for me were not. Being sick sucked, but being told it was my own fault because I was psychologically fucked up and that my disease wasn't worth studying was enraging.

The whole ME/CFS community was stewing in that sea of rage, and every long-term patient had to work out how to deal with it. For myself, I found it helpful to study the entire mess like an anthropologist, moving beyond repugnance at individuals like Wessely into a detached analysis of our medical and scientific systems.

I saw the same pattern unfold with other poorly understood diseases. Ulcers, for example, were viewed as the result of a driven personality until the bacteria that causes them was discovered. Multiple sclerosis was viewed as the result of neuroticism until imaging showed the breakdown in the sheaths protecting the nerves. And other diseases we currently do not understand well—post-treatment Lyme disease, fibromyalgia, multiple chemical sensitivity, Gulf War illness, mitochondrial diseases— developed the same kind of political problems that ME/CFS had.

My conclusion was that the messiness of these diseases confounded many ordinary scientific processes. And then scientists, who are commonly drawn to their fields because they like clarity and certainty, often respond by pushing the illness into the semi-scientific realm of psychosomatic illness. That dismissal sets up a self-reinforcing network of interactions. Researchers, doctors, and the public all view the illness with scorn; research funding isn't made available; academic researchers become disinterested; medical societies spread bad information; doctors don't know how to best treat their patients. Each element weaves around the others, tightening into an inescapable knot.

The most likely solution, as I saw it, was to gradually, patiently work on each rope in the knot, digging in fingernails to produce tiny movements, tiny bits of space that might eventually allow everything to start moving again. I started creating that space internally, just by working to bring acceptance and compassion and understanding to the whole mess. Each infuriating situation I read about became an opportunity to digest my own rage, to absorb the energy contained within it and to let its poison move through and past me. I thought of my mother's notion that our tiny, personal struggles are cosmically linked to planetary ones. I wouldn't say that my efforts to deal with teasing in fifth grade had had any effect on the Soviet war in Afghanistan. But if nothing else, I took comfort in the idea that this personal work, which I felt I needed to do in any case, might in some way extend beyond the confines of the trailer I was lying in, day after day.

And in a concrete way, independent of any cosmic connection, that internal work had readied me to write this article for *Slate*. I could bring the compassion and understanding I had worked so hard to build inside myself to my readers.

ANNETTE WHITTEMORE found her own way to turn her rage and desperation into treasure for others. For 20 years, her 32-year-old daughter had suffered from ME/CFS bad enough to leave her housebound, with frequent seizures. Whittemore faced the same Gordian knot I and other patients did, with her beloved daughter strangling at its core.

The wealth and connections she had developed as a real estate and gas developer gave her a sword that she hoped just might, if she wielded it carefully enough, slice through the whole tangle. She established a scientific institute to blast past the lack of governmental support and find some answers. She named it the Whittemore Peterson Institute, honoring Dan Peterson, the pioneering clinician from Tahoe, who collaborated with her on the project.*

Just three years after the institute opened, in 2009, Whittemore's greatest dream seemed to come true when Judy Mikovits, the institute's lead researcher, found the retrovirus XMRV in most ME/CFS patients and a few healthy controls. She published the finding in *Science*.

* In 2016, it was renamed the Nevada Center for Biomedical Research.

The result had a stunning implication: The nation's blood supply might be at risk. Retroviruses, the best known of which is HIV, spread through blood—which means they can infect anyone, not just crazy, psychosomatic people. And because retroviruses infiltrate the DNA of their victims, scientists know of no way to cure them. Doctors can at best keep them at bay. XMRV might be an enormous threat to the health of everyone.

Many patients exulted, especially those who had suspected a virus or retrovirus for decades. Although my illness had crept up on me, many people seem to get a sudden, terrible bug they never recover from. Naturally, many patients longed to know if they themselves were infected with XMRV, and they clamored for testing. The Whittemore Peterson Institute obliged. A laboratory linked to them produced a $500 commercial test, and patients began raiding their social security checks to send in their blood.

In the meantime, the threat to the blood supply opened the taps of research funding, and scientists rushed to replicate Mikovits's finding. But they soon got inconsistent results. Mikovits belligerently defended her work, and the laboratory continued to sell its unvalidated XMRV tests to patients.

Finally, a definitive study showed that the XMRV in the blood samples came from laboratory contamination rather than an infection in patients.*

Then things really got messy. The Whittemore Peterson Institute fired Mikovits in a dispute over who controlled her lab samples. Soon after, Mikovits's former research assistant, on her request, secreted critical lab notebooks out of the building to her. The institute pressed charges against her for theft and she was arrested, appearing in chains in a California courtroom. She ultimately returned the notebooks, and the charges were dropped.

Of course, this was media catnip, and as usual, most of the coverage made me groan. A *Wired* article that appeared shortly before mine yet again trotted out the claims that Wessely and others had received death threats and concluded that while Mikovits and ME/CFS patients had behaved badly, science had functioned beautifully. Governmental scientific institutions, journals, outside researchers—all deserved a big clap on the back. The article ended without so much as a thought for the patients

---

* On December 22, 2011, three weeks after my *Slate* story appeared, Mikovits's *Science* article was formally retracted.

still ailing, still without answers, still without serious research. A dagger of rage toward my fellow journalists regarding the PACE trial had grown inside me, and it twisted painfully as I read this.

To me, the toxic history led directly to the current mess. I pointed out in my own article that many patients felt that Mikovits wasn't just an ordinary scientist, trying to do the extremely difficult task of wrenching answers from nature's grasp. She was their redeemer, the sole defender of the theory that might rescue more than a million desperately ill Americans. In the context of such need and desperation, both some patients and many in the press conflated the legitimacy of the retrovirus research with public acceptance of ME/CFS as a "real" disease. Patients without deep familiarity with the scientific process had little idea how essential and uncertain replication was.

It seemed likely that being the object of such desperate adulation had an intoxicating effect on Mikovits. Patients' fervor may well have fueled that of Mikovits, convincing her that she was the only one left standing up for patients and supercharging her initial enthusiasm for the work into self-righteous certainty. It was easy to imagine how her sense of obligation to produce results quickly for desperate patients, and the polarized atmosphere around ME/CFS research, could have greased the slide she took from cautious science into reckless overreaching.

I argued in my story that whatever the failings of Mikovits, Whittemore's institute, or the patients who trusted them, they weren't the point. With a disease this debilitating and marginalized, some patients are bound to make leaps of faith; some researchers might start to believe their own press; and a mother might overextend herself in her quest to save her child. But the alienation of the patient community only arose because of the mishandling of ME/CFS by the public agencies.

I ended the piece with this: "The best way to avoid this kind of fiasco would be for researchers and public health officials to follow their obligation to protect public health, be faithful to the science from the beginning, and fund and pursue ME/CFS research."

WRITING THE PIECE NEARLY killed me. My editor was convinced that the disease was a "real, psychiatric illness" and didn't understand why patients were so resistant to that idea. At one point, he threatened to hire someone to rebut my piece if I didn't make the tone less polemical—which nearly made me despair, since I'd already asked several writer buddies to read my draft to help me excise any angry notes in it. The editor insisted that I add a mention of the death threats, and when I pointed out that these death threats were little more than a rumor since they were entirely unsubstantiated, he told me I nevertheless had to include them to make the piece appear "fair-minded and balanced."

And naturally, I had to disclose that I was a patient, so readers could judge how that influenced my perspective. I'd never hesitated to tell people individually of my diagnosis—being open felt like a good way of counteracting the shame that attached itself to the illness—but publishing it meant I'd lose all control of that information. Still, I agreed.

I pounded out frustrated e-mails to my friends each time I got a revision back from the editor filled with absurd changes and obtuse questions, but in the end, the hard-nosed editing made the piece stronger and less vulnerable to attacks. Once the piece was out, I appreciated it, and I felt enormously proud of the end product. At that time, there was almost no reporting that reflected the full reality of this disease, and I felt like my piece could, perhaps, nudge the strand of public ignorance and scorn in the ME/CFS knot just a bit looser.

But after working on the piece for five days, I barely got out of bed for the next week, except to go to the bathroom.

Many of the comments on the piece were dreadful—a typical one was, "People who claim they have CFS rant, accuse, judge, whine, compete for who hurts the most, and hold on for dear life to that one thing that makes them feel special and deserving of sympathy: chronic fatigue syndrome." But informed and generally polite patients came out to rebut the haters, and I felt far less alone with the illness than I ever had before.

Despite the cost, writing the piece transformed me. I'd come out publicly about having the illness. I'd reframed my illness for myself from an individual to a collective battle. I'd spoken the truth at a time when that truth had mostly been silenced, and in the process, I'd claimed my own power.

I might be sick, I might never recover, but I could still make a difference in this world.

CHAPTER 11

AN UNLIKELY HYPOTHESIS

I started getting a stream of Facebook friend requests from ME/CFS patients after the *Slate* article came out. I accepted them all—seemed the friendly thing to do.

My attitude toward my fellow patients had already started to soften as I had been exploring the forum more, and on Facebook, I found them endearing, even inspiring. I saw how they turned to one another not just for advice, as on the forum, but for a community and support and a social life after they'd been abandoned by so much of the world. They were creating meaningful lives for themselves at whatever level they could: knitting hats that they sold to one another; taking cello lessons even if it took all their energy for the day; celebrating grandchildren; strategizing about how to get research funding and improve doctor training; acting as watchdogs on the federal health agencies; even founding start-ups to help the chronically ill.

One neighborhood of this teeming world consisted of folks who called themselves "moldies." They believed that toxic mold was the source of their illness and that avoiding even tiny quantities of toxic mold had improved their health. Many of them abandoned all their possessions and lived in the desert for months or years on end. *Holy cow! Yet one more whacked-out theory,* I thought. *May they somehow derive comfort from it.*

Then I came across the blog post of a young man, Joey, who reported that after two months of doing "extreme mold avoidance" by living in a cargo trailer in the desert, he was able to exercise vigorously without ill effects. Tears stung my eyes by the time I finished reading: I missed exercise *so much*. I felt as if I had been forced to act like a hypochondriac old lady, obsessing on minute signs of fatigue so that I might stop in time to avoid a relapse. "Exercise" consisted of my five- or ten-minute swims to get my legs working again when I was paralyzed, or some brief strength exercises I did at home when I was feeling capable, which I hoped might keep my body from liquefying and melding with the bed. But true exercise—pushing my body against its limits with abandon—was out of the question. So I read Joey's post over and over, feeling a crack open in the wall I'd built up against my seemingly impossible desire to exercise, to be well, to again run in the mountains.

Around the same time, I was chatting with my primary care doctor in Santa Fe, who also happened to be my next-door neighbor and a friend. I'd long ago given up going to him for my ME/CFS, but he'd kept looking for things that might help me. He mentioned that he'd heard Dr. Ritchie Shoemaker, a pioneering mold specialist, speak at a medical conference. Shoemaker's talk had made him think of me, and he thought he might be onto something. He gave me Shoemaker's book *Surviving Mold*.

I was intrigued. I was pretty sure there was some scientific respectability to the idea that mold could do bad things to you, though I had also picked up a bad smell around it, like perhaps the science had been stretched past the breaking point. The book, though, claimed it had solid scientific backing. I skimmed it in search of the obvious, basic information: How can you know if mold is making you sick? And what do you do about it if it is? Almost all I could find in the book, though, were meandering stories and self-congratulations. Many of the scientific assertions didn't sound right to me, but I didn't trust my knowledge of biology enough to be sure. Within minutes of picking it up, my poor swollen brain would overload, and I'd put it down again.

Still, the combination of the Facebook posts, Joey's tantalizing story, and Shoemaker's claims got me interested enough that I reached out to one of the patients on Facebook who was so excited about mold. I explained that I'd never had any indication that mold was a problem for me, but that I was intrigued by Joey's improvement and wanted to know more. I got back several documents, including one that was an astonishing 900 pages, and an invitation to join an e-mail list for "moldies."

I started with the shortest one, a 25-page biography of an ME/CFS patient named Erik Johnson, who dubbed himself "Erik the Mold Warrior." He had been a victim of the Lake Tahoe epidemic in the late 1980s, and the CDC had chosen Erik as a model patient, or "prototype," for the apparently new syndrome.

Erik soon suspected that mold might be contributing to his illness. Since childhood, just picking up an old book could leave him so weak he could barely stand—and then if he went into the fresh air, he'd feel fine again. Also, when Erik had been a student at Truckee High School near Lake Tahoe in the early 1970s, going through the front doors left him so headachy and confused that he ended up using a side entrance. And the epidemic had affected a huge number of teachers at the high school—plus, many of them described the teachers' lounge making them feel ill.

Erik decided to apply techniques he'd learned in the army to survive chemical or biological warfare. Treating mold as if it were nerve gas seemed to work: six months later, Erik climbed Mount Whitney.

La la la, I thought. *Nice story.* People occasionally recovered in all kinds of weird ways: cough medicine, a device that zaps electricity through your wrist, homeopathy. Anyone who managed to get better attributed their success to *something,* and then they often became convinced that that something was the cure for everyone with the disease.

And this particular something didn't sound like it would apply to me at all. I'd certainly never been suddenly sickened after picking up a moldy box or walking into a building. I'd gotten sick in very dry New Mexico, which surely didn't have much mold. One house I'd lived in had a small patch of mold, but I'd moved there long after I'd first gotten sick. Plus, I'd lived in perhaps a dozen different houses over the course of my illness, none of which had visible mold, and moving never seemed to make me better or worse.

So I wrote to the e-mail list, introducing myself and also expressing my doubts that the theory applied to me (keeping any doubts about the theory as a whole to myself).

The patients were unfazed. If I had lived in just one moldy house along the way, they said, my belongings would have picked up mold that was sufficient to continue my exposure. One of them argued that mold sensitivity operates a bit like a peanut allergy: Just as a very few peanut molecules can set off a person who is severely allergic, so a very few mold molecules could set off a person who is severely mold sensitive. The patient argued, though, that it's a toxic rather than an allergic response—that is, rather than causing an overreaction of the immune system, it destroys the immune system and other parts of the body. And if you're constantly surrounded by mold, the patients claimed, your body becomes so overwhelmed that it may not have an additional reaction to a particularly moldy building.

On their request, I provided a detailed history of my illness, and one patient wrote back fingering the culprit: Berkeley. She pointed out that it was only after I moved to Berkeley that my illness got really serious—*true enough*. And Berkeley, she said, is an especially bad place for moldies. She was convinced that Berkeley had some toxin in the outside air that people who are sensitive to mold are also susceptible to—but since no one had studied it, she explained, no one knew just what this toxin might be. *Hmmph*, I thought. *That sounds pretty crackpot. But hey, the Bay Area is awfully damp. Wouldn't surprise me if there were plenty of moldy houses there.* Hilariously, the moldies called this toxin "ick." One patient made a valiant effort to make it sound more scientific and less embarrassing by renaming it IC for "idiopathic contaminant"—pronounced "ick"—but this rebranding never took.

The patients also pointed out that when my first, relatively mild symptoms appeared, I was living in my trailers while I was building my house. Almost all old trailers, they said, are moldy—they're essentially tin cans lined with particle board, so condensation inevitably soaks into the wood, causing rot.

I patted the wall of the trailer as I read that, frowning. I *liked* my trailers. I'd put in hardwood floors, replaced the furnace and the refrigerator and the stove and the toilet, painted them a clean white. Surely my old friends hadn't been making me sick!

But the patients were united in their verdict. Since I had been stewing in mold for years, they agreed, it wasn't surprising that I hadn't noticed changes from place to place. Only by "getting clear," removing myself from mold completely for a long enough time for my body to adjust, would I start to notice the effects of moldy environments.

Then, to recover, I'd need three things: a location with good, clean air; a safe, mold-free home; and uncontaminated possessions. And I'd need to do an extended program of detoxification. The theory here was that we store the toxins that molds produce—called mycotoxins—in the tissues of our body, and that once we've become sensitized to them, we need to get rid of them to fully recover.

One patient had gotten rid of her stuff and had been living in a fiberglass RV for the previous four years, finding locations that felt good to her, and she'd gone from being sicker than I'd been, she said, to nearly recovered. While I'd heard of severely ill ME/CFS patients sometimes getting a bit better, *recovery* was so rare for this group that I'd never heard anyone claim it before. A patient said that she'd talked to dozens of people who had recovered from moderate to severe ME/CFS, and mold avoidance played some role for almost all of them.

The patients agreed about what I needed to do to find out if mold was an issue for me: I had to go to a particularly pristine desert for two weeks with none of my own belongings. I might or might not feel better while I was there, they said, but if mold was indeed my problem, then when I came back, I very likely wouldn't be able to tolerate my own living space. They warned me that I needed to have a plan to deal with that possibility—if I stayed in my home, I might get very ill indeed. Some people, they said, had even committed suicide when they returned to a moldy house.

This all seemed a little crazy, particularly that suicide bit. Still, I was intrigued. It was a more coherent theory than anything else I'd heard—even Klimas had offered only a thin explanation for what pushed patients into the valley of ME/CFS. Also, a bunch of these folks were smart and impressive. One was a Harvard-trained lawyer, another was an MIT computer scientist, another had been an art history professor.

But the alluring prospect of recovery came with a nasty kick. If mold was indeed my problem, I would have to get rid of everything I owned and move to a new house—if I could find one I could tolerate. Many moldies couldn't, and some people in the group were living in tents or RVs, or even in their cars, indefinitely.

Also, odds were that I would have to leave Santa Fe. While Santa Fe wasn't nearly as bad as Berkeley, the outdoor air, oddly enough, carried too many toxins for someone as sick as me to recover, the patients said. One fingered fire retardants used on forest fires in the area as the problem. She believed that natural molds consumed the remnants of the fire retardants and that this changed the toxins they ordinarily produced, making them far more dangerous. I didn't get her reasoning for concluding this, but the upshot was clear: I might never again be able to live in the house I'd built.

I dipped into the 900-page tome I had been sent, which turned out to be a compilation of Erik the Mold Warrior's posts in various online forums. But as I read more of the book and the e-mail list, I often thought these people sounded like total wackos. For one thing, their theories got unbelievably elaborate. Mold, they said, occurred in plumes outside, so that you could suddenly be hit by one just walking down the street. Mold sometimes couldn't be seen or smelled or detected in any way, except that it could make people sick. "Ick" was apparently undetectable to scientific instruments (but not to moldies!). There were suggestions that mold might cause nearly every malady known to man. People described reacting to their husbands, to their hair, to their own sweat. At one point, the patients began discussing the evils of airplane contrails and vaccines, and I felt a surge of anger at the universe. *Really? I'm reduced to seriously considering the ideas of people who believe crap like this?*

I thought back to my early distaste for the forum and my worry that I'd go down the garden path in pursuit of some nice-sounding theory and end up in a crazy, unscientific wasteland. Then, I had slammed that garden gate shut, but now I was standing just outside it, eyeing the path warily and peering at where it disappeared in the distance.

I was so much sicker now, and so much more desperate. Science sure as hell wasn't likely to provide answers anytime soon, I had come to accept. And I knew I couldn't continue the way I was going—I was running out of money, for one thing. It felt better to try something than to lie in bed and rot.

I did think that if I was going to pursue an unproven treatment as a Hail Mary pass, I wished it could be something with a solid scientific story behind it. Couldn't I find my version of Lorenzo's oil? Camp out in medical libraries and decode the illness, persisting in spite of the skepticism of researchers to save not just myself but everyone else too? I'd much rather be a scientific hero, rather than fairly well abandoning science altogether.

When I read the scientific literature, though, it felt like tissue paper to me, the findings fragile, with great gaps between them. There were thousands of studies out there, many of which identified abnormalities—but the abnormalities seemed barely related, and the studies were generally so small I didn't trust them anyway. Plus, I was a mathematician, not a biologist; beating through the thickets of jargon was way more than my brain could handle, especially when my quarry—an effective treatment—seemed wily and distant. So my Hail Mary pass was going to have to be an idea generated by someone else.

I had zillions to choose from, of course: swallowing supplements or sticking to diets or pilgrimaging to "alternative" doctors. But I'd already tried a zillion supplements, and they never seemed to do a damn thing for me—no side effects, no intended effects. Special diets had been similarly useless, and most doctors had only taken my money. Even Klimas seemed out of ideas. All the other alternatives I contemplated seemed random and hopeless. I certainly wasn't tempted by the several-hundred-dollar device to zap my wrist and somehow rewire my nervous system.

Also, if I could pull it off, spending a couple of weeks alone in the desert sounded pretty cool. I was feeling a bit better than I had over the summer and fall, though I had no explanation for why—*all hail the Greek gods!* It seemed like I might just be able to pull it off. Once I got set up, I figured it wouldn't be too demanding, and I loved the idea of having an adventure even while I was so damn sick. Even if the theory turned out to be totally loony, at least I'd have a good story to tell from it.

I was struck by the key role a "good story" had in my decision making. Go to the desert for a while, retreat from society, have an adventure even while goddamn fucking sick: Nice story, I'll take it. Conceive of the world as toxic and dangerous, see myself as unusually sensitive and susceptible, be constantly vigilant for (real or imagined) contamination: lousy story, obviously ridiculous. My enthusiasm for this venture wobbled as one interpretation or the other gained prominence in my mind.

But of course, a good story wasn't necessarily true, and a nasty story wasn't necessarily false. So I warned myself against getting so wrapped up in the value of the story that I blinded myself to the simple facts of the situation: Mold either was or was not contributing to my illness, whether I liked it or not.

At the same time, though, part of what made it a good story for me was that it cast me as adventurer rather than victim, and I figured an adventurer was much more likely to forge a satisfying life than a victim, regardless of the underlying reality.

I also noticed that when I contemplated this expedition to the desert, a sort of current ran through me, an energy that felt different from personal excitement. Ignoring it felt not just unwise, but somehow wrong, like I'd be going against some structure of the universe I was feeling.

At the same time, the insistence that I leave all my possessions behind struck me as outrageous, and buying everything brand new—a new tent, new camp stove, new clothes, new cell phone, new computer, even a new toothbrush—was going to be a ridiculous burden on my already eviscerated bank account. So I decided to go for some middle ground, taking as little of my own stuff as possible without breaking the bank.

The patients in the discussion group didn't like that idea at all, and one of them recommended that I ask Erik the Mold Warrior about making that compromise. I hesitated: Erik's writings had a strident tone, and he ascribed an unbelievably wide range of evil powers to mold. It wasn't just unusually susceptible people who were affected, Erik argued. No, mold was a creeping menace that caused heart attacks, traffic accidents, cancer clusters. Erik had been warning the authorities of this great evil for years, decades even, but they hadn't listened to him, and now, he said, he was giving up. When the menace had spread far enough, people would finally come to him and listen—no, they'd beg for his advice. The only question in his mind was whether by then it would be too late.

Christ on a cracker!

But in for a penny, in for a pound, I figured. I did as instructed and wrote to Erik, running my history past him and asking him if washing my stuff from Berkeley might be sufficient. I got this response:

> Parts of Berkeley are so bad that anything that passes through has the potential to be a slammer. You just never know. Did you hear my story of getting sick at the UCB campus by a plume event, and having a friend die of a heart attack at the same time and place?
>
> Washing stuff there might not be a good idea, and you can't trust new possessions to be free of this special contamination.
>
> This whole paradigm is just as brutal as the bio-warfare scenario I was trained for.

I groaned when I got his response. For one thing, he didn't even seem to understand what I'd told him: I wasn't planning to wash things in Berkeley, since I didn't even live there anymore! Also, how could *new* stuff be contaminated—and if that was true, how the hell was I supposed to do this? Not to mention the suggestion that his friend's heart attack was caused by a "mold plume"—I didn't even want to go there.

I wrote him back with a clarification, and he said:

> This is a tricky deal. The experiment only works if you happen to be lucky enough to break free of this contamination . . .
>
> The real way to learn this is to go places with a moldie and have it demonstrated.

He explained that you have to learn to recognize a very subtle sensation as a sign that you've been exposed to mold, and initially, people tend to dismiss it as insignificant. That's why it's so helpful to have a moldie like him along:

> I literally have to insist, "You feel that? You feel that?" and when someone admits there is a slight perception, I say, "Remember it, for that feeling is plutonium to you."

This did *nothing* to reassure me. Erik was advocating a completely different approach from the one my Facebook group moldies had: Instead of going to the desert to get clear, I should find a moldie to demonstrate the effect to me—an effect that might be so subtle I could barely detect it, and then the moldie would hound me into admitting some slight perception. *Holy crap, this whole thing is dumb*, I thought. *Sounds like brainwashing.*

I decided to share my doubts with the folks in the group. I started by saying, "Okay, I'm going to be totally honest with you guys: I'm starting to get a little creeped out." I described the exchange with Erik and then said:

> Here's what I'm left feeling: NOTHING I do will ever be enough to be sure there's no contamination. After all, my nose hairs could be contaminated! New things I buy could be contaminated! A car I rent could be contaminated! Someone could drive by in a car carrying mold spores! If one really accepts that *any* exposure continues the reaction—even to the point where you may not be able to tell whether mold is relevant for you—I think you've just dived into complete impossibility.
>
> Overall, this seems like a hypothesis that can't be refuted, and that's pretty creepy to me.

The patients talked me down a bit, partly by admitting how ludicrous the whole theory sounded. One of them quoted Erik: "I didn't make up the rules to this stupid game—I just learned how to play it." They also said that "ick" is rare and that other biotoxins are less virulent and less inclined to cross-contaminate, so that my concerns about the complete impossibility of getting away from it were overblown.

And, someone in the group claimed, everyone who had tried mold avoidance "according to Erik's instructions" had gotten better—though I took that with a grain of salt because it seemed like the only way to really follow Erik's instructions was to walk naked into the desert, with no supplies of any kind. Anything short of that would leave room to say that someone who didn't get better hadn't done it well enough.

But I kept going back to Joey's blog post, and each time, I'd cry. One memory in particular haunted me during this time, coming into my mind like a vision: When I was a teenager, my mother and I often hiked through the Santa Fe watershed with our dog, Ruby Jean. My mom would lean forward and swing her arms as she walked fast up the hills, and then on the gentle stretches, we'd walk hand-in-hand, sharing stories or simply listening to the birds and the wind. In the wintertime, Ruby would loop circles across the frozen reservoir like an ecstatic ice skater, and I'd be dazzled by the ice-crystal forest on top of the snow, sparkling like a glass palace. Officially, hikers weren't allowed to go there at all, but lots of people broke the rules along with us. After my mother died, I spread her ashes in the watershed at an aspen-covered spot by the stream, marked only by a small branch I carved for her. A couple of years later, I was delighted to see that beavers had built a dam right at that spot. But for years now, I'd been too sick to hike to her grave, or to any of the other spots in the Sangre de Cristo Mountains that were so sacred for me. Over and over, I thought, *If I don't get better, I'll never be able to visit her grave again.*

Each time I reread Joey's post, I would end up ruminating on how to pull off this ridiculous experiment. Bit by bit I acceded to the outrageous requirements. I swapped cars with a friend, borrowed camping gear, bought new clothes. The only things that I brought with me of my own were my credit cards and cell phone (in Ziploc bags) and my mother's necklace (because I wore it all the time and simply forgot about it). I bought a wireless keyboard to use with my phone so that I could write, and a solar panel and marine battery so I'd have power. Of course, any of those things *could* be contaminated—how the hell would I know?—but I gave it my best shot.

I gathered items from various friends, bringing them like talismans: a wool sweater from George, a camp chair from Bruce. I borrowed a tent from Geoff—though he'd left Santa Fe long ago, he still had a storage locker there filled with forlorn, abandoned stuff left over from our marriage. If my friends thought I was crazy, they were polite enough not to say so. In gathering my supplies, I chose friends whose houses didn't seem moldy, and in any case, I figured, it was far less likely that their stuff was contaminated with "ick." The great bulk of the stuff came from

William's brother Gary, who lived in Santa Fe. It had been seven months since William and I had split up, but Gary and I were still friendly. He swapped cars with me, lent me most of the camping stuff, let me use his house as a staging area, and was gracious enough not to sneer at the embarrassing lengths I went to not to contaminate my new gear, such as washing my hair and Frances with vinegar and putting on new clothes before handling any of it.

Gary even helped me with things I couldn't easily do myself. For example, the boxes for the items I had ordered online had been in my trailers and car, and hence were (presumably) contaminated. I couldn't figure out how to deal with this, because if I unpacked the boxes in my contaminated clothes, I might contaminate my new stuff, but if I showered and got into uncontaminated clothes, then handling the contaminated boxes could mess up my few uncontaminated clothes. So Gary did it for me, taking the stuff out, disposing of the boxes, and storing the stuff for me in his (hopefully) uncontaminated garage. As I watched Gary unpack boxes, my breath caught as the profile of his nose reminded me so much of William. But William had never managed such easy, unmetered helpfulness.

I spent weeks preparing for the trip whenever I was capable, and at each day's end, I would lie in bed, barely able to move. Talking to a friend on the phone one night, I heard a hysterical edge creep into my laughter. *Ha ha ha, I can't lift my head, I'm going to arrange for all new equipment and go to the desert for two weeks by myself, ha ha ha ha ha ha!* I assured myself that my state varied so much that surely I'd have a moment when I could stagger to my car and get back to civilization if I really had to.

And anyway, absurd or no, I felt carried along by some unstoppable tide. I was doing it.

I had to decide where to go. People on the group often discussed Death Valley, since it is particularly pristine. But I had spent time there with William, and I wanted to avoid those memories.

Most other deserts weren't warm enough in February for comfort. Southern New Mexico was 10 degrees colder than Death Valley. I considered the Mojave, but it wasn't clear whether I'd be able to camp at low elevation there, and higher elevations would be cold.

Anza Borrego near San Diego appealed to me—it held no baggage for me, was likely to be warm, was beautiful, and allowed backcountry camping. There were no direct reports on Anza Borrego from any moldies, but I figured it must be okay, being a desert and all.

Remarkably, one of the moldies volunteered to drive there herself to check it out for me. I appreciated that but also found it a bit creepy—why was a stranger going to so much trouble for me?

Her report wasn't good: The prevailing winds blow crap from San Diego into Anza Borrego, she said, so the air there wasn't very good after all. That seemed to leave me with no choice. *More outrageous demands!* I thought. But I acceded to that too, and I resigned myself to Death Valley.

In a poetic way, going to Death Valley felt so appropriate as to be inevitable. I felt as though I were going to the desert to die. Not literally—I fully expected to be breathing at the end of the trip. But it felt like the end of the road, a giving-up, a surrender. All the external structures of my life had fallen away: My relationship with William had ended; I'd moved away from Berkeley, where I'd spent five years building a life and community; my *Science News* math column had ended; I was too sick to work much anyway. I'd worked so hard to keep everything together in spite of the illness for years, but I knew I couldn't keep it together anymore.

As I struggled with the decision about whether to go or not, pondered whether the moldies were crazy or sane, wondered how much I could trust them, and got the willies at how far I was straying from science, I also felt inexorably drawn to the desert. All that thinking almost seemed like it was just a way of keeping my brain busy with its imagined control and decision making while I was being carried along by greater forces than my mind could comprehend.

PART 3

IN THE WOMB
OF THE EARTH

CHAPTER 12

DEATH VALLEY

I cracked an eye open and oriented myself. I was in Death Valley, in a tent, on a camping pad, in a sleeping bag, with Frances curled up next to me. *I've made it.*

Then it came flooding back: The wind. Geoff's tent that was so manly that testicles seemed to be required to erect it. The wrestling match. The physical limits I so totally blew past.

Can I move? I stretched my fingers, rolled my shoulders, and finally bent my legs. Everything moved. I was creaky and achy, but okay.

Maybe the experiment is succeeding already!

I scooted to the door of the tent, let Frances zoom out to explore her new surroundings, and looked out, still tucked cozily in my sleeping bag. The sun labored to crest the Amargosa Mountains, and light beams glowed as they shot above my head in an angelic fan, their endpoints reaching lower as the day slowly brightened. They finally fell upon me like a sacrament.

I moved to my chair up by the car for the full grand view, each step painful and slow, but manageable. Frances sat like a sentry nearby, and I breathed deeply. *I made it!*

The wind had died down overnight, and the silence felt thick, enveloping me. I couldn't hear a single sound coming from a human. That great, empty expanse thrilled me, opening an answering space within. I felt no need to *do* anything. Just sitting, feeling the cool desert air, looking across that astonishing, bare valley, was plenty.

I checked my phone and found that it picked up a weak signal, not strong enough for more than an emergency call but sufficient for e-mail. I was relieved—if something went wrong, I could get help—but also a bit sad. *I know I won't be able to resist checking my e-mail. Will it dilute the experience?*

I watched a single car inching along the undulating black pen line of the one road, the only sign of humans I could see. I whooped, just to hear the sound of my own voice. The sound was swallowed, not even returning to me in an echo.

I am alone.

Aloneness had been my companion for years, though not so vividly as at this moment. I remembered the night after my mother died, lying in bed alone in our house, shocked by the fury that had come up in me: *How dare you make me work that hard to save you, and then just die!* Just under the rage was a fear so profound I recoiled before I could become fully aware of it: I felt as though my mother's death proved that when tested, the people I loved most would abandon me or fall apart.

And that fear seemed to prove true over the years that followed. Geoff had fallen apart. William couldn't handle my illness, at least not in a way that I could live with. And now I was utterly alone in the desert, not entirely sure I could take care of myself and with no one to help me if I couldn't.

I laughed, looking at the moonscape of sand and rocks that surrounded me for miles, with neither a human nor even a single tree or spot of green. *I sure know how to bring my worst fear to life!*

The air was cool as it passed through my nostrils and filled my lungs. The slight breeze carressed me like velvet. Outrageous streaks of purple and yellow and green in the mountains across the valley were sparkling into life as the sun grew higher. Frances nuzzled her nose against my leg, and her ears felt soft as whipped cream under my hand.

Right at the moment, that aloneness didn't feel so bad. In fact, it felt pretty fucking magnificent.

I SPENT THE DAY slowly setting up my camp. Before I'd left home, I cooked dinners for myself for the whole trip, frozen them in individual containers, and loaded them into an electric cooler. I had also bought an 80-watt solar panel and a battery to charge the cooler and my phone. I set up a little kitchen for myself on a folding table, with a two-burner, white gas camping stove.

The work took me most of the day, and by the time I was done, I didn't have energy for the walk I'd hoped for. But still, I felt very satisfied with myself. I watched the sky streak gold and red as I sat in my camp chair with my dinner in my lap.

The next day, I took a slow, cautious walk up the jeep trail. *Does it feel better than it would have before I left?* Each step, I tried to assess, not sure. But the next day I crashed and was stuck lying on my camping pad. *Okay, well, it's probably too soon for much improvement. No reason for discouragement.*

Over the following days, I continued pushing my walks a bit longer, hoping each time that I'd break through to free, easy movement and get a clear signal of recovery. I occasionally got optimistic, but even on the good days, I typically spent several hours crashed out, feeling as will-less as a sack of potatoes, listening to the wind drum the sides of the tent and ring the zipper pulls like prayer bells.

I spent time training Frances: drilling recalls, teaching her right and left, practicing loose-leash walking. Frances spent a lot of time on a rock at the top of the ravine above the tent, crouching up there like a mountain lion. She learned that the tiny ragged bushes often contained hidden lizards, so she scurried from bush to bush on our walks. I discouraged her from celebrating the rare passing car with a chase.

One night she heard a visiting critter outside the tent, one that even had the gall to drink water from her water bowl, mere inches away on the other side of the fabric. I was as curious as she about who our visitor was—a coyote, perhaps?—but the zipped-up tent blocked our view. The critter returned nightly, even when I brought her water bowl in. One night was warm enough to just have the mesh door closed, and I hoped we'd be able to get a glimpse of our friend. I awoke in the middle of the night to a commotion: Frances was trying to crash through the mesh. I settled her back down, but then she tried again—and succeeded, ripping a hole right through the mesh and zooming off into the night. I heard her excited yips receding into the blackness, and my heart pounded until she came back, panting and delighted. I kept the solid doors mostly zipped up after that and cringed at the thought of telling Geoff that she'd destroyed his tent. Though she may have discovered who our visitor was, I never did.

I found that I had no desire to see or talk to people face-to-face. From time to time, the wind or the sun got so intense that I'd briefly reenter civilization to seek refuge in the blessed dim coolness of the café in Furnace Creek, a building my moldie friends assured me was okay. I'd fill my eight one-gallon jugs of water there along with my five-gallon solar shower, and the staff quickly embraced me as a regular. But that was only every few days, and the human contact felt incidental: It was the coolness, stillness, and water that drew me.

Nearly a week into the trip, I took a walk up the road and felt better than I had previously. I wrote exultantly to friends, "I have had the first indication that this experiment might be working. I just went for a walk in which I think I would have kept up with your sedentary Great Aunt Thelma, who rarely gets out of her barcalounger. I might even have outpaced her." And the next day, I felt okay—*woohoo!*

I got more ambitious and took Frances to nearby Golden Canyon, a gentle hike along a twisting ravine through fantastically colored badlands. I managed to go two-and-a-half miles in a couple of hours, but I had that usual feeling of draaaagging my body along, and the next day my eyes were swollen and moving was difficult.

Another day, I drove to Ubehebe Crater, a great round hole in the earth created when magma crept up close enough to the surface to meet up with underground water, which turned to steam so fast that the ground exploded, leaving a 650-foot-deep crater. William and I had visited it together, and we had ventured beyond the crater across the hills. The solitude had been intense, the landscape extreme, its unremitting dryness heart-expanding.

When I arrived this time, however, hordes of people were crawling all over the crater. I knew that the crowd would peter out once I got beyond the crater itself, but as I climbed up the hill toward peace, my body dragged, each step grinding. Frances had to be on leash around the crater, but she kept pulling—strictly forbidden on our service-dog training program—and I was too exhausted to deal with her and get up the hill too. I could feel my frustration with her bubbling toward the surface to meet the pool of loss I kept hidden underground: the loss of my strong body, the loss of my relationship, the loss of much of my career, the loss of my sense of control. I felt the danger that all that grief might erupt as rage at Frances, so I allowed my legs to creak to a halt and my body to sag down to the ground. I sat peering down into the crater, imagining the explosion that had so suddenly ripped a vast hole into this landscape, perhaps only 300 years earlier. I felt a glum kinship with it, feeling the crater in my own ripped-apart life.

I gave up my ambitions after that. After all, my moldie friends had told me that I might or might not feel better while I was in Death Valley. The real key was to see if I reacted to my trailers and stuff when I got home. As much as I wanted to know if the experiment was working, there was no point in pushing myself.

So then I stayed by my campsite, and contentment returned. Just being there, taking little walks, sitting in my chair watching the colors of the desert change as the sun moved across the sky—it felt like enough to me. A full life.

I could just stay here forever.

The contentment felt unfamiliar, even a bit shocking. An anxious internal drive had prodded me forever—but I only noticed it in the desert, once it was gone. That striving had started with the need to save my mother, but when she died, it had transmuted itself into a feeling that I was obliged to be a success myself in order to redeem her life. I had always imagined that contentment would come as the natural end product of accomplishing my goals, but I never quite seemed to get there.

Now, though, plunked in my camp chair in Death Valley, achieving "success" seemed absurdly beyond my capabilities. *So much effort,* I thought. *I quit!* Just taking one breath after another, managing to heat up my food and wash my dishes, occasionally sweeping the sand out of the tent—that felt like success enough for me. With all my assumed obligations removed, life seemed unimaginably spacious. Just being alive was a thrill, a blessing, a tiny miracle beyond my expectation or control. Anything I managed to accomplish above that was a gift.

One day a few months before my mother died, she told me, "I'm not worried about you anymore. You've learned everything you needed to from me. Now, I just want you to be happy. That's the only thing I'm not sure of—that you'll be happy." I'd been stunned. Happy? I'd never heard her talk much about happiness before. A statement that might be banal from most people was, from her, astonishing, a benediction.

But the truth was, she'd been right to be concerned about me on that score—I hadn't been very happy. Oddly, now that I was abandoning my perceived obligation to my mother, I was at last fulfilling her final wish for me.

I thought about that strange feeling I'd had that I was going to the desert to die. Perhaps now I knew what that feeling had meant. Yes, I was still breathing, but I had reached the end of everything I had worked so hard for all my life. The path I'd been following had evaporated beneath my feet, carrying the world I had known with it. I was now standing in a vast blankness, trusting that the world would form itself beneath me as I walked forward.

And I liked it.

MY THOUGHTS WANDERED TO the future occasionally, though the unknowns were so enormous that it felt almost beyond contemplation. Since the moldies said that the outside air in Santa Fe wasn't good enough to heal in, I figured that if the mold hypothesis held out for me, I'd end up living out in the desert wilds for a while.

I came up with the image of buying a Volkswagen Vanagon, which could be stripped down to bare, mold-free metal if necessary. The minimalism appealed to me. I imagined Frances and me in southern Utah in our Vanagon, watching the colors change there, just as we were doing in Death Valley. I could write from anywhere, of course, if I was well enough. But mostly I imagined just being, the way we were just being right then, far from people, out in nature, with nothing to do or accomplish or strive for.

These fantasies, I noticed, didn't include anyone else, not even on the sidelines. I figured that eventually I'd have a partner again, but in an immediate way, I felt like I just wanted to pull away, far away from a society in which I no longer seemed to be capable of functioning.

But then, of course, this experiment could simply not work. Maybe mold had nothing to do with my illness. Maybe I'd get home and have no reaction to my trailers whatsoever. What then?

One thing was clear, whether the experiment worked or not: I was going to need money. My savings were close to gone. If the experiment worked, I was going to need to get rid of everything I owned, and if I were living off in the wilderness, I had no clue if I'd be able to make much money, or how quickly I'd be well enough to do so. And if the experiment didn't work, well . . .

A little more than a week into the trip, I decided to e-mail Lenny, my undergraduate advisor, to ask for help. Of course, he hadn't the slightest obligation to help me—it felt kind of outrageous to even ask—but I hoped he might be willing. He didn't have kids, and in some small way, I felt like I played that role in his life. I explained the situation and ended the e-mail with, "If it did feel like something you could be comfortable with, my gosh would it make a difference for me, and I'd do my damnedest to use your generosity to bring riches into the world." I sent the e-mail off fast, before I lost my nerve, and then I tried hard to put it out of my mind. The next day I got a response—Lenny simply offered to send me $10,000, no strings attached. I sobbed.

I also got another small financial reprieve: The tenant in my house asked to stay one more month, changing her earlier plan of breaking the lease with thirty days' notice. I suspended my efforts to arrange showings from afar, with relief.

TWELVE DAYS INTO MY TRIP, I watched a bee discover Frances's water bowl, buzzing around it as if drunk. I poured the water out to get rid of the bee, and within minutes, it returned with hundreds of recruits in a great invasion, sucking every drop out of the ground where I'd spilled the water, as well as from a damp sponge and my drying clothes.

How do the bees survive out here anyway? There are no flowers and no water! Surely they don't get by on a few hapless campers like me.

The sun had addled my brain, I was feeling poorly, and I wanted to get the hell away from the bees, so I decided to head down to the dim, cool, bee-less café in Furnace Creek. As I took long licks from an ice cream cone, I realized that despite my casual dismissals of the whole thing as crazy, I desperately wanted this mold hypothesis to be true. And over the course of my time in Death Valley, the hypothesis had come to feel true. Emotionally, it felt like it fit somehow, like it made sense in the overall trajectory of my life. The theory had brought me here, to this extraordinary place, to this extraordinary suspended moment. I felt emptied out, as though everything I had once thought of as me had vanished. To go through such an experience, only to get to the end and conclude that the whole expedition had been a crock of shit— it seemed almost inconceivable.

But of course, that didn't mean that the mold hypothesis was true.

When I looked at the situation dispassionately, the results seemed unsettlingly ambiguous. I felt better than I had right before I left, not having any of the days where I woke up unable to move for no apparent reason. I didn't, however, feel as well as I had during a good spell in the middle of January. With just a couple of days remaining, it looked like my experiment was coming out just as I had worried it would: a meaningless muddle. How I felt ordinarily varied so much that it was impossible to pull any signal from the noise to know what the experiment was telling me. I had feared squishiness and uncertainty, and that seemed to be just what I was getting.

I reminded myself, though, that my moldie friends had warned me that I might not feel all that much better in the desert. The real test would only come once I got home, when I'd find out if I reacted to my trailers and stuff. Every single patient who'd made an effort like mine, they claimed, reacted strongly once they returned home, no namby-pamby, maybe-maybe-not stuff. So I just had to hope that when I got home, I'd get really, really sick.

One of Erik the Mold Warrior's comments from before the trip niggled at me, though. He'd pointed out how hard it can be to get completely free of contamination—and honestly, I had no way of knowing if I had succeeded. Then he'd said, "The real way to learn this is to go places with a moldie and have it demonstrated."

I had been annoyed and dismissed his comment, but now that my time in Death Valley was wrapping up, I worried about it. Erik was supposed to be the great guru in this whole moldie game, and I wasn't following his advice. I'd be goddamned if I was going to go to all this trouble and not be sure I'd given it a full shot.

The obvious moldie to demonstrate the effect to me was Erik. Reno, where Erik lived, was only a six-hour drive away. I could meet the Mold Warrior himself and have him take me to famously moldy locations that had sickened people during the Tahoe epidemic (or at least so he said). I'd be going from the best possible place, Death Valley, to the worst possible place, Lake Tahoe, and if anything would make me react, I figured, it would be that. The idea intrigued me journalistically as well. *That guy seems like such a freak that I'd love to meet him!*

But when I e-mailed Erik to ask for a "mold tour," he said no, in his typically extreme way:

> I conducted a tour for someone who really wanted to see it for themselves, without having an adequate backup plan. I made a huge mistake and almost killed her . . . Before I do any more tours, I want to have a decontamination facility within fifteen minutes' time of exposure available. Otherwise a mold tour is almost certain to cause harm. So . . . sorry, I'm still working on it, but it won't be ready for a while.

I wrote to my moldie friends about his response, and one said that she knew the situation Erik referred to: That patient had been extremely sick and had also ignored Erik's instructions, charging into a very moldy building. For me, she said, Erik's concerns were overblown. She said she'd try to talk him into it—and the next morning, I heard that she'd succeeded. *Woohoo!*

I packed up my tent, my solar panel, and my mini-kitchen, and when I was done, the only sign I'd ever been at my camping spot was the soon-to-evaporate moisture in the sand from where I'd just emptied Frances's water bowl.

As I drove away, the land returned to its silence.

CHAPTER 13

THE MOLD TOUR

As I drove out of Death Valley, I sent a somewhat sheepish e-mail to Gary, who owned the little Subaru I was borrowing: "I'm now on my way to Reno—hope you don't mind."

After a few hours, I stopped at a campground, and as soon as I got out of the car, a swarm of midges surrounded my head—midges in my eyes, midges whizzing past my ears, dozens on my arms moments after I wiped them off. I ran around, but they followed me. I went into the bathroom but didn't elude them. Even getting in my car didn't allow me to escape the insufferable buzzing.

With no nearby lake to jump into, the only solution I saw was to kill the little bastards. That plan presented two problems: One was that I had no insect repellent with me, and the other was that, even if I had some, I'd been warned that if I was indeed a moldie, I'd likely have developed chemical sensitivities by now.

A possible solution to the first problem presented itself when a van pulled up. My halo of midges and I walked over to say hello, and I asked the bright-eyed, white-haired couple inside if they had any insect repellent I could use. They had an extra bottle—I could keep it, they said.

So that left the question of these supposed chemical sensitivities. I was skeptical, never having had the slightest hint of chemical sensitivities in my life. Plenty of chemical smells were unpleasant to me, but aren't they to everyone? It was easy to imagine someone letting their imagination run away with them, focusing on that dislike so much they started feeling ill. And anyway, I had no intention of accepting that I had chemical sensitivities without even testing it. Now was my chance!

So I smeared the blessed stuff over all my exposed skin, and instantly, the midges vanished. *Ah . . .* Still, I couldn't deny that a mild anxiety prickled at me as I waited to see if the spray would make me sick.

An hour later, I felt completely fine.

I found it rather gratifying. People's worries about toxicity often struck me as unscientific and ridiculous, driven by an emotional longing for purity rather than logical thought. People had pushed so many stupid ideas on me over the years: The problem was electromagnetic fields! I was irresponsible to use Wi-Fi, and I should be turning off the power in my house every night! It was my microwave! Sometimes I ate nonorganic produce! I used Roundup on the poison ivy on my land a couple times! All those niggling insistences made me want to dive into the damn bug spray, feel just fine afterward, and tell everyone to go screw themselves.

On the other hand, I was quite hoping there was something to this one little corner of the toxicity hypothesis that would hold true, about mold. *Does my lack of reaction to the bug spray indicate I might not be a moldie after all?*

I heard from Erik that the next day would be a "horrifying day for a mold tour." Mold releases more mycotoxins when the weather is bad, Erik claimed, particularly when a storm is first coming in and the barometric pressure is dropping. But he suggested that whenever I arrived, we should get together and talk. I was arriving on a Wednesday. *How is this guy so flexible with his schedule? Does he have a job?*

I asked him for advice on a mold-free hotel in Reno, but he said he didn't know. That also seemed odd to me. So I chose a hotel randomly, having no way to distinguish a good one from a bad one.

When I walked into the hotel room and closed the door on the wind, any worries about that wafted away: Being indoors felt miraculous. I took my first full shower in two weeks, and the endless outpouring of hot water amazed me. While camping, I'd used my solar shower to wash my body, but it had been too difficult to wash my very long, thick hair. I'd kept my hair braided constantly to protect it from the wind, and it had gotten so thick with accumulated dirt that it had practically rebraided itself each morning. When I stepped out of the shower, my hair sleeking down my back like a seal, I felt reborn.

I also used the shower to wash all my clothes, which were as stiff with dirt as my hair had been, and then I draped them up to dry. It didn't even occur to me that I was risking contaminating my clothes in the process if the room was moldy.

I couldn't get a solid commitment from Erik about when he was coming. I could only reach him by Facebook messaging—his e-mail inbox had gotten full years ago, he said, and he didn't have a telephone—and now he wasn't responding. So I waited around in the hotel room, hoping he'd show up soon, getting increasingly hungry but not wanting to go get food in case I missed him.

Just as my hunger was growing miserable, Erik showed up. He was in his late fifties, with a disheveled mop of curly gray hair and a diffident manner, riding a bicycle with a homemade trailer rigged behind it. We said hello, rather awkwardly, as he locked his bike outside my hotel room.

I asked him if he'd eaten lunch and he said he hadn't, though he didn't seem to care much about eating. Since I certainly did care about eating, we went to my car to drive to a restaurant.

I asked him to check out my stuff in the car for mold. I kind of figured he'd declare everything "horrifically bad"—one of his favorite phrases—and thus condemn my whole experiment. That would certainly preserve his theory, given that I hadn't, so far, gotten much better. *Yeah, yeah,* I thought to myself. *I know that's not supposed to mean anything, and it all depends on what happens on the mold tour. But still.*

He sniffed around in my trunk. "Seems okay," he said casually.

Wow, so this experiment is still on!

Erik only knew one place to suggest for lunch—he never ate out, he said—and it turned out to be out of business, so we went back to the restaurant attached to the hotel. A funny look passed over his face as we walked in. "You okay?" I asked. He said no, that he was feeling a hit of mold. I suggested we go someplace else, but he declined. *Okay . . .* When we sat down, though, he said the space felt acceptable to him.

I asked Erik about when he'd first gotten sick, and those turned out to be nearly the last words from my mouth for an hour and a half.

It all started, Erik said, with an algal bloom on Lake Tahoe in the winter of 1984. Large portions of the water and the sand on the shore-front were covered with a dull-green, wispy algae. That had been happening more and more, but that winter, Erik noticed something stranger: In places, the sand was neon green, "Halloween-corpse green," as if it might glow in the dark. Millions of crawdads, he said, washed up dead on the lakeshore. The prevailing winds blew across the lake, and he was convinced they were picking up toxins from the algae and this neon-green stuff and spreading them through the north shore of Lake Tahoe.

His second clue was that although he had been susceptible to mold since he was a little kid—Truckee High School had been especially bad—suddenly, every building that had ever bothered him felt vastly worse. And it wasn't just him, he said. Other people, people who had no idea they could be susceptible to mold, were being sickened in the same spots he was.

Then a particularly nasty flu passed through town, "the China flu," Erik called it. Some people who caught it never recovered. Their faces and lips went numb. Their eyelids sometimes drooped uncontrollably, and in order to see, they had to hold them open. Patients' legs or arms grew suddenly weak. They reported feeling as though an electric current was rolling through their skin. They would try to reach for something and find that their arms wouldn't move unless they concentrated so hard that they broke out in a sweat. They couldn't coordinate their muscles well enough to guide a spoon to their mouths. If they lay down, their heads spun with wild vertigo, but if they stood or even sat up, they passed out.

Then Erik caught it. He was so ill he had to slide to the bathroom on his belly. His brother spoon-fed him. When he tried to speak, sometimes what came out was incomprehensible, as if he were speaking in tongues, and others' words sounded like gibberish to him.

All of this was similar to what other victims were experiencing, but he noticed something else too: His vulnerability to mold skyrocketed, even beyond its already heightened level. An exposure could leave him feeling that he was fighting for his life. His house had a couple of spots of mold, and he felt so much better outside that he ended up living in the camper of his truck. He recovered enough to go out some, and he found that particular spots reliably did him in—a sewer grate outside the

7-Eleven where his girlfriend worked was especially bad. And if he took others who had gotten the China flu to the spots that felt worst to him, they fell apart too. Furthermore, the areas that felt worst to Erik also tended to get clusters of people sick with the mystery illness.

Erik became convinced that mold was combining with other toxins and weakening people's nervous and immune systems. He knew that molds go to war with one another, producing poisons to try to kill one another off. The United States once accused the Soviet Union of attacking Hmong tribesmen in Laos and Cambodia with one of these poisons, and Iraqis under Saddam Hussein filled warheads with another. Erik went a step further, reasoning that if molds are exposed to other chemicals, it might make the poisons they spray about worse than usual. Perhaps that neon-green stuff by the water had somehow activated the mold, making it far more dangerous.

Erik had turned for help to Dr. Paul Cheney, who, with his partner Dr. Dan Peterson, diligently probed the mystery illness. They didn't have any effective treatments to offer, but they collected so much data on the illness's odd effects that they convinced the Centers for Disease Control and Prevention to come investigate. At one point, Cheney called Erik in and asked him to be a "prototype" for the syndrome—that is, a model patient that the description of the syndrome would be based on.

Erik recounted that he'd said no, and Cheney had said, "You have to." Erik had responded, "What do you mean 'I have to'? Of course I don't have to." And Cheney had said, "Yes, you have to." Erik repeated Cheney's insistence and his own refusal so many times that I was tempted to join in as a call-and-response: "You have to!" NO! "You have to!" NO!

Eventually, Erik continued, Cheney explained that Erik was the only patient who had all the characteristic problems with the immune system but was negative for the Epstein-Barr virus. If Erik served as a prototype, the theory that the mystery illness was caused by a chronic infection with Epstein-Barr would be discarded. I anticipated Erik's response and again wanted to join in on the chorus: NO!

Finally, Cheney said that as a prototype, researchers would listen to him.

Those were the magic words: Erik agreed. If he was a prototype, they'd have to investigate the role of mold and toxins in the illness, Erik figured. He'd tell them about his experiences, and they'd unravel the whole illness.

But no researcher had ever come to talk to him, Erik reported bitterly.

With no treatments available, Erik focused on avoiding mold, and he got somewhat better. But in 1994, his house became moldy and he again got desperately ill. He went to see Dr. Peterson—Cheney had by then moved to North Carolina—who approved him for a clinical trial of the drug Ampligen, which was only available to the sickest patients. "This can save your life," Peterson said. The catch was that patients had to pay for it, and it cost $60,000 a year, Erik said. The company was funding a trial for patients who were bedridden, but because of Erik's mold avoidance efforts, he was able to get out of bed occasionally and therefore didn't qualify.

Erik couldn't afford it, and he was in despair. He decided to shoot himself. First, though, he went on a farewell camping trip in the desert with his family.

And in the desert, he felt better. Much better.

As he tried to make sense of his improvement, he remembered an experience he'd had in the army. His captain was disciplining him, yelling in his face, and Erik was doing the "Yes sir, no sir, no excuse sir" routine. Suddenly, the captain collapsed, and his lackey ran over and asked Erik, "What did you have for lunch?" Erik was totally confused—the captain seemed to be having a heart attack, and this guy wanted to know what he had for lunch? But Erik stammered out that he'd had a peanut butter sandwich. It turned out that the captain had a severe peanut allergy.

After the captain had recovered, Erik said, he didn't discipline Erik further, and he begged Erik not to let his secret out, lest the other soldiers realize the power they had over him. Erik said he kept his mouth shut—and he escaped punishment for whatever infraction had gotten him in trouble in the first place.

This experience made him wonder if in a similar way, his sensitivity to mold had increased so much that minuscule quantities were now enough to make him sick.

So he went extreme. He treated mold like tear gas, using the methods he'd learned in the army. The lessons from the army about cross-contamination were indelible: He still remembered how soldiers occasionally got lazy and stored their unwashed field jackets in their lockers after a very slight exposure to tear gas. Later, he saw them running back to the showers because their pants, which had merely touched their jackets in the locker, had started burning them.

Erik pursued his theory by spending time in the desert with all new belongings to completely escape toxic mold. He felt better, but then he found that when he returned to civilization, places that had bothered him before felt even worse.

So he taught himself to recognize early signs of mold exposure, paying minute attention to how his body felt. He'd get mild heart palpitations, he said, or his skin would burn, or he'd suddenly feel depressed. If he recognized the exposure quickly and then took a shower and changed his clothes, washing the clothes before the contamination could spread, he could avoid the worst symptoms.

He figured out that his house was a problem, and after attempts to remediate it were insufficient, he sold it and bought an RV. Over time, though, his RV grew moldy too. He replaced it with another, then another. Finally, he built his own from the ground up, using only metal and foam. Even that eventually gave him problems, he said, which he ended up tracing to the cardboard hidden inside the construction of his refrigerator. He tore that out, and since then, it had felt good to him.

He recovered enormously—enough that he'd climbed Mount Whitney, the highest mountain in the continental United States, each year for the previous decade.

But recovery for himself didn't satisfy him. To him, his recovery only proved that his theory was right, and he was still furious that those researchers had never materialized to talk with him. He desperately wanted some doctor or researcher to work on it with him.

His efforts to persuade them, however, were less than successful. He alienated Peterson even before he figured out how to successfully avoid mold by throwing a temper tantrum in Peterson's office. He showed up for an appointment and the receptionist said it had been canceled because Peterson was at a conference. Erik was furious at the lack of notification. He screamed so loudly that Peterson himself came out to investigate, and Erik saw that he was treating another patient, not at a conference after all.

"They were all liars!" Erik yelled in the restaurant. He reported that he'd chewed Peterson out too. Then he'd said to him, "I just need to know: Are you going to help me figure out this mold thing or not?" And Peterson said no.

"Can you believe that?" he asked me. I gave a vague grunt. *Hmm, somehow, yes, I think I can believe that . . .*

Even after that, Erik wouldn't leave Peterson alone. He kept dropping notes off with the receptionist, reporting on his experiments and experiences. Eventually, Erik said, Peterson told his patients not to talk to Erik. Erik fulminated on the outrageousness of this, the utter lack of integrity. "It's a clue!" Erik's eyes threatened to pop from his skull. "They should be following up on clues!"

Erik certainly wasn't going to stop just because he couldn't get Peterson interested. He told me about going to conferences and "stalking" the researchers, cornering them to get them to talk to him. None of them would listen. "Can you believe it?" he exclaimed, over and over.

If I weren't so goddamn desperate, I wouldn't be listening to you either, I thought. I imagined my science-writer friends eavesdropping on the conversation and being astonished that I would pay attention to a madman like this. Internally, I retorted, *Hey! I'm just being a journalist! It's not like I actually believe the crap this guy is spewing!*

But I couldn't deny that when I was sitting in my camp chair in Death Valley, fantasizing about living in a Vanagon in the desert with Frances, I'd felt a sense of not just hope but calling, as if the future were reaching back and pulling me into it. Remembering that, I felt moronic. *Maybe my desperation has rotted my brain,* I thought. My mouth tasted acrid, and I reached for my water glass.

Erik prattled on. Years ago, he said, he'd been most interested in what was going on with mold and ME/CFS. But at this point, he reported, his voice rising, he thought the far more interesting story was about how all these researchers wouldn't listen to him. I closed my eyes to make their rolling invisible to him.

After lunch, Erik said we should go to a nearby Whole Foods, which had a history of feeling moldy to him. It wasn't as bad as the places he'd take me the next day, he said, when the weather would be better, but still, I might experience the effect.

As we left the restaurant, Erik finally paused his diatribe to ask his first question of me: "So who are you? Are you a journalist, a researcher, or what?"

I almost laughed: He'd been talking to me for an hour and a half and hadn't even bothered to ask who I was? We'd never really talked before. I explained that I was a journalist, but at the moment, I was just a patient trying to get better. Any writing about it was a question for another day.

When we got into the car, Erik asked me why I thought all these researchers wouldn't listen to him. I said, mildly, "Well, I think presentation really matters with these things." Erik responded that early on, he'd been very mild-mannered, and he'd only gotten more strident when that hadn't worked. "And you know," he said, "the more strident I got, it seemed like the less they listened!" I almost laughed, but I also felt sad for him, devoting such energy to his cause with so little reward. *Why can't he recognize that his strategy is backfiring?*

When we pulled into Whole Foods, Erik paused to warn me, "If you haven't been hypervigilant, then you may not feel anything on an exposure."

I wanted to strangle the bastard. The *whole point* of this exercise was to maximize the chances that I would react. How the hell was I supposed to be hypervigilant if I didn't know what to be vigilant for? And hadn't I just spent two weeks in Death Valley to make sure I wasn't getting exposed, so that I'd be able to feel something? Yet again, the whole theory seemed to be unfalsifiable.

"So I can only find out what I need to be aware of if I'm already hyperaware of it?" I asked.

"Yep!" Erik nodded. "This is a hell of a paradigm."

Then he had me look at the veins in my hands: When I got exposed, he said, they'd be more prominent, so I should remember how they looked beforehand.

We walked around the store, and I felt astonished by the bright lights, the endless aisles of food, the well-dressed people. At home, I often shopped at a Whole Foods not so different from this one, but now, it felt like a different planet from the rocks and sand of Death Valley where I now felt like I belonged.

Suddenly Erik stopped, his eyes focusing into the mid-distance. "Oh yeah, I feel it. It's heeeeeere!"

Am I in a poltergeist movie? I resisted an urge to snicker. *But, okay, I haven't come this far to give this stupid theory anything less than a full shot.* So I paid close attention to my body: Could I feel anything differ- ent? Was that a constriction in my heart? Perhaps a slight pain, maybe the needle-in-the-heart feeling I'd heard my online moldie friends describe? *Could be,* I thought, *but then again, it could be a random sensation I would never even have noticed if I weren't paying such close attention.*

Erik had me check the veins in my hands again, but I wasn't sure whether there was a difference.

After we left the Whole Foods, he pulled down his sock and noted the indentation from it, and sagely said that this was a sign of exposure. He had me push my sock down: I had an indentation too! I pointed out that I would expect that, exposure or no, and he said that he might have thought that as well, but when he'd gotten clear in the desert, that didn't happen. "But I was just in the desert for two weeks!" I cried. He didn't have much to say.

We got in the car, and I felt like I could sob. *This is exactly as ridicu- lous as it all sounds. What the hell am I going to do now?*

Erik broke in: I shouldn't give up hope, he said. Every ME/CFS patient he'd taken to Truckee High School, where we were going the next day, had reacted.

He then carried on about all the reasons I might not have detected the mold even if mold was indeed sickening me. "You've just got to give the theory a chance!" he said.

At this point, my irritation overwhelmed me. "Look, Erik," I said. "I am here specifically to give your theory a chance—I've just spent a bunch of money, spent two weeks in the desert, and have now driven up to Reno, all for the express purpose of proving you right. Now it just has to work."

He blinked. "Thank you," he said. And then he carried on some more.

BEFORE HE PEDALED AWAY on his bicycle, Erik instructed me to pick him up on a street corner the next morning for our Truckee High School expedi- tion. I was so annoyed with him I felt like I was going to jump out of my skin. I spent hours working to calm down, pacing around my hotel room. *What an idiot! What a fucking waste of time!*

I recognized that my anger was coming largely from disappointment—and shame. I knew that I could tell my science-writer friends that it had all been a lark, that I'd never really believed in the theory, but I also knew that wasn't quite true. My fantasies of living with Frances in a Vanagon in the desert taunted me.

Finally, it was late enough that I could go to bed. Erik told me I should be sure to shower before bed, but I didn't. It was pretty clear to me at this point that mold wasn't my problem. And anyway, I wasn't trying to avoid a reaction; I was trying to create it.

I WOKE UP in the middle of the night needing to pee. I felt awful. When I got up, I found that not only could I barely walk, I couldn't even stand up straight. I hadn't had trouble walking since I'd left Santa Fe.

Oh my god! It might be true! I might be a moldie!

I staggered to the toilet, my excitement battling against a feeling of nauseating, aching, swollen illness. *I feel so, so awful. This is amazing!*

I felt the wall of skepticism within me crumbling, a wall I'd erected to protect myself against my desire that this ridiculous theory be true for me. And through the cracks in the wall, relief began flooding in: After so many years of nothing working, maybe this was the answer. I lurched back to bed and fired off e-mails to a bunch of my friends who had been following my saga: "Woohoo! I'm having trouble walking!"

As I lay in bed, too worked up to go back to sleep, I tried to put my scientist hat back on. This was just one data point, hardly conclusive proof that mold was my problem. Intriguing, but nothing more. I had to make sure I didn't get carried away and let myself be misled by my own hopes. Was I just setting myself up for all the bitter feelings I'd had after we'd left Whole Foods and it hadn't seemed to affect me—but worse?

After a while, I took a shower, and I was amazed to find that I felt much better afterward, walking fairly normally. Showers had never made a whit of difference in the past. And when I woke up in the morning, I felt quite okay. *Astonishing!*

As Erik and I drove to Truckee, I told him what had happened during the night. He seemed surprisingly blasé about this, saying little in response.

It was as windy and cold as it had been the day before, and I wondered if Erik would again declare it a "horrifically bad" day for a mold tour. But Erik said the mold only goes really out of control when the weather first deteriorates. That day, he expected it to be bad but not dangerously so—perfect.

Erik pointed out the area where he'd seen that strange, neon-green mold growing on the lakeshore just before the epidemic had broken out. We drove past Cheney and Peterson's old office and then headed toward the dreaded Truckee High School, where so many teachers had gotten sick. As soon we pulled off the highway toward the high school, Erik said he felt the mold already: "It's a killer!" I, naturally, felt nothing.

We parked across the street from the high school, lest the car get contaminated just by being nearby. The high school was closed for a snow day, and workers were shoveling outside it. We stood outside the front doors, and Erik said he felt it, but not as powerfully as along the road. I tried to tune in to what I was feeling, but it was hard to detect anything beyond the cold making my body clench. Again, maybe I had a slight feeling of a needle in the heart, maybe a feeling that my brain was being compressed. I certainly didn't have the heart palpitations or burning skin that Erik was describing, and the moments I might have been feeling something didn't correspond well with the moments Erik said he did. We stood outside for just a couple of minutes and then dashed back to the car for warmth.

Next, we drove a few blocks to the Henness Flats Apartments, a public housing complex where, Erik said, a lot of people had gotten sick and testing showed high levels of toxic mold. When we drove up, I thought the apartments looked quite nice, seeming newer than they were. We walked through the complex of small, interconnected buildings, and I still felt pretty much nothing.

We went inside one of the buildings, into a little common area between the apartments. "It's heeeere!" Erik said, making me silently giggle again at poltergeists. I paid very close attention to my body. I felt nothing.

Then I felt a wave of lightheadedness, and I started feeling rather out of it. *Big whoop*, I thought. *The illness itself sometimes makes me feel lightheaded and out of it, so that means precisely nothing.* I was also getting hungry, which could have the same effect. When we got back to the car, I pulled out an energy bar.

We started heading back toward Reno, stopping along the way at another area he said was bad that we could just drive through. Again, I could identify some slight funny sensations, maybe a feeling of brain compression, but they didn't correspond well to when Erik said he was feeling it.

I was getting tired, I was still hungry, I was feeling grouchy, this whole thing was clearly a waste of time, and I wanted it to be over. But I felt like I should do something to thank Erik for his time, so I invited him to lunch.

Over lunch, I was so out of it that holding a conversation was painful. Erik continued bloviating about how ignored he had been, how unethical the researchers were, how terrible mold is. I desperately wanted him to shut up. I wanted to put my head down on the table, I wanted my food, I wanted to go to bed, and I never wanted to see this annoying man again in my life.

I apologized for not being much of a conversationalist. "It's from the mold," he said, and I thought, *Yeah, well, maybe. It could also be from the hunger, or the illness, or the god-awful annoying company.*

WHEN I GOT BACK to the hotel, I napped, and when I woke up an hour later, I couldn't walk.

I couldn't even come anywhere close to standing up straight. I had to support my upper body by resting my hands on my knees to stagger to the bathroom. I felt indescribably awful, even worse than the night before. The awfulness was a bit different from what I was used to—what came to mind was that I felt poisoned, as if every cell in my body wanted to throw up.

I took a shower, following instructions, and was again astonished to find that the awful, awful, awful feeling went away. It seemed surreal, especially since showers had never helped before. Swimming had certainly helped, and I'd always showered first, but I'd staggered out of the showers just like I staggered in. *But now I'm pretty much fine!*

The next morning, I sat in bed, cuddling with Frances and trying to figure out what to make of the previous day's events. *Wow. Crazy Erik the Mold Warrior seems to be right.* It all felt like a dream, as if the story were living me rather than the reverse. This outcome felt simultaneously absurdly unlikely and inevitable, and nearly impossible to fully absorb: All these years of suffering may have a simple explanation. It had all just been a microbe poisoning me, a single, external, physical factor. Maybe.

There was something bewildering, though, about having the explanation delivered by a raving guy with the disaffected air of a homeless person, rather than by a white-coated doctor.

The stories Erik had told me started to resonate differently in my mind and heart. What would it be like to figure out something that might be the key to the suffering of millions of people and have nearly no one listen to you?

Of course, it was a huge leap to go from mold being the problem for Erik, and a few other people, and now maybe me, to it being the problem for everyone with ME/CFS. And his strategies for bringing attention to his "clue" violated pretty much every norm in the scientific community. It was no surprise they hadn't worked. Still, when I imagined it from Erik's point of view, my heart broke a bit.

Don't get ahead of yourself, Julie, I thought, putting my scientist hat back on. I needed to do a lot more experimentation before I was fully convinced that the effect was real—two data points were clearly insufficient. I winced a bit, imagining how disappointed I'd feel if the hypothesis didn't hold up at this point—but one way or the other, I needed to know the truth. I didn't think it made sense to do more in Reno, though, because with the exposures I'd had, I couldn't be sure that any symptoms were from new exposures anyway.

So it was time to go home, for the real test: Would my trailers and belongings cripple me?

CHAPTER 14

HOMECOMING

As I crested the big hill on I-25, I got my first view of Santa Fe. Its familiar ridgeline zigzagged across the horizon, and the smooth white hump of Baldy shone in the winter sun. *Home!*

Ordinarily, my heart swelled when I saw those mountains I knew so well. But this time, I felt like a band was constricting around my chest. So much hung on what happened in the next 24 hours. I was counting on my trailers triggering a dramatic reaction and vindicating the moldies, and my Reno experiences had left me expecting that—sort of. *It just seems so far-fetched,* I thought. *I've been in and out of my trailers so many times without a problem.* I knew the moldies said they could explain that away, but still . . .

I felt trapped, like whatever happened, I couldn't escape the fear and uncertainty. If I got back and felt just fine in my trailers, then my crazy experiment would be over, I'd still be terribly ill, and I'd have no idea what to do next. And in the "happy" case that my trailers did me in, I'd likely lose the straw-bale house I'd put my soul into along with all my belongings, and I might not be able to live in Santa Fe for years, if ever. And even then, I didn't know whether I'd end up feeling better—my Reno experiments had only suggested that mold could make me feel worse.

I did hold out some hope that I might be able to live in my house if the mold hypothesis turned out to be true. Just before I'd left Death Valley, I'd heard from a nearby moldie that the area around my house—20 minutes north of Santa Fe—had good air, much better than Santa Fe itself. So as long as my house wasn't moldy, perhaps I could live there after all.

Oddly, though, even that news had only reinforced my uncertainty, making me feel peculiarly let down. I'd grown attached to my image of me and Frances in a Vanagon in the desert, a bit like Thelma and Louise retreating from society (where Louise just happened to be a dog). The silence, the stillness, the expansiveness of the desert drew me. Something profound had happened to me while I was in Death Valley, and I worried it might get sucked out of me if I returned to ordinary life.

At the same time, the possibility of returning had awakened a longing to be in my house again, a longing so intense it frightened me. I had built a barricade inside myself against that desire—the only way I'd been able to stand being away for so long—and now I felt that barricade cracking. *Once I return, will I ever be able to bring myself to leave again? And am I ready for that?*

The idea of returning to the house like this—sick, poor, and alone—made me feel oddly ashamed. When I'd driven away to Santa Cruz nearly seven years earlier to start a grand new career, I certainly hadn't imagined returning to my house with my life this much of a mess. I knew my illness wasn't my fault, but still, the feeling niggled at me that I'd failed—and that if only I could restore my life to productive order before returning home, my illness would stay dreamlike, unreal, not fully attached to me.

My breath felt like a caged hummingbird. *Working myself into a frenzy is certainly not going to help matters,* I thought, and I consciously breathed in slowly, expanding my chest and belly, feeling the gaps grow between my ribs.

Suddenly, the band I'd felt cinched around my chest seemed to snap, and my lungs expanded easily. A thought fell into my mind, as gentle as rosewater: *I died out there in the desert. This is all extra. So who cares about what happens next? It's all bonus, all wonderful, an unearned gift no matter how it works out.*

I felt as if I were sitting in my camp chair in Death Valley again, feeling the seeds of the desert's spaciousness blossoming inside me. The valley's huge and ancient stillness seemed to unfurl within my cells, quieting my body as it opened my skin, connecting me with the piñon-pocked hills around me, with the air above the town stretching off to the mountains.

There's nothing I have to accomplish. Simply breathing in and out counts as success. Everything I had ever worried about in my life now seemed dinky, absurd, as if I'd been obsessing about a battle among my own tin soldiers.

Astonished tears pricked at my eyes. The breath went in; the breath went out.

But then a sinuous whisper penetrated the wonder: *Life certainly doesn't feel like such a blessing when the pain is so bad you can only endure it moment by moment, breath by breath. And you might have to bear miseries far worse, like plenty of other patients do. Sure your nice little epiphany won't disintegrate when tested?*

I let the thought enter, felt its sting, and didn't allow myself to clench up against it. I had to acknowledge that all that was true. I had no idea of the agonies awaiting me, or how robust this feeling would turn out to be. But I found that thinking about that didn't squash the spaciousness pumping through my body like freshly oxygenated red blood cells. I felt as though a forgotten but inalienable birthright had returned to me.

I looked again at the Sangre de Cristo Mountains. *Thank you for being here for me to love,* I thought. *Whether I'm able to make my home here again or not.*

MY PLAN WAS TO STAY at my friend George's house that night. I'd save the big test—going into the trailers—for the next day, when I was fresh. Or, actually, I'd save it for the next night, when I planned to sleep there. Although my moldie friends had said that just a few minutes would be enough for me to know if the trailers were bad for me, I found that hard to believe. When I'd gotten exposed in Tahoe, I hadn't been at all sure at the time, and it had taken hours before I'd really felt the mold hit me. If I slept in my trailers, I figured, I'd be sure to react—if I was going to react at all.

Since I was arriving earlier in the day than I expected, I decided to head out to my land just to say hello. I missed it. While I was there, I could get my tent set up as a retreat from the mold if the trailers indeed sickened me the following night.

Frances perked up from her slumber as we rumbled down our one-lane road, and when I rolled down the window for her, she wiggled her nose out it with intense concentration. As I pulled onto my land, I gave the ponderosas, oaks, and willows my usual silent greeting, but I found that I felt unborn, as if my individual self had dissolved and what was left of it was too undeveloped to commune with these great beings that had once been my intimate friends. I opened the door, putting my feet on the pine duff and letting Frances out of the car. Frances leapt out and sped after a squirrel, schooling it for its impudence.

Just below the trailers was a beautiful camping spot with a deep, soft bed of composted oak leaves, protected by overhanging oak branches. I'd have to clip a barbed wire fence to get there, which was easy enough— except that the wire clippers were in the trailers, and I had planned to stay out of the trailers until the next day. I took a deep breath outside, held it, dashed in, grabbed the clippers, and fled. Then I got to work.

Once the tent was up, I leaned against a ponderosa, smelling its deep butterscotch scent, listening to the stream. I felt all the possible futures projecting out from this moment like spreading tendrils, heading toward different universes, different lives, each inviting my thoughts to slide out along them, imagining their potential and uncertainties.

I don't know. I can't know. I stopped my thoughts from trying to fill the void of unknowing, and instead, I centered myself in it, feeling the spaciousness from my drive, feeling this precise unknowing moment as a space to occupy. I watched a bird pecking between the dead leaves in the driveway, felt a pine needle poking at my leg, rested my head against the knobbly bark of the ponderosa.

Afterward, as I drove toward George's house, I found that I was unable to get my breath, panting, and I felt mild heart pains. I had never felt that way before. *Could the trailers have really done this to me, even though I hardly spent any time in them?* But I knew that the mere expectation of nasty symptoms might be enough to create them. This was the placebo effect's evil twin, which scientists call the nocebo effect. *But, I didn't expect that such a short exposure would cause problems. I was much more nervous when I used that bug spray after I was supposedly going to become chemically sensitive, and the bug spray didn't do a thing to me.*

Still, I had to acknowledge that I'd invested so much now in this idea that my trailers would make me sick that my brain could be playing tricks on me. That idea made a lot of sense, really, so I focused on chilling out.

Come on, Julie! I thought. *You're getting worked up over nothing. You've built this up so much: "Oh my god, the mold is so bad bad bad!" Take a deep breath, relax, everything is just fine.*

And that did help, a little bit, calming me down even though my heart still sped. A shower at George's house had a much bigger effect, settling my breath into an even rhythm and slowing my heart rate. I put it out of my mind, figuring it was just anxiety, or nocebo, or a temporarily overactive imagination, or whatever. Nothing to worry about, especially since that had to be way too brief an exposure to cause problems.

But when I woke in the middle of the night to pee, I had trouble walking.

This time, the nocebo effect didn't seem like such a compelling explanation. I'd felt totally relaxed by the time I'd gone to bed, not feeling concerned about my strange little reaction at all. And I'd been sleeping soundly.

Oh my god, this really may be true!

I fired off another round of e-mails to my friends: "Holy crap! . . . I keep thinking that this won't pan out, or it will be so subtle I won't be sure. But this ain't subtle. I guess I'm turning into one of those crazy moldie people!"

Over the next week, I tested the hypothesis further. I spent 10 minutes in my trailers, and although they smelled a bit musty after being shut up for weeks, I felt no unusual physical sensations. *Oh man,* I thought. *Here we go. This looked so promising, but now it's going to fall apart.* Less than two hours later, though, I couldn't walk. And again, taking a shower immediately made me feel almost entirely better.

It wasn't just the trailers that did me in either. Sitting in a restaurant two days later, I felt as though I were gradually turning to stone. I gimped out of the building, sat in the fresh air, and within minutes was able to walk fine, though I still felt somewhat crappy. Fresh air clearly wasn't as powerful as a shower and change of clothes.

Another day, I needed some papers from the trailers, so I asked a friend to get them for me and I took them to Kinko's to copy. I had a whisper of a bad feeling when I held the papers, but I dismissed it as paranoia. Within an hour, I was crippled, and yet again, a shower restored me instantly. *That's freaky.* I thought back to Erik's story about his sergeant collapsing from Erik's peanut breath because of allergies and his claim that mold operates similarly, with tiny quantities being enough to do in the susceptible. *Maybe Crazy Erik was right.*

My car offered further confirmation. I tested it in the hope that I could return Gary's little Impreza to him. Though I felt ridiculous as I sat in it—*of course it's fine!*—I could barely get out after five minutes and staggered away.

All of this felt persuasive, but I longed for evidence that was more rigorous. I started thinking about how I could design a randomized, placebo-controlled, double-blind experiment: I could, say, expose myself to a bunch of washcloths, half of which had been in a moldy building and half of which hadn't, to see if I could distinguish them. But such an experiment seemed too complicated to take on at the moment, and I kept it as a possibility for the future. For the moment, I just cultivated my skepticism, figuring that if mold wasn't truly the problem, over time I'd see evidence against it—as long as I didn't let myself become too gullible.

I pursued one more avenue for rigorous evidence. Ritchie Shoemaker, the crusading mold doctor whose book I'd found so impenetrable, had a set of blood tests he recommended that he claimed offered strong evidence about whether you were sickened by mold. Given that many of his claims in his book had struck me as scientific word soup, I was doubtful about the significance of the tests, but hey, they were covered by my health insurance, so what the heck. And indeed, my results did broadly fit with Shoemaker's predictions for someone with mold illness.

Interesting, I thought, *but I still don't trust this guy. I'm more persuaded by my own reactions.*

MY VARIOUS TESTS INCREASED my confidence. When I was sitting in a café a week after I got back from Death Valley and found myself feeling so awful I could barely keep my head up, I didn't hesitate—time to get out.

I sat outside, addled and achy, trying to figure out what to do next. Leaving had helped, but I still felt fairly terrible. I decided to try driving out to my land to see if the rumor I'd heard was right and the outside air on my land was indeed better for me than in town.

I sat well away from the trailers with Frances, bundled up and soaking in the sunshine. After about an hour, I felt quite a lot better. *Maybe the moldies are right again.* A familiar skeptical whisper piped up, though: *It could just be from the rest. It might have nothing to do with the air or with mold.*

After another hour, I thought, *Wow, I really do feel better!* I decided to try taking Frances for a bit of a walk. *We'll just stroll up the arroyo a tiny bit. Don't want to overdo it.*

I ambled while Frances screeched up and down the hillside. I cringed as she careened toward trees, her strong, lithe body dodging them at the last possible moment. With every step, I assessed my body's state: *Do I need to turn around now? Now?*

I treasured each familiar detail in the arroyo; the smooth, gray, dolphin-shaped rock with the alabaster intrusion; the twisting, wind-scoured dead juniper branch; the graceful curves the water had traced in the sand. I especially delighted to see tiny grasses growing in dirt that had accumulated behind dead branches I had put across the drainage years before, in an effort to slow the water down. A hundred years ago, these hills had all been covered with grass that had stabilized the earth and kept these arroyos from scarring the landscape, but too many sheep and cows had nibbled the grass away. Each new blade felt like a tiny healing.

I was astonished to reach the saddle at the top of the arroyo—I hadn't imagined I would walk nearly so far, a good half mile of climbing. *You should really stop here,* I thought, but my body felt strong and fluid, and I couldn't help myself: I turned left and started tromping up the ridgeline. *I'll turn back at that next tree,* I thought. And then when I got there, *Maybe that tree there instead.*

Soon I found myself at the top of the 350-foot hill behind my house.

My breath caught in my chest, as if it couldn't decide whether to be a sob or a laugh or a whoop. I hadn't been able to climb that hill for a year and a half. *This can't be real,* I thought. *This can't be real.*

To my right, the Nambe reservoir dam cut a sharp, curved line across the land. In front of it, the mud-hill barrancas undulated and crinkled. Snow gleamed on the peaks of the Jemez across the valley, and to the left, the Sandias humped up like a breaching whale. Even further to the left, the buildings of Santa Fe dotted the plain. Frances ran up to me and I pulled her in, burying my face in her neck as I said, *It's true, it's true, it's true!* But she backed away, confused by my intensity. I told her to go play, and I looked around greedily, wiping the tears from my eyes.

I pulled out my phone, snapped a picture, and e-mailed it to a bunch of my friends, with the subject line: "Oh. My. God."

When I had no payback for my exercise the next day, my worries about whether the mold hypothesis was true or not started feeling feeble. *If this is the placebo effect,* I thought, *it's good enough for me.*

Instead, I started fantasizing about what I might be capable of now. *Could I hike to the waterfall? Could I even start running again?* I didn't want to wonder and test and assess anymore—I wanted to put my energy into getting better.

I knew I didn't have the kind of evidence I'd publish in *Science,* but I wasn't trying to prove any scientific theory. I was just trying to manage my own little life. And something incredible had happened on that hike, something incredible enough to whoosh away my doubts. If I was wrong about this mold thing, I'd figure it out soon enough when things stopped making sense. For now, I had enough evidence to place my own bets. I was finally all in on the mold theory.

What that meant for my future still wasn't clear, though. For one thing, I didn't know whether I'd be able to live in the house I'd built. Perhaps some water had found its way into the bales and caused some rot, or perhaps a tenant had carried some nasty toxin in with their stuff. I felt okay in the house for short periods, and my tenant even let me sleep in the house one night, which to my enormous relief seemed to go fine. But one night wasn't enough to be sure—for that, I had to be there longer, after my tenant left in three weeks. Then I'd know whether it was time to shop for a Vanagon or to settle down in Santa Fe.

In the meantime, I focused on practicalities: I was homeless, I needed to buy a car, my computer had died just before I left for Death Valley, I had very few clothes, and even if I had more, I had no place to put them.

Unwilling to drop a couple thousand dollars on a new Mac, I bought a used one. My moldie friends had warned that computers could pick up contamination and then spray it all around when their fans turned on, but that struck me as unlikely. I felt torn—on the one hand, the moldies had been dramatically right about improbable things in the past, but on the other, fear ruled the lives of many of them as they endlessly ran from exposures. Accepting that the mold theory was broadly true didn't mean that everything that any moldie had ever imagined affected them would necessarily affect me too—after all, I hadn't developed chemical sensitivities as predicted (*at least not so far!* I thought, crossing my fingers). I didn't want to let mere rumors rule my life.

Each time I used the computer I bought, though, I felt slightly off afterward, and over the next few days, I found myself feeling worse overall: My back hurt, my eyes swelled, I felt exhausted. I stopped using the computer and felt better. *I'm getting rid of this computer. Maybe I'm being ridiculous, but ridiculous is better than sick.* The fellow I bought the computer from took it back, though he clearly thought my explanation about mold sounded crazy. I could hardly argue with him on that score. I bought the least expensive new MacBook Air I could find, and I had no problems with it.

Another practical problem was money. If I had to replace everything I owned, the $10,000 Lenny had given me wasn't going to last long. And from what I'd read from my moldie friends, learning to avoid mold was likely to take most of my attention for some months, so I probably wasn't going to be earning much money anytime soon.

My thoughts went to Geoff's family, who had treated me with extraordinary generosity and love throughout our relationship. After Geoff and I split up, he had lived at home for several years while doctors continued to fiddle with his medications and he worked to rebuild his life, shielded by his family from destitution or abandonment. We talked occasionally, so I knew that he now had an excellent job and seemed basically content with his life, though his illness had cost him dearly. *Maybe his parents would be willing to help me like they helped him—not as much, of course, but maybe some.*

I e-mailed Geoff to ask what he thought, and he volunteered to ask them for me. I, of course, worried that they might find my asking for money outrageous when I'd left their son, and I also worried that his dad, a transplant surgeon, might find my mold theory dopey and ridiculous. But in fact, Geoff's dad e-mailed within a few hours, letting me know that they would be happy to send me $2,000 a month for as long as I needed it and they could afford it. He also said he had a colleague at the medical school who was convinced she'd recovered from a similar illness by eating lots of kale, and "personally, I find a bad effect of mold much more likely than a miraculous healing effect of kale." He told me that Geoff's mother insisted that I consider it a gift, not a loan, and ended his e-mail by saying, "You are still a daughter-in-law in our accounting of family members."

I bawled. My muscle fibers seemed to loosen a couple of ratchets as the relief flooded through me. At the same time, all the grief at my loss of them, grief I couldn't let myself feel at the time, poured in. I reread his last sentence over and over, and I sobbed and sobbed and sobbed.

I DECIDED I WAS READY to get rid of all the stuff in my trailers. I worried that if I didn't, I might walk past the trailers and get small exposures to "ick," the (purported) toxin endemic to Berkeley. I also hoped that once I removed my belongings, the trailers would prove to be no moldier than many buildings in town. Then they would be safe enough for a non-moldie to live in, and I could rent them out for some income.

The symbolism of getting rid of everything and starting over seemed almost embarrassingly crude. Life seemed to be making a little joke for me, as it had with my going to *Death Valley* of all places. If my life were a novel I was editing, I would scratch those things out, saying, "Be a little more subtle, please."

I bought a hooded white Tyvek suit like the ones asbestos removal workers wear, along with a respirator that made me look like an insect, rubber gloves, goggles, and booties. In the full getup, I felt like a cross between a clown and Darth Vader. I walked into the trailers cautiously, as if waiting for a lightning bolt of mold to strike me from the heavens. I tentatively concluded that I was okay.

A friend helped me go through everything. Just a few months before, I'd paid to have all this carefully collected stuff brought out from Berkeley. Now, though, it was almost all destined for Goodwill. I figured I'd store a few things that were really meaningful in the hope that I might be able to tolerate them years down the line, but everything else was a goner. Out went the down pillow I'd had since I was a teenager, its cover yellow with age; my copy of *Osler's Web,* the history of chronic fatigue syndrome that had so horrified me; food and toiletries and printer paper and clothes. I kept the sweater I'd knitted for my mother, with nearly 60 different yarns in it, in shades of black and silver to match her hair. I also kept a wooden mask William and I had bought together in South Africa, its empty eyes peering through ropes that hung like dreadlocks from above its forehead.

After a couple of hours, I felt as if I were the tin man in the rain, my joints gradually rusting shut. I was a bit shocked that being in the trailers did me in even through this whole getup. I pulled off my protective gear, sat outside, and breathed the fresh air. An invisible oil can seemed to go to work, restoring my mobility. I figured I'd taken enough of a hit for one day and quit, skedaddling back to George's house to shower and change.

The next day, I felt like crap and took the day off, lolling about stuporously. Each day I felt capable, I suited up again. I mostly stayed outside the trailers while my friend brought me stuff to sort outside, but still, after a couple of hours I rusted to a halt. Getting crippled each day made getting rid of everything I owned surprisingly straightforward, because it felt so apparent that my stuff was doing me in. Plus, every few days, I walked up the hill behind my house again, and my future beckoned. A pair of blue jeans or a tchotchke or some books couldn't compare.

The only exception I made was for objects that were only metal, glass, or ceramic. I had been told that those materials didn't seem to absorb toxins the way others could. So I scrubbed my glasses and pots and plates and cutlery and set them aside to use, well, once I had somewhere to use them. I was particularly pleased to keep those things, since they had mostly come from my mother. The knives were the Henckels I'd bought her for Christmas when I was 15, and she had received the pots as wedding presents.

Every once in a while, I got stuck, like when I picked up my fanny pack: *This is the perfect fanny pack! If I get rid of this fanny pack, I'll just have to go buy another one exactly like it, and that's ridiculous! Surely there is some way of saving this. Wouldn't it be okay if I just washed it?* I knew my moldie friends would say no to that—any fabric so deeply steeped in my personal kryptonite, ick, wasn't worth saving, they'd say.

Suddenly, I snapped to: It was just a fanny pack. It was nothing compared to my health. I tossed it in a Goodwill box and moved on.

ONE DAY SOON AFTER I finished clearing out the trailers, I walked up the trail along the stream. I greeted all the familiar spots I hadn't been able to go to in so long: the ponderosa grove with lush willows on one side and cholla cactus on the other; a high log bridge I used to run across; the stream bank where Frances loved to squish her toes in the silt. The north-facing slopes were snowy, and the south-facing ones were dry and sunny.

My body carried me happily up the trail nearly two miles, where I entered a narrow canyon with cliffs on either side. The first time I'd come here was when I was a teenager, and the entrance to the canyon had been so grown over that I'd missed it. I'd climbed up up up with the main trail, peered over the edge of the cliff, and glimpsed a waterfall. *There's got to be some way to get there,* I'd thought, so I backtracked and bushwhacked my way to a tiny trail that crossed and recrossed the stream. In a couple of places, I had to make tricky leaps between rocks, but in the end, I was rewarded with a 20-foot waterfall that thundered and sprayed its grotto with mist. Since then, the forest service had cleared the trail and lots of people came to the waterfall on beautiful summer days, but it still felt like my personal treasure.

Late winter ice now slicked over some of the rocks and made the tricky section of the trail even trickier. I felt like a goat as I leapt between them and made it dry-footed. *Nice job, body!*

Even before I got to the waterfall, I could hear that its thunder was muffled: It was encased in ice. At its base, the column was a dozen feet around, narrowing at the top. Light sparkled among the fractal filigrees of ice, small columns filling in between bigger columns, and behind it, I could see the water flickering, the waterfall's heartbeat.

At the very top of the ice column, a small slit had melted, and an occasional splash of water bounded out of it. Spring was arriving. Tears sprang to my eyes. *Yes, winter is ending, the ice is melting, everything is coming back to life. Including me.*

I carefully clambered over the frozen pool to peek inside the slit and see the water flying on its way. When I got back to solid ground, I play-jumped at Frances and she ran and ran, sliding out on the ice, leaping over the rocks, threading between the trees. I threw my arms in the air and whooped. *Thank you! Thank you! Thank you! Thank you! Thank you!*

CHAPTER 15

AN EMBRYONIC LIFE

I could hardly absorb the new reality of my life. I felt like a kid in a candy store: I could start running again! I could try biking! I could hike in all the places I so loved!

I hiked into a box canyon near where the artist Georgia O'Keeffe made her home in New Mexico. I followed a tiny stream through the cottonwood trees with cliffs on either side that grew closer and taller. After two miles, the trail dead-ended at a giant box of cliffs, with water seeping straight through the sandstone to form the stream. On one side, the cliff blazed incandescent orange as the sun struck it; on the other, the shadows glowered a deep red. I raised my arms and turned my face to the sky, where blue seemed to seep from every molecule. *I died out there in the desert. This is all extra, an unearned gift.*

At the end of the four-mile hike, I felt like a squirmy puppy unable to keep my tail from wagging. I was barely tired. I knew that I couldn't possibly live the rest of my life in a state of giddy delight, but at that moment, it seemed nearly inconceivable that I could ever feel any other way.

I WAS STILL STAYING with friends as I waited for my tenant to leave, but during one four-day period, none of my friends had free bedrooms to offer me, so I found a good deal on a vacation rental. The manager, an older Hispanic fellow, showed me the casita, which was lovely, clean, bright, totally renovated, not a whiff of mustiness.

But just after entering it, I felt a peculiar sense of internal heaviness—just the kind of sensation Erik the Mold Warrior had tutored me to pay attention to. Still, I couldn't bring myself to leave on the basis of such a wisp of a feeling. *Maybe it'll pass.* Then I felt an unfamiliar wave of light-headedness. If this place was indeed moldy, I knew the likely cost of staying: a day of feeling poisoned, with a bone-deep ache, swollen eyes, a fuzzy brain. *Not worth the risk.*

But telling this fellow that his lovely little house was moldy, when the evidence I had for it was so weird . . . The words stuck in my throat.

Time to get used to trusting weird little feelings like this, I told myself. I coughed out an apologetic explanation that I was "allergic" to mold and didn't feel well here.

The man's weathered chestnut face stayed impassive, as if he were used to bizarre statements from these rich white folks he dealt with all the time. "I have another casita," he told me, his voice rising and falling with a classic northern New Mexico accent. "Do you want to see it?"

Indeed I did. But again, within moments of being inside, I felt light-headed. I apologized again and fled.

I tried a hotel next and was relieved to feel fine there. I felt torn between being thrilled that I seemed to be developing some weird and much-needed sixth sense and horrified that I was entering a warped parallel universe. *Am I becoming Super Mold Girl, or am I turning into a muttering bum on the street, flailing my arms at invisible airborne tormentors?*

MY TENANT LEFT, and I moved back into my house—that is, I carried in my camping gear. It was time to find out if my future was in Santa Fe or in a Vanagon.

I put the two flimsy pots I'd borrowed from Gary in the cabinet where I'd once kept the Revere Ware saucepans my mother had gotten as a wedding present 50 years earlier. I set my one dish, a big white plastic soup/salad bowl, into the empty mahogany dish rack above the sink. I'd designed that rack just the right size for my dishes, so I could wash them, put them away, and let them drip straight into the sink as they dried. The soup bowl looked cheap and lonely there.

The house echoed as I walked around. I unrolled my camping pad and sleeping bag in my empty bedroom and put Frances's bed next to them. I saw the scratches in the walls left by various tenants, the torn window screens, the stains in the toilets, and I felt as though I'd neglected the house over the last six-and-a-half years. I swept cobwebs from the bas-relief in the stairwell that showed our two dogs, now long dead, playing in the snow. Geoff's sister had created it for us using natural clays, back when we still imagined that someday our children would run up and down the stairs. Ghosts seemed to be brushing past me.

Every time I turned around, I discovered something I didn't have. No trash can. No trash bags. No couch. No telephone. I couldn't bring my router over from the trailers in case it was contaminated, so I huddled in the one corner of the house where the Wi-Fi reached. I knew I shouldn't run out and buy a router or trash can, since I didn't know yet if the house would work for me. I wouldn't need such stuff in a Vanagon.

I sat on the brick floor leaning against a cabinet, monitoring my body for unusual feelings. It *seemed* like I was okay, but I felt acutely aware that at any moment, a stray sensation could divert the course of the next several years of my life. I focused on my breath, on the pressure of the floor against my butt, on the faint whisper of the stream outside. The evening light shone through the stained-glass window that my mother had found in a consignment shop years ago, a remnant of a torn-down church. My eye traced the curves of the kiva fireplace tucked under the stairs and the undulating adobe wall along the oak stairway, covered in chocolate-colored earth plaster. *You done good, Julie. This is a beautiful house.*

But an overwhelming loneliness prodded and shoved at me. In Death Valley, the aloneness had felt expansive, but now, it came with a flutter in my breath I recognized as fright. *What am I scared of? I have no idea.* I watched the emotion like a scientist studying cells in a petri dish, feeling it move in my body. It seemed like a primal impulse, an instinct far deeper than consciousness: Must Be Part of Tribe!

Hello, fear and loneliness, I thought. *You are part of me too.*

The air went into my lungs, out of my lungs. Into my lungs, out of my lungs.

I SLEPT BADLY. I was using a borrowed child-size sleeping bag for Frances's bed, and every time she shifted, the nylon made a scritch-scratch noise. The neighbor dog barked off and on through the night, sometimes while sitting just below my window. As I watched time snail past, I worried: Was I failing to sleep because of mold? I didn't feel poisoned, but my moldie friends had told me that sleeplessness could be a sign of mold exposure. *But then, they say practically anything could be a sign of mold exposure! It's far more likely that you're not sleeping because you're anxious. Calm the fuck down, Julie.* It struck me that "Calm the Fuck Down" was a good motto for living, and I pondered getting "CTFD" tattooed on my wrist.

But still, I didn't sleep.

The next day, I was unsurprisingly exhausted. I tried taking Frances for a walk, but I was so tired and draggy that I cut it short. The tiredness made sense after the poor sleep, but the dragginess—was that really normal? I didn't know anymore. After I took several naps that didn't make me feel much better, my worries grew teeth.

I tried to reason through it: Maybe a bad night's sleep could make even a healthy person feel this way. Or maybe it wasn't normal, but I was reacting to mold from the restaurant I went to the previous day, not the house. Or maybe neither of those things were true, but after so many years of illness, sleeplessness was more stress than my body could handle gracefully. Or maybe my house was moldy and I was fucked. *How the hell am I supposed to figure out what's going on?* I thought. *There are too many variables at once!*

That night, I put a non-crinkly blanket down for Frances's bed, curled up next to her, threw a prayer to the mold and barking dog and sleep gods, and closed my eyes. I slept straight through to the morning, and when I woke up, I didn't feel poisoned or exhausted. I got up tentatively, stretched, and walked to the bathroom, feeling how each muscle and joint moved. Frances offered me her head for scratching as I peed. "I think I feel okay, cutie pie," I whispered into her ear. "I think I feel okay!" I got up from the toilet and, naked, chased her around the empty office. "I think I feel okay! I think I feel okay! I think I feel okay!" Frances danced her delight.

All that day, I felt better than I had in a year and a half. When that continued for the next two days, I began buying stuff: a router, a trash can, a telephone.

I'm home.

IT WAS THE BEGINNING of a monetary diaspora that shocked me, about $200 a day scattering as I gathered the basics. Frances saw no need for furniture: With the house empty, it was a giant doggy playground, ideal for running laps and tearing up and down the stairs. I disagreed. Happily, I had left some of my furniture in Santa Fe, so it seemed likely to be safe. Bit by bit, I moved in my mother's claw-foot dining table, some chairs, a clothes cabinet, and a desk. But with almost no living-room furniture and no rugs, the house still echoed.

I hired my cleaning lady to rout out all the dust in the house, removing any mold fragments along with it. She had cleaned the trailers and chopped my vegetables and helped me up the stairs when I couldn't walk, so I felt a loyalty to her. The truth was, though, that she wasn't a very thorough housecleaner. Plus, she didn't speak English, and I knew only a little Spanish, so communication was difficult. Since I wanted it cleaned well, I worked beside her, the two of us scrubbing side by side. She was astonished: "*¿No estás enferma nunca más?*" You aren't sick anymore?

We spent five hours cleaning the downstairs alone. My dusting cloth seemed to be wiping away separation and neglect along with the dirt, renewing a sacred bond between me and my house.

I was thrilled to be able to trust my body to accomplish the task, but I ached the next day and my limbs trembled. I knew I must have breathed in whatever mold bits were hanging out in the dust. Still, I found it unnerving to feel so shaky and weak. I couldn't help but worry: Could the house not be so good for me after all? I wished I could just stay home for a week to thoroughly convince myself my house was okay, but tasks called, and every time I went into a store to buy something, I risked getting whacked from mold. I finally managed to hire a truck to haul the stuff from the trailers away, so I once again donned my Darth Vader clown suit and loaded it all up—and I got whacked. My cleaning lady and I cleaned the upstairs together, leaving me whacked. Each time, I spent the next day catatonic, lolling outside in the sun on my camping pad, feeling like an unstrung marionette.

But my good days overflowed with productivity and joy. Every task I accomplished, every hike I took, every day that I just sat in my very own home—they all felt like small miracles. On one level, I felt like a rat scuttling at the edges: small, cautious, uncertain, dangers all around in a world no longer designed for me. But at the same time, I felt a strong current carrying me, as if a boat cradled me like cupped hands.

It reminded me of how I'd felt before my mother died: Just below the surface, mythic currents had seemed to be propelling me toward my destiny of saving her. But those currents had vanished with her death, leaving me suspended in a void filled only with my ignorance of what my life might hold without her. For years, I had allowed for the possibility that my childhood feeling was largely fantasy, but I now felt that same deep knowing, the same mythic quality breathing itself into my life. The feeling had transformed in the intervening decades, though. As a child, I'd seen myself as the hero, accomplishing my destiny through great effort and individual fortitude. Now, though, I felt as though my core "I" had vanished, replaced with a flowing spaciousness. Effort felt beside the point.

At the same time, I felt a bit like I had when I'd first started doing math and knew less than all of my classmates: I had to learn as fast as I could to survive. Now, my ability to function, apparently, depended entirely on my ability to detect and avoid mold—and to diagnose the problem when I failed.

So I started accumulating tools and habits to keep myself safe. I bought a dozen baseball caps, and whenever I went into a building I was unsure of, I tied my hair into a bun and put on a cap. I kept spare shirts and caps in my car along with bottles of water, and whenever I got exposed, I swapped caps, rinsed my face and hands, and changed my top, aiming to get rid of the contamination as fast as possible. Then, when I got home, I immediately stripped my clothes off and showered, depositing my clothes straight into the laundry basket. If I'd taken Frances with me, I took her straight to the bathroom and washed her too. Happily, I had taught her to like baths, and she'd rest her head on my knee and close her eyes as I rubbed shampoo into her throat.

I felt like I spent half my life scrubbing away mold. I'd been told that washing machines were prone to getting moldy, especially front-loaders like mine, so I was doing all my laundry by hand. At the end of each day, I faced a dishearteningly big pile of dirty clothes, with all the clothes-changing I was doing. I wanted to test my washing machine, but I had only one tool for doing so: my body. I couldn't bear a self-inflicted hit on top of all the others I was taking, so I kept wringing and scrubbing.

Even with all my washing and effort, I didn't always get it right. One night, I woke up in the middle of the night feeling poisoned. I quickly realized why: I hadn't showered before bed. I'd gone to town, but since I hadn't gone anywhere that seemed moldy, I'd thought I could get away without taking one more damned shower. *Wrong, wrong, wrong.*

I staggered up to wash off and considered the consequences of my mistake. My body had almost certainly cross-contaminated my sleeping bag and blanket, just as Erik had seen field jackets cross-contaminate his fellow soldiers' clothes in their lockers. The only solution was to wash them—*ugh*. The sleeping bag and blanket were so big and heavy that it exhausted me just to consider washing them in the tub. Instead, I decided to lug them into town to wash them at a friend's house.

But the next night, I again woke up feeling poisoned. *What the hell is the problem now?* I washed the bedding by hand, figuring that since I'd washed all the bedding in a single big load, it might have been packed too tightly to get thoroughly clean.

But the third night, yet again, I woke up feeling awful, though less so. I panicked a bit—*Is the house no good after all?* I decided to try sleeping with the windows open, and finally, I slept.

My mind spun a thousand alternate hypotheses to explain what had happened. Maybe the bedding was still mildly contaminated but the fresh air made it tolerable; maybe the house was moldy; maybe I had it all wrong and something else entirely was happening. The uncertainty unnerved me, but hey, I was feeling good again. That was what really mattered.

One thing was undeniable: When I felt good, I really felt good. One day, I even tried going for a run. I moved pathetically slowly, stopping frequently to walk, but nevertheless, Frances and I capered and danced when we got home. *A run! I went for a run!*

I worked up my courage and washed a T-shirt in the washing machine to test it. I cautiously held it up to my face, breathing through the fabric, waiting for the mold gods to strike me down. *Seems okay . . .* So I wore the T-shirt for the evening. *Still seems okay . . .* I wore the T-shirt to bed, with the windows closed against the cold. I woke up feeling mildly poisoned. I pulled off the T-shirt, showered, changed my bedding, opened the windows again (cold be damned), and slept fine. So, what to conclude? Was it the T-shirt, the window, the run? I didn't know.

Wouldn't it be great, I thought, *if I could train Frances to detect mold?* I had heard of "Molly the Mold Dog," whom you could hire to go into a house to find any moldy places. I had a vision: I'd go to an unknown building and send Frances in without me. She'd run around sniffing, run back to me, and scratch at my leg if she found any mold. And maybe I could even hold up the questionable T-shirt for her to assess. Frances might be able to hugely expand my world. And I'd have a mold-detecting sidekick to go with the new mold-detecting superpower I was acquiring!

I could think of a bunch of reasons this might not work. The truth was that I didn't even know what it was that made me sick. I was using "mold" as a stand-in for some environmental something that did me in. Water-damaged buildings contained a stew of toxins, from mold, bacteria, particulates . . . Plus, if "ick" was part of the problem, no one knew what the hell it was. Could Frances sniff out "ick"? Maybe, but I probably wouldn't be able to find out without doing a huge amount of possibly fruitless work. It seemed even less likely that she'd be able to tell me if the T-shirt was problematic—how much mold could possibly be on it? And there were bazillions of types of mold, most of which, I guessed, weren't a problem for me at all. Cheese, for example, is made with mold, and I didn't seem to have any problem with cheese. Would she end up telling me about lots of stuff that didn't matter?

Still, I sent e-mails to several dog trainers. They pointed out that, in addition to the worries I already had, the process of training her might kill me. Frances would need samples to sniff during training, which would require me being in alarmingly close proximity to bad stuff. She might even get enough of the bad stuff on her snout just sniffing it to make me sick.

Hmm, I thought. *This sounds too hard to take on right now. But maybe eventually I'll find a way . . .* In the meantime, I continued the service-dog training we'd been doing for months.

I TOOK ON THE TASK of buying a car, feeling bad about keeping Gary's car for so long. I found a Subaru an hour away in Albuquerque around the age of my own car. Carfax showed that it had spent almost its entire life in Albuquerque, with just one oil change in Portland—a bit worrisome, since Portland had a moldy reputation with all its dampness, but it seemed like it had only been there briefly.

As I test-drove it, I had a few alarming tinges, including the shooting-pain-in-the-heart feeling that I had been told was an indication of the evil "ick." But it was so mild that I didn't make much of it. *Jesus Christ, if you're really paying attention, you can feel all kinds of weird things, right?* I arranged to have the car overnight so that my mechanic in Santa Fe could check it out and so that I could have a more extended period to test it. As I was driving home, I had a tight feeling in my lower back that could be an indication of walking troubles. I pulled over and found I could barely get out of the car.

So I turned around and skedaddled on back. I rolled all the windows down, trying to get as much fresh air as possible. When I arrived at the lot, I staggered out of the car, bracing my arms on my knees, scuttling like a slow, loud, groaning crab. The salesmen were agog. One came over to help, and I asked him to get me a trash bag to sit on, because I was worried about cross-contamination. He looked at me like I was crazy, but he did it.

I called an acquaintance in Albuquerque to ask if I could use his shower. When I arrived and staggered out of the car, his jaw dropped. I felt the shower do its work within seconds, like a sheath of immobility was washing right off me. I was walking fine when I got out. When my friend saw me walking normally after the shower, he cried, "Nooo! You're not serious!" And later he said, "You live a weird life."

I felt disbelieving myself. I'd had that experience many times before, but I hadn't gotten over the nonsensical bizarreness of it. What mechanism could possibly explain that? I could imagine the mycotoxins causing some kind of neuroinflammatory response, but a shower wouldn't immediately stop the inflammation entirely, would it?

Later, I tried a second car in Albuquerque, and this time, my body gave no alarm signals. I drove it home without difficulty too. But when I drove it to the garage to get it inspected the next day, I started feeling bad within minutes. *How can this be? Yesterday, I drove it all the way from Albuquerque without a problem.* Soon breathing became difficult. *Okay, okay! I'll take it back! Just let me get there before I asphyxiate!* I drove with the windows down, wondering if I'd have to pull over and lie down in the weeds on the side of the highway in the rain, waiting for some cop to come along and rescue me—or if I'd pass out, have a wreck, and kill myself, or worse, somebody else. I arrived intact, but staggering. When I got back into Gary's little Impreza, I patted the dashboard gratefully.

OVER THE NEXT SEVERAL WEEKS, I found that my responses to buildings became clearer, stronger, easier to assess. Plus, I'd found key buildings I could trust, along with ones to avoid, so I less frequently had to test unknown buildings. My worries about my house had faded, and I even started doing some work again, for the first time in months. I settled into a pattern of regular short runs, building up my distance slowly, thrilling at every expedition.

When I made it through an entire week with nary a day of catatonia, I felt as if I'd just aced a final exam.

CHAPTER 16

A WAKE AND A BAPTISM

After one run in early May, I felt exhausted. Even worse, I felt lousy the next day, and the same thing happened the next time I ran. Plus, my overall energy had sagged a bit. It was frighteningly similar to the end of my remission in Berkeley. *Maybe this is all just a chance improvement, and now the Greek gods are revealing their prank.*

I took a deep breath, trying to breathe away my growing panic. Then I thought, *I died out there in the desert. This is all extra, an unearned gift no matter how it works out.* I breathed in, long and slow, and felt as though Death Valley filled my chest.

I wrote to my moldie friends, who quickly offered a diagnosis: Now that I'd been out of mold for long enough, my body was starting to detoxify, pulling mycotoxins and other toxins out of my tissues and getting rid of them. That was a good and necessary thing, but it came with a downside—as the mycotoxins traveled through the bloodstream before getting filtered out, they poisoned me afresh, like a pinball lighting up a pinball machine anywhere it touches. When I first started avoidance, this detox process hadn't ramped up, so although I had plenty of toxins stored in my tissues, they weren't moving into my bloodstream and hence weren't making me feel bad. Without fresh exposures, my blood levels of mycotoxins were low, and I felt good. Now that the toxins were seeping out of my tissues, there were more of them in my blood and it was making me feel worse.

Detox . . . groan. My skepticism about the mold hypothesis as a whole had been so enormous that I'd held my abundant skepticism about detox in reserve. The first I'd heard of detox was years earlier at a spa, when I'd overheard a young man flirtatiously telling a nubile girl that she should jump into the cold plunge because it would squeeeeeeze the toxins right out of her. The notion of these invisible bad actors squirreling themselves away in our bodies, causing all kinds of untraceable damage, struck me as laughable, and the multiplicity of supposed detox cures was absurd. Drink lemon juice with cayenne! Brush your skin! Go on a juice cleanse! Sweat in a sauna! But not just any sauna—a far-infrared sauna. Wait, no, make that a near-infrared sauna!

But I no longer had the luxury of sneering at such ideas. Since I had already made the leap to believing that mold and its invisible buddies were causing me damage, it was a short step to imagining that some of them were capable of squirreling themselves away in my body and making me feel bad as they came out. I swallowed my disdain and listened up.

The most common recommendation was that I take cholestyramine, a drug which was more commonly used to reduce cholesterol but which Ritchie Shoemaker, the crusading mold doctor whose books I'd found incomprehensible, claimed also binds with mycotoxins. The idea was that mycotoxins float in and out of the gut from the rest of the body, so cholestyramine could mop them up as they passed through. The drug was low-risk, so I started taking it. I also took other low-risk steps that seemed sensible in any case: I continued exercise at whatever level my body was up for; I started eating huge quantities of vegetables; I made my own kefir for its probiotics. But I hesitated before doing more. Which of the zillion possible methods were effective, which were kooky, and which were downright dangerous?

I took a step, which, given my accumulated experiences, felt almost radical: I asked a doctor. For years, I'd heard about a doctor in Santa Fe who specialized in environmental illness, Erica Elliott, and I figured it would be good to get a perspective outside the weird little world of my moldie friends. Her MD didn't carry much weight for me, though—even Klimas, as wonderful as she was, hadn't been able to help me. I figured I'd just have to hear what Elliott said and then decide whether it seemed worth listening to.

The first question Elliott asked me when I went into her office was,

"Does it feel okay in here to you?" I had never been asked that before—and by a doctor! I was delighted to be able to say yes.

She listened intently as I told her my story, occasionally jumping with motherly enthusiasm: "That's exactly right!" "You figured that out all by yourself?" "You're doing such a good job!" And she said that yes, detox was indeed the next step. "These are toxic times!" she declared. "It's not like the 1940s. We're all loaded with toxins in our bodies." So, she said, we've got to give our bodies some help getting rid of them.

Internally, I rolled my eyes at this a bit. I wasn't so sure that our world was much more toxic than it was in the 1940s. I thought of the Cuyahoga River, which caught fire 13 times starting in the mid-1800s but was now full of fish, thanks to the Clean Water Act. I also thought of the moths in Manchester, England, that had evolved to become black during the mid-1800s because the industrial pollution was so bad that the white moths became glaring targets for birds. After the air became cleaner a century later, the white moths came back. I didn't like or much believe the story that the world was a polluted, threatening place, constantly endangering my health. Plus, I thought, our bodies are built to get rid of dangerous chemicals—that's what we have livers and kidneys for.

But I shut up my internal dialogue and listened. Saunas were Elliott's first recommendation. It was well documented, she said, that we sweat out a huge variety of toxins, including heavy metals, polychlorinated biphenyls (PCBs), and mycotoxins. (I later checked on this, and she was right.) One patient of hers, she said, reported that her sweat smelled like the dry cleaners she had lived upstairs from as a kid—she was excreting the dry-cleaning chemical PERC (perchlorethylene). Elliott warned me to start slowly, since the heat from the sauna moves toxins stored in fat into the bloodstream, and if more are produced than my body could handle, I could poison myself.

She also explained that the liver uses five different pathways in its second phase to clean the blood. Depending on your genetics and your lifetime experiences, some of those pathways might not be working so well. Pathway by pathway, she recommended supplements that could help.

Diet, she said, was essential, and a faddish short-term cleanse wouldn't cut it. I needed to eat a very clean, paleo-type diet with lots of organic vegetables and healthy fats, for life.

Hesitantly, I asked about a detox approach my moldie friends discussed with particular enthusiasm, one that seemed so bizarre and disgusting that I could hardly believe anyone did it, much less that anyone had thought it up in the first place: coffee enemas.

"Oh yeah! Lots of my patients do great with those!" she said, her face brightening. I asked her what on earth a coffee enema does—wouldn't using water be just as good? No, she said. Nobody really knew exactly what they did, but one way or another, it seemed that coffee compounds supercharge the liver. She preferred the theory that the compounds cause the liver to excrete bile, which is the substance the liver puts the toxins into after it pulls them out of the blood. The liver works more efficiently, she said, when it produces more bile. But some people thought that the compounds in coffee increase production of the exceedingly important antioxidant glutathione, which the liver relies on for detoxification. Because mainstream scientists tended to sneer at the idea of coffee enemas, they had barely been studied. In any case, she said, they were very safe, and many of her patients found them to be a lifesaver.

I asked her about testing—couldn't I check and see if I really did have enough toxins in me to be causing problems? Not so easily, she said. For one thing, no one knew what levels were safe, and some people might be more vulnerable than others. Plus, commercial tests weren't available for most toxins, so I'd have to find some research laboratory willing to do it for me, and she didn't know of any. There was a commercial test for mycotoxins, but it was questionable and expensive—$700. Heavy metals were the one thing I could test for at reasonable cost, and while the test couldn't determine total levels, it could at least give some indication of changes over time.

She also pointed out that the results wouldn't affect my treatment. My symptoms were enough to convince her that toxins were part of the issue, and the methods for getting rid of mycotoxins or heavy metals or pesticides were all the same. So beyond curiosity, there wasn't much point. I decided to do the test for heavy metals, but nothing more.

I left Elliott's office warmed but uncertain. I liked her, but she spoke with an awful lot of confidence when I wasn't sure there was a solid scientific basis for her claims. Of course, she had studied the experiences of many patients over many years, and that offered a valuable expertise on a different level. But I worried that her belief in the pernicious effects of toxins was so strong that she would interpret anything as supporting that view.

I ran her suggestions by my moldie group, and they approved. So once again, I swallowed my discomfort and took another step down this path, ordering hundreds of dollars' worth of supplements, buying a used sauna from one of Elliott's patients, and picking up an enema kit at Walgreens. At least none of it sounded dangerous.

One evening when I was feeling draggy and muddled, I brewed up some coffee and pulled out my enema kit. I sat on a towel on the bathroom floor, lubed the tip of the enema bag with oil, and, shuddering, slowly inserted it. I let the coffee stream in slowly, stopping each time my gut cramped its objection to this violation of the ordinary direction of flow. I breathed and twisted, telling my gut that everything was okay, even though neither it nor I were entirely convinced. When the cramping stopped, I reopened the valve.

Once the bag was empty, I lay on the floor, feeling ridiculous, reading the news on my phone and checking the time over and over.

Seven minutes in, I felt a sort of wave pass through me. My brain suddenly felt clearer, my body lighter. *Wow.* I didn't know what had actually happened, but the sensation felt very much like some unpleasant substance had been filtered out of my body—though the suddenness of it was surprising.

After my 15 minutes were up, I moved to the toilet, and, as the Web site I was following so delicately described it, "released" the enema. My nose revolted at the roasty-toasty coffee smell combining with that of shit. But there was no denying that I felt better—much better. *Yet again, my crazy moldie friends had some pretty good advice.*

I settled into a pattern of doing coffee enemas first thing in the morning, since I typically felt muddleheaded and achy when I first woke up. Over and over, I was amazed to find that an enema (or two or three) brought me fully to the world again. *I don't know if this is really detoxifying me, but it sure as hell is doing something remarkable.*

I found this so astonishing that I spent some time looking for scientific papers about it. I found a reference to a study of coffee enemas in rats. *Really? They were injecting coffee up rats' butts?* It turned out that they gave 15 rats suppositories with one of the many compounds that occur in coffee and found that their livers produced more bile afterward. *Okay,* I thought, *but it's tiny, it's in rats, it's not really a coffee enema, and it hasn't been followed up on. Big whoop.* A study of 11 patients with inoperable pancreatic cancer found that a program of coffee enemas along with bazillions of supplements extended their lives dramatically, but a follow-up study by an outside group catastrophically failed to replicate the result. That was pretty much all I found. So the benefits of coffee enemas were certainly scientifically unproven—but then, they were also almost entirely untested.

I encountered emphatic denunciations of coffee enemas from Web sites claiming the mantle of being scientific, like Quackwatch and Science-Based Medicine. The latter said flatly, "Given the lack of benefit and potential harms, there is no plausible justification to undergo these treatments." But when I investigated those harms, I found only about a dozen reports, generally from disapproving doctors. Several were about people who did so many coffee enemas they became dehydrated and electrolyte-depleted; one was about someone who used boiling water (cringe); another managed to puncture his colon (double cringe); a couple used amoeba-infected water; others were people so sick that the problem may or may not have been caused by the enemas at all. The only reports I found disturbing were two in which people acquired colon infections after doing a single enema—but given how many people seemed to be doing them, and how few reports there were of that, I couldn't work up too much alarm.

So basically, science failed to shed any light. And the evidence that the enemas made me personally feel better was extremely strong—though I had no idea whether the mechanism was indeed through detoxification. Over time, my preferred theory was that they somehow reduced inflammation, but with no scientific studies to go on, I was (ahem) talking out of my butt. I could have strengthened the evidence by testing it against a placebo (say, comparing it with a water enema), but with no objective way to measure improvement, it would shed no light on the mechanism. And frankly, I didn't much care. The effect was so profound that even if it was a placebo, that was good enough for me—though if so, I did wish my brain had chosen a more convenient and less embarrassing treatment for its preferred placebo.

The uncertainty took a toll on me, though. Each time I inserted that nozzle into my butt or sweated in a sauna or downed supplements with uncertain efficacy, I felt like I was taking one more step away from the world my science-writer friends lived in, and one step further into this new, warped universe.

I DECIDED THAT IT was important to resist the sense of isolation I felt in pursuing such an odd course of treatment, so I invited friends out to my house to celebrate my spectacular recovery. I figured I'd hold it mostly outside to protect my house from possible contamination, and I asked friends to bring items like serving utensils and chairs that I no longer owned. I dubbed it my "Wake/Baptism Party": We'd celebrate the death of the old me and the birth of the new.

As I prepared for the party, I couldn't help but think of William. We'd held a bunch of parties, and they'd always felt like a ratification of our life and relationship. Now, my house contained little indication that he'd ever been part of my life—nearly everything was lost in the Great Purge. A small, all-metal sculpture we'd gotten together in South Africa was one of the few exceptions. On top of that, William had come to feel bitter about the end of our relationship, and we barely had a friendship anymore.

Tall weeds had sprouted between the flagstones of the patio. I pulled them to tidy up for the party, thinking about how I'd intended to plant creeping thyme there for a good decade. Heck, I'd intended to landscape the whole front yard for more than a decade. Some yellow-flowered chamisa bushes had popped up on their own, but otherwise, the yard was only dirt and weeds. *So much love in this place, and so much brokenness.*

I had invited my ex-husband Geoff to the party, never imagining he'd come all the way from Minneapolis but wanting to include him. To my delight, he came. We hadn't seen each other in five years, and he hadn't been back to the house since shortly after we finished it more than a decade earlier.

When he arrived and I opened the door, it was hard to recognize the lithe and graceful young man I'd known. I immediately knew what had happened: The medication he relied on to keep hold of his mind had brought weight gain. His belly jutted forward farther than his frame seemed designed to accommodate, his upper eyelids had grown sleepy-looking, and his hair was pulled into a thin, graying ponytail. We'd once been a matched set, with long, thick blond hair, squinty eyes, and heavy eyebrows. I almost had to look away: I felt as though my own body were being stretched and aged.

But when he said hello, his voice snapped him into the person I knew. He hugged me, and although we fit together differently than we had before, he smelled the same.

I showed him around, studying his face to figure out how he felt, being there for the first time in a decade. *He's brave to come,* I thought. Did he get a twinge, seeing the huge, empty bookshelf his math library had lived on? I couldn't tell. He commented on the mud plaster on the range hood, which had been a plywood box when he'd last seen it, and he stopped in the stairwell, smiling at his sister's bas relief of our two long-dead dogs. As we walked around, I felt as though we were shadowed by the ghosts of our younger selves, watching us and grieving.

A couple dozen friends came over the course of the afternoon, sitting under a shade tent on my patio. I watched Geoff's face as he chatted, and for all the changes, I saw the same compassion and kindness I had loved in him years ago shining through. And I picked up on no bitterness from him that I was living in this house we'd both invested so much in, just pleasure that I was back in it. *I chose a good man, all those years ago.*

He hadn't been in a relationship since we'd broken up, and I felt a pulse of longing that he find someone to love, someone to be loved by. I thought of him lying alone night after night, year after year, when he'd been such a skillful and tender lover to me. I didn't want to be the one lying beside him, but I wished someone were there.

I told my friends my stories about how astonishingly ill I had been and how astonishingly I had recovered, and they all seemed to accept them with undoubting delight. I felt myself managing to weave my strange experiences back into ordinary existence. The conversation rolled through a variety of rich topics, the sun warmed the back of my neck, the birds chirped, the cicadas buzzed, the stream burbled, and I felt as though I were expanding beyond the limits of my body, into the house, the land, the community.

I had a sudden urge to reach out and take Geoff's hand. When I noticed, I felt a burst of shock, the same feeling I'd had as a small child when I'd reached up toward my mom's hand, only to realize that the leg next to me led not to my mom but to a stranger. The urge I was feeling, I knew, was arising from how I was wired to share my expansiveness and pleasure with a partner. Since Geoff had once been that partner, the feeling naturally and mistakenly flowed toward him. I put my hands in my lap.

This pleasure is for me alone, I thought. *This is what it feels like to throw a party all by myself. Perhaps someday I'll share my life with a partner again, but for right now, this is good. It is enough.*

PART 4

EMERGENCE

CHAPTER 17

CONNECTION

Even though I felt more comfortable being alone than I ever had before, I thought it'd be fun to date a little bit. Nothing serious—my bizarre task of learning to avoid mold left little room for that. But I liked the idea of meeting some new people, maybe going for some hikes, pushing the edges of my little moldie world.

I wrote up a profile on OkCupid, briefly describing my illness and dramatic improvement and commenting that "I feel, quite literally, like I've been reborn." I said that the experience had brought me "a deep acceptance of the world and appreciation for it, and a quiet joy at being alive that is independent of whether I get what I want." I felt a little funny "selling" myself by talking about my illness, but not doing so felt misleading. *And heck, it's got to be more interesting than saying I like romantic candlelit dinners.*

I was pleasantly surprised to meet several interesting guys and no creeps—but no romantic prospects either. I quickly ran through OkCupid's small pool of men in Santa Fe, so I searched Boulder. *A weekend fling with some Colorado mountain man could be fun! Maybe in a nice, mold-free tent . . .*

One profile caught my eye, for a man who was a runner, poet, hiker, admirer of Jung, and cook. "I know that I'm responsible for my happiness," he wrote, "and that I have to know what I need and ask for it." The words sent a wave of relaxation through me. He was striking too, with silver hair and blazing blue eyes, looking at home in the Rocky Mountain wilderness.

Soon, we were exchanging long e-mail messages. John had lived in rural New Mexico for five years, had run hundred-mile races, wrote for a living, and practiced Sufism. The latter brought up images in my mind of black-bearded men in long robes whirling ecstatically, but he said his version of it was quiet and internal. "I'm probably most attracted to Sufism because the answers are within, the teacher is within, grace is key, and love is the greatest power. It is also not about gaining anything, but losing everything—an experience I know you have tasted." I laughed, looking around at my empty house. *I'll bet Sufis don't usually mean that so literally!*

His e-mail went on: "I feel a steady presence of love in my life, a love beyond me but in me. I try to stay aligned to that every waking moment, remember it is there, feel it through my breath, and in my heart." I thought of the spaciousness that had bloomed in me in Death Valley. *I died out there in the desert. This is all extra, an unearned gift.* I felt it within me just as strongly now—through my breath, and in my heart, as John had written. I cradled an emptiness at my core.

Four days after I first saw his profile, we talked on the phone for nearly two hours. At the end of the call, he said, "I thought about it before I called, and the only time I could come down to Santa Fe in the next three weeks is . . . right now. Could I stay with you tonight?"

My mind fluttered. *Is that safe? Will I be able to get rid of him if I don't like him? Will he contaminate my house? Will he assume I'm going to have sex with him? But . . . do I really want to wait three weeks to meet him?*

"Um, uh, yeah, I guess so," I said, and then paused. "But you'll have to bring a sleeping bag, because I don't have any beds."

He arrived at 11:30 that night. I ushered him straight to the shower—before he came, I'd warned him that would be necessary and asked him to bring unworn clothes to change into. I wished I had clothes I knew were uncontaminated on hand for him, but I didn't think my clothes would fit him. I just had to hope his house and clothes weren't moldy.

We talked into the wee hours of the morning. He told me about growing up in suburban Denver in an upwardly mobile but inwardly hollow family; I told him about being an only child with seven siblings. I studied the curve of his eyebrows, the veins on his hands, the laugh lines around his eyes. I liked him—but I also felt as if my immune system had expanded beyond my body and was on alert against an intruder into my house.

By the time he ran his fingers through my hair and pressed his lips to mine, though, my only thought was, *Soft.*

When we finally went to bed, he unrolled his sleeping bag next to mine. I wondered if I'd be able to sleep—I'd grown uncivilized, waking and sleeping at random hours, cuddling with Frances or flopping about— but when he wrapped his arms around me, my body relaxed, the way it had when I'd read his words about being responsible for his own happiness. I slept, and when I awoke, my apprehensiveness had vanished. My immune system, it seemed, had accepted him.

I was exhausted after so little sleep. After breakfast, John suggested that I nap, using his lap as a pillow while he read on the couch. When I awoke, he massaged my back and shoulders, moving up to the bare skin on my neck. A shiver traveled from my skin through the core of my body. I sat up to kiss him.

Then I suggested we go upstairs. I eyed the camping pads with an internal groan. I'd gotten used to sleeping on mine, but for this purpose . . . I had bought a futon recently, hoping to move up in the world from my camping pad, but over the week I'd slept on it, I'd felt worse and worse and had given it up as moldy. *But surely the futon can't do much to me in just an hour or so . . .*

I pulled John onto it with me, and the exuberance I'd been feeling about life as a whole flowed right into lovemaking. As his body fit with mine, a circuit seemed to snap closed, allowing a flow of energy far bigger than us to travel through us and beyond. *And I thought being alive was good when I was all alone in Death Valley!* Afterward, I lay with my head on his shoulder as he stroked my hair, feeling as though every cell in my body had settled into its right place.

But then the feeling shifted, something within subtly not right. *Ugh, this futon.* I had warned John that the futon might cause me problems, so

I knew he wouldn't be completely shocked if I limped on my way to the shower. *But man, what a way to impress a new lover!*

John pulled away slightly and looked at me. "We need to get you off this futon," he declared. *How did he figure that out?*

I nodded and then groaned as I got up and staggered a bit, feeling lightheaded and weak. *I hope this isn't a response to making love!* I got to the bathroom counter and braced myself on it while John stroked my back. My head swam and I sagged further, ending up in a fetal position on the floor.

John kept stroking. "How can I help?" he asked. His voice was calm and steady.

"I'll be okay once I shower," I whispered. "I just have to get up the oomph to get there." A couple of minutes later, he helped me into the shower, and once again, strength flowed back into me shockingly fast as the water flowed over me.

John hauled the futon outside for me, took a shower himself, joined me on the camping pads, and made love to me again. Afterward, we hiked up the stream together. *Guess it wasn't the lovemaking that did me in!* I thought as I capered up the trail. The trail was too narrow to walk side by side, but we held hands when we could. Each time we paused to admire something, we ended up embracing, and his scent mingled with the familiar oak and pine and earth smells. John goggled at the trees and the stream. He squeezed my hand. "This feels . . . enchanted."

AFTER JOHN LEFT, I went to a craft store and bought some Sculpey clay. He had invited me to his birthday party in Boulder a few days later, and I had an idea for a birthday present, inspired by a story of his that had impressed me.

He'd grown up as a fat kid, he'd told me, and some bit of him that felt unworthy was whispering that I'd reject him. Even having run hundred-mile races through the Colorado high country and knowing that it would take a fine scalpel to scrape any lard off his frame, the fat kid still dominated his own self-image.

His childhood weight had been all the more agonizing because it came with a mind-fuck: His mom, who had her own food issues, would give him a Metrecal diet shake instead of dinner and then bake a cake he wasn't allowed to eat—but, bright-eyed, she'd offer him a mixing bowl with icing to lick.

When he was in eighth grade, he came up with a plan to wriggle out of this emotional trap: He joined the wrestling team. "Sorry, gotta make weight tomorrow!" he'd say, pushing away his plate. He not only lost weight, he found his power. He started getting good grades, gained friends, and became downright skinny. *Wow, that kid had strength!* I thought. *Way to outmaneuver your parents.*

I had the idea of sculpting a model of John as a fat kid as a symbol of my embrace of the child inside the man. I asked him for pictures of himself as a little boy, and then I sculpted him with chubby cheeks and blue eyes, wearing a shirt with huge polka dots like in one of the pictures. Squeezing the clay, I felt like a kid in art class, as though childhood-me had come back to life to make a gift for childhood-John.

I found myself almost purring as our 19 hours together and our twice-a-day Skype calls rolled through my mind. I kept pondering one particularly amazing thing he'd said: "Even if your health doesn't get better than this, that's okay with me." *Could that really be true?* I thought. *Feeling that way now doesn't mean he'd feel that way if it happened. Regardless, it sure is an amazing thing to say.* I shaped a clay ear as I pondered. *But let's not find out if his statement holds up. I'll get better instead.*

I drove up to Boulder for his party, bringing my sleeping bag and tent with me so I could camp out in his backyard if his house didn't work for me. My moldie friends had warned me that I might encounter "mold plumes" as I drove and advised me to put all my belongings in my car in plastic bags just in case. "That's ridiculous" flicked through my mind, but it was no more than a flick by now. *In for a penny, in for a pound.* Anyway, it wasn't much of an imposition: I had no suitcases, so I would have used trash bags even without the threat of mold plumes.

Fortunately, the precaution seemed unnecessary—I felt fine the whole drive. John greeted me with a dozen red roses and a hug and kiss so huge that I ended up giggling. When I walked into his house, my senses were bristling. *Seems okay, I think. I hope.*

Later in the evening, I pulled out his birthday present. As he unwrapped it, I suddenly felt so nervous that I wanted to grab the box, stuff it under my shirt, and pretend I'd never mentioned it. *Why didn't it occur to me what a bad idea this was? He could think it's ridiculous!*

As he pulled the sculpture out of the box, I started babbling against my will. "It's you as a fat kid. See his chubby cheeks? I'm not much of an artist or anything, but I don't know, I just . . . I kind of just wanted to reach back in time and let that kid know that I'm waiting for him."

John kissed me, looked again at the sculpture, looked at me. He had tears in his eyes.

I WOKE UP the next morning feeling awful. Moving my legs in bed was hard.

My mind spun: *I've been so stupid! Why didn't I sleep outside like I'd planned?* John had been willing but hesitant—his house was a duplex and he worried about his neighbor's reaction. *He would have agreed if you'd pushed for it. You didn't take care of yourself the way you should have, Julie.*

Even worse, I'd brought all my clothes into the house, so I had no uncontaminated clothes to put on. And his birthday party was that day. I was going to meet a bunch of John's friends, along with his dad. *Shit. Shit, shit, shit.*

I tried to calm down and strategize. *A step at a time, Julie.* It wasn't clear that the problem was John's house, I realized. I'd eaten dinner on my way at a place with an outside patio, but I'd had to walk through the building, and it had been moldy. I hadn't been able to shower for some hours afterward. So maybe my clothes weren't all contaminated from John's house, and maybe I'd recover just fine.

Regardless, I needed to deal with the immediate situation, which meant taking a shower and doing detox. But doing a bunch of bizarre things under the eye of a guy I was falling for but still didn't know all that well . . . *Ugh.*

I braced myself, fessed up to John about how awful I was feeling, and ran through my theories about what was going on. I told him I'd probably stagger as I got to the shower and that I'd need to do at least one coffee enema. I spoke in even, matter-of-fact tones to cover up my embarrassment. Then I admitted that I was scared, that I may have really screwed up and didn't know what it would take for me to recover. John listened calmly. If he was shocked to see my slow, painful movements to the shower, he didn't show it. He just asked if he could make me some coffee.

The shower and enemas brought me back pretty much fully. *Thank god, thank god, thank god.*

I put on the only pretty dress I owned, and John's friends greeted me with such enthusiasm that I knew he must have been telling them all about me. John showed off the little sculpture I'd made him. His face was shining all afternoon, and I was struck by how much his friends seemed to love him. *Just like I'm starting to do.*

Over the next couple of days, I persuaded myself that his house was reasonably okay for me. Not only that, but his car was fine too—amazing, since the half-dozen used cars I'd tried had all crippled me.

The mold gods, it seemed, were blessing our union.

A FEW DAYS AFTER I returned from Boulder, John came down to spend nine days in Santa Fe with me. He'd already scheduled time off from work to go to a workshop, and he canceled it to spend the week with me.

"Fruit trees!" John cried, when I mentioned that I wanted some but hadn't gotten around to landscaping my house. "Let's plant them while I'm here!" As he dug the holes for them a couple of days later, I laughed to myself. *This guy plans to stick around!*

We took a half-day hike off trail through the hills around my house, going places I hadn't gone in close to a decade. He gave me tips on my running form. We left stores and restaurants over and over when I declared them moldy. We soaked at a Japanese spa. We climbed together at a rock-climbing gym.

I felt as though there had been a John-shaped hole in my life, and I hadn't even known it.

As John packed to go back to Boulder, I told him, teasing, "I just had the crazy idea that I could hop in the car and go with you."

John said, not teasing, "You should!"

So I did.

WE HAD ONE CHALLENGE we had to work out, though: John had a cat and I had a dog. Frances was very excited about Lao and wanted to be friends, and she had clear ideas about how to do it: "I'll chase you and it'll be fun!" Lao, an affectionate, feisty gray tabby with strong opinions, clearly considered this behavior ghastly.

The first time I brought Frances to John's house, I closed Lao in a bedroom first. Frances immediately bashed the door in—I apparently hadn't gotten it properly latched—and chased poor Lao under the bed. As I hauled a scrabbling, yipping Frances away from the bed, I thought, *Oh my god, John is going to think my dog is a monster.*

In fact, though, John was both confident in Lao's ability to defend himself and eager to collaborate on training Frances. We bought a baby gate to put across the stairs to give Lao a safe zone upstairs. Several times a day, Frances and I would stand at the bottom of the stairs and then John would appear at the top with Lao in his arms. Instantly, I would start cramming bits of cheese in Frances's mouth. Frances had only one duty, to eat the cheese.

Whenever I wandered toward the bottom of the stairs, Frances would trot over with a wagging tail, making her verdict clear: "This is an *awesome* game!"

After many repetitions, I threw in a twist. When Lao and John appeared, I waited. Frances twisted her head my way: "Hey, where's my cheese?" Instantly, I commenced cheese-cramming.

That tiny moment was the beginning of victory. We had created a new neural pathway. Rather than *cat* being instantly linked to *chase!* and then to a brain explosion, it was now linked to a new idea, *cheese!*, which was in turn linked to me.

From there, John and I designed a thousand variations. I made Frances wait a bit longer before getting her cheese. I asked her to sit first, or lie down, or shake, or stay and then come. John brought Lao closer. I held Frances in my lap and John set Lao down downstairs. We tied Frances up outside and let Lao use his cat door to go out. We brought Lao to Santa Fe for the first time—by then, we'd begun splitting our time between the two towns—and we started the whole process from scratch in the new location.

Eventually, Frances learned to use the cheese to modulate her own excitement. She would watch Lao, her intensity growing, and just before she lost it and lunged at him, she'd turn to me for cheese, calming down as she licked it from my fingers. When she did especially well, she'd prance toward me with head high, as if saying, "Look at me, I'm so good! Cheese, please!"

Lao apparently held out hope for Frances's redemption despite her appalling conduct, and he initiated his own training program as well. He would come partway down the stairs to observe Frances, to her fascination and delight. As long as she was reasonably calm, he stayed, studying her. But as soon as she started jumping or barking, he split. Some time later, when she had calmed down, he'd appear again. Mellowness, she learned, was the only way to keep him around.

Each step of progress—*Look, Frances saw Lao through the screen door and didn't freak out! Lao got within five feet of Frances while she was tied up!*—felt to John and me like a ratification of our relationship.

We also celebrated my physical progress. After more than a year of being stuck in bed much of the time, I thought my muscles would have withered into dental floss, but my ability to run came back astonishingly fast. Week by week, I could run further, climb higher, go faster.

At the end of the summer, John ran a 50-kilometer race in Silverton, most of it above 10,000 feet. After he'd been running five hours, I started from the end and ran the course in reverse until I met up with him. I ended up running a total of nearly eight miles, and I even managed to keep up with John to the finish. *Just make John run five hours more than I do and we're kind of equal!* I started dreaming of running a half-marathon.

AT THE SAME TIME, I was reacting to mold more strongly and bizarrely, so much so that I could hardly believe my own experiences. I picked John up at the airport after he had traveled to Berkeley, and to protect myself against Berkeley "ick," I brought him fresh clothes to change into in the airport and a trash bag to enclose his suitcase. My precautions only went so far—I sure as heck wasn't going to keep from hugging him when he first arrived, and he couldn't shower before changing his clothes—but any exposure would be far too minuscule to matter, I figured.

About 10 minutes from home, I could feel the paralysis starting in my lower back. I was also unreasonably hungry, and a strange, foreign crankiness had invaded my delight at having John home. Both unreasonable hunger and unreasonable crankiness, I'd learned, were signs of exposure.

We arrived home and John stripped his clothes outside as I gimped into the house, going up the stairs on hands and feet. John came up from behind me, scooped me up, and deposited me straight into the shower as I giggled.

The shower restored me as usual, but my worries didn't end there. We had to decontaminate his stuff, and, I now realized, even absurdly tiny amounts of it mattered. Plus, from what I'd heard, "ick" was far harder to get rid of than ordinary mold and spread more easily to other objects. My moldie friends had told preposterous stories about cross contamination—one said she had to move out of her house after a pair of shoes contaminated the whole thing.

We washed John's clothes at a friend's house and then hung them outside to dry in the sun. A day later, I tested his jeans by draping them over my face for 10 minutes—and then I couldn't walk. As far as I could tell, that never happened anymore unless I'd just been exposed to something bad. *But how much mold, or ick, or whatever, could possibly be on his jeans after they've been washed? This just seems crazy!* But it was hard for me to argue with my body's responses.

I hadn't worried too much about that bizarre story about the shoes until now: *Could one trip to Berkeley ruin my house for me forever?* I tried to reason with myself to keep my anxiety from running wild, reminding myself that John had visited Berkeley many times before we met without taking any precautions, and I was able to tolerate his house. So it must be that whatever bothered me dissipated over time. *Don't go borrowing trouble, Julie.*

Another wash, a few more days in the sun, and John's clothes felt fine to me. I felt some of the tension drain from my body. *Maybe I won't have to dive quite that deep into the craziness of the moldie world.*

Despite my extreme caution, I felt like I careened from one hit to the next like a pinball. I seemed to be especially susceptible to any exposure while I slept. John and I bought a bed together, and while sleeping in it felt like an unimaginable luxury, over the next few days, I found myself feeling less good. I generated a bunch of hypotheses about what might be going wrong, but day by day, I felt worse.

When I got crippled after a short nap on the bed, the verdict seemed clear: The bed was doing me in. My reactions, it seemed, got stronger and faster as an exposure was repeated.

At that point, I moved back to the camping pads and immediately improved—but not completely. *What's the problem now?* I guessed that perhaps the pillows had gotten contaminated by their extended period on the bed, so the next night, I used a freshly washed, folded towel for a pillow. I woke up feeling fine. Later that day, I tested my pillow theory by holding one to my face, and I felt myself deteriorating. *I guess I figured it out right.* I washed the pillows, retested them, and concluded all was okay.

That episode passed, but later, I woke up in the middle of the night paralyzed again and had to sleuth out the problem. If one of us went into town and simply sat briefly on the bed, that was enough to do me in. Even setting a backpack that had been through a contaminated building onto the bed briefly was enough. Once, Frances went to doggy daycare, and although the building was all concrete and felt fine to me, I reacted to the bed after she'd been on it. I figured that she might have played with a dog from a moldy house and picked it up on her coat.

John and I developed a routine: I'd wake him when I woke up feeling poisoned, and he'd help me to the shower. Then he'd pull the sheets off and go shower while I, freshly decontaminated, would put new sheets on. Then back to bed, fingers crossed that we'd exorcised the mold demon. Usually it worked, but on unlucky nights, I awoke paralyzed again, and we had to come up with a new theory: The pillows were contaminated, or perhaps it was the comforter underneath its cover. We repeated the whole routine of shower and sheets, taking one more step of replacing the pillow with a towel or using a different comforter. Eventually, I slept.

I wouldn't have sworn that all the stories I concocted to explain these middle-of-the-night adventures were true. After all, I came up with theory after theory until the problem went away. Perhaps I felt better only because the Greek gods had smiled upon me, and I took that as evidence for whatever theory happened to be in play at that moment.

But that skepticism couldn't carry me far enough to dismiss the overarching idea that some kind of contamination was sickening me.

Every time I woke up feeling poorly in the night and ignored it, hoping I'd be okay, I only felt worse. Every time I took a shower, I felt dramatically better. When I ignored a clue—say, I forgot and put my backpack on the bed, and I didn't change the sheets because really, how the hell could that cause a problem?—I paid the price.

I watched for inconsistencies that might reveal cracks in my stories, but I didn't find any revealing flaws. I shopped in Trader Joe's several times, each time hoping it wouldn't bother me, and each time I had to flee without getting groceries. I went to the Department of Motor Vehicles in Boulder to renew John's registration and stayed after it started feeling bad to me because I was determined to finish the errand. I got paralyzed, and only afterward did I remember that a fellow moldie in Boulder had warned me about it—I'd forgotten, figuring I wouldn't have reason to go there anyway. Often, when I found that a part of a friend's house bothered me, the friend would say, "Oh, yeah, we did have a roof leak there . . ." A friend who was shocked that her house bothered me discovered mold throughout her roof insulation a few months later.

The evidence that something environmental was doing me in was so strong that I couldn't seriously doubt it—but I constantly prodded at the boundaries of my knowledge. Certainly, something in water-damaged buildings was bad for me, but it could have been mold itself, or the toxins molds produce, or bacteria or particulates or volatile organic compounds or who-knows-what. And who the hell knew what ick was, if it even existed. Given how good I felt when I felt good, avoiding anything that seemed to bother me was clearly the right path. But still, I struggled with how implausible it all seemed.

I felt a little better about it some time later when I talked to someone who had worked in a "clean room" manufacturing computer chips. As he described the endless precautions—HEPA filter ceiling tiles, fans that pull air through the ceiling tiles down through a raised floor and outside, Gore-Tex suits and double layers of gloves and on and on and on—I had an urge to move into one. Then he described how at one point, the quality of the chips deteriorated despite all this. They determined that the chips were contaminated with minute quantities of boron—which was bizarre, since they didn't use boron in their entire manufacturing process. They eventually traced it to one of the workers, who was washing her new baby's diapers with boron (but not her own clothes). The boron had found its way onto her clothes, through all her protective gear, past the elaborate filtration system, and onto the chips. The sleuthing process he described sounded so familiar that I didn't feel quite as crazy.

One morning during a bad period of middle-of-the-night poisonings, I asked John if he ever wondered if the whole theory was a bunch of hooey. He certainly never expressed anything along those lines to me, but really, how could he not? I certainly did!

"That's not important," John said. "All that matters is how you feel."

I pushed further—but what if my explanation for how I felt was all a nasty fantasy I'd been beguiled by?

"I made the decision from the beginning to never question it," he said. "It just would make it more complicated and harder for both of us. If it's true and I doubt you, I'm going to make it harder on you. And if it's not true, well, you believe it is. Either way, I'm going to have to do the same thing, which is to change the sheets and take a shower. And ultimately, when you don't feel good, and you have an idea about what might make you feel better, why not do it?"

For him, that was that. Along with countless showers and endless laundry, he helped me get to the bathroom, left buildings on my say-so, rubbed my back, made me coffee, cooked me meals, reassured me when I got discouraged. "What can I do to make your life more wonderful?" he'd ask.

While he left it to me to figure out when my theories were right and wrong, he sometimes sleuthed out problems that eluded me. Driving to a friend's house for dinner, I found myself deteriorating so fast that by the time I realized there was a problem, I could hardly hold my torso up and couldn't speak at all. My thoughts moved so slowly they were barely decipherable, like a 78 rpm record played at 33.

John asked if I was okay, and when I didn't respond, he pulled over. "Take that sweater off!" he barked. I had borrowed it from him, and he realized he hadn't washed it in ages. When I could barely move my arms, he pulled it off me.

I instantly improved, enough so that I could hold my torso up and talk and think. I staggered into the shower at our friend's house, and then we had dinner as planned.

That experience left me haunted by a nightmare of being out alone, going into a badly moldy building, getting paralyzed and unable to speak, and being taken to a hospital that turned out to be moldy. What would happen if I didn't get away from mold? Would anyone be able to figure out that they should contact John?

I ended up getting a medical ID bracelet that said:

SEVERE MOLD ALLERGY
GET ME TO FRESH AIR
RINSE BODY AND HAIR
CALL JOHN: XXX-XXX-XXXX

Anytime I went into town without John, I made sure I had it on.

Standing in line at the grocery store on my own one day, the bracelet caught my eye, a black nylon strap against my wrist with an etched metal plate. I read and reread the last line: "CALL JOHN."

Call John, I thought. *If something happens to me, call John.*

I wasn't alone anymore.

CHAPTER 18

THE DEVIL DISEASE

We were only a few weeks into our relationship when John first asked: "I'd like to take you to Tasmania. Will you go with me?" He was already planning a trip himself—his dad had gotten remarried to a Tasmanian woman, and they split their time between Tasmania and Denver. Now that I was in John's life, he wanted it to be our first trip together.

When I confused Tasmania with Tanzania, John had to explain to me that Tasmania was an island state off the southern end of Australia, very far from Tanzania, a country in east Africa. He showed me pictures from his previous trip to Tasmania. Some showed white sand beaches edging aquamarine water that looked like the Caribbean; others showed neon-green, grassy hillsides that looked like Ireland; and others showed impenetrable, fern-filled bush that looked like Middle-earth. Instead of deer and squirrels and coyotes, it had wallabies and Tasmanian devils and potoroos. To me, it sounded only a small notch less exotic than Timbuktu.

So I desperately wanted to say, "YES! Duh." I had just one wee concern: Flying to Tasmania might kill me.

What if the plane was moldy? What if I couldn't tolerate his dad and stepmom's house? What if the outside air was filled with the dreaded "ick"? What if I was sick the whole time, while trying to make a good impression on John's folks? Also, as crazy as I was about John, I'd only met him weeks before—was it really wise for us to be planning international travel together, months away?

So I made a vague grunt into which I tried to pack interest and openness with a sprinkling of uncertainty and doubt.

Every few weeks, John brought it up again. When I responded with my various worries, he started brainstorming energetically. If the plane was moldy, I could use my respirator, he suggested. His stepmom's house was just above a beach where they set up a campsite—if the house was moldy, I could sleep there. If I was sick while we were there, well, then I was sick: He wanted me with him, sick or well, he said.

His enthusiasm was contagious. I read on my moldie list about a carbon blanket that acted a bit like a magic shield, trapping all manner of crap in the air, and John bought me one and got a beautiful cover made for it. We started looking into flights that avoided airports with terrible reputations among moldies. Together, we came up with (and giggled over) the idea that we could bring strap-on roller skates with us, so that if I got paralyzed, John could push me to safety.

Carrying that latter idea out turned out to be complicated, because we discovered that no one manufactured adult-size strap-on roller skates anymore. I did manage to find a version that went under your heels only, and you were supposed to lift your toes to scoot forward, spinning groovy, flashing, multicolored lights. I bought a pair to try out. I strapped them on at a moment when I was crippled, and as soon as I stood up, both legs swept out from underneath me, my ass careening toward the floor. John caught me inches above the ground, and then we laughed until we cried. We gave up on that approach and tracked down some antique metal clunkers on eBay.

Part of me still thought it was insane to fly to the other side of the world when I was barely keeping myself functional while living a tiny life, avoiding unknown buildings whenever possible. Just going into a random Starbucks was a game of Russian roulette. My entire life was organized around my body's needs, and I still wasn't even well enough consistently to do much in the way of work. But John swept me up in his enthusiasm so much that I couldn't imagine saying no, especially as he proved himself so capable of handling the disasters that were an ordinary part of my life.

John's the one who will have to pick up the pieces if I fall apart. If he's up for it, why shouldn't I be?

The trip started seeming more plausible to me in the early fall, when I achieved enough stability that I could start working again. I revived my math column for *Science News,* and I found it utterly soothing to talk to a game theorist about his advice to climate negotiators or to an economist about the problems with Medicare's auction for durable medical goods. Massaging words on a page was like massaging balm into my soul. *There is nothing, nothing in the world as grounding as simply doing my work.*

That got me thinking about how awesome it would be to report a big feature story while we were in Tasmania. When William and I had gone to Peru a few years earlier, I'd had a ball writing two little stories from the trip, talking to researchers and getting an insider's view of the country.

But now I had grander visions of a long, deep, narrative feature article. I found a story I was excited to write about: Over the previous several years, scientists had come to realize that a newly discovered contagious cancer might wipe out Tasmanian devils entirely—and, because devils play such a key role in the ecosystem, a whole raft of other species could disappear along with them. I chose *Discover* to pitch the story to, because a friend of mine was an editor there, and I knew she'd be sympathetic if my health gave me trouble. They bought the story. *Woohoo! I'm going to Tasmania! To write a story on assignment!*

A COUPLE WEEKS BEFORE we left for Australia, I started reacting to the carpet in the bedroom of John's house in Boulder, where we were spending half our time. We retreated to sleeping on camping pads in the living room and tried every trick I could think of to fix the bedroom—ozonating, sprinkling the carpet with baking soda and vacuuming, steam cleaning. But my reactions only grew more intense. When I carried some clothes that had been on the carpet to the washing machine, my face started frowning involuntarily, the corners of my lips pulling down into a bizarre grimace. I felt like calling out, *Hey! Who's frowning my face? Cut it out!*

I knew the only solution was to get the hell away from whatever was doing this to me, and soon we returned to Santa Fe. But even there, I found little respite. John had previously brought down one of his beautiful oriental rugs, which had once sat on the carpet. Though I'd had no trouble with it before, now just walking past it crippled me. Even worse, Lao and Frances both liked to lie on that carpet and had spread the contamination around the house, including to the couch and, worst of all, the bed. I took shower after shower, only to get whacked almost immediately after emerging. I huddled in the bathtub, the only place I felt safe.

We threw everything we possibly could into the new washing machine I had bought, including the couch cushion covers. But I found myself reacting even to freshly washed items. I wanted to cry. *My brand new washing machine is contaminated!* Other moldies had reported that could happen. We threw borax and vinegar and every other decontaminant we could think of in the machine, ran it on its self-clean cycle, and crossed our fingers. Then we ran a test load and I draped a T-shirt from it across my face, breathing through it for 10 minutes, waiting for my nervous system to freak out. Thankfully, I was okay.

Even that didn't end the nightmare: I ended up mysteriously crippled again. I was near despair, but John figured out that we'd mixed up some contaminated clothes with some freshly washed ones. We began scouring the house for unexploded ordnance, washing anything conceivably contaminated or that had touched anything conceivably contaminated.

Eventually, I was okay again—but rattled. *Seriously? I'm this vulnerable, and I'm going to fly to Australia? Am I nuts?*

DESPITE MY WORRIES, we headed to the Denver airport on November 14, 2012, on our way to Tasmania. Just walking through the airport felt transgressive. Ever since I'd gone to Death Valley nine months before, unknown buildings had been landmine-studded fields for me, to be stepped through with utmost care. *But here I am, walking through the airport tra la la la like a normal person!*

Well, truth be told, not quite like a normal person—I had my carbon blanket wrapped around me, and I had a backpack filled with a respirator, a carbon mask, roller skates, two fresh shirts, and two fresh baseball caps. Still, it was normal enough to blow my mind.

I walked onto the plane with my Spidey sense on alert, but all seemed to be fine. I made it through the Los Angeles airport without problems.

The next step was the scary one: boarding a 737 for a 16-hour ride, with no exit available. *Seems okay. I think it's okay. Is it really okay?* It really was okay.

The Melbourne airport was fine too, though I felt freakish, wrapped in my carbon blanket in full Australian summer. I was fine through the next hour-and-a-half flight to Hobart, and then in John's dad's car. It felt like a miracle.

Just before I faded off to sleep in the car, John's stepmom, Sue, pointed to a dark hump in the road. "That's a Tasmanian devil," she said. "Roadkill. They get hit all the time. They're scavengers, so they come out onto the roads at night to eat other roadkill, and then the next car takes them out." We veered around the small, furry shape, about the size of a beagle.

"They haven't become less common, with this cancer?" I asked.

"Not yet," Sue said. "They're rare in the northeast corner of the island, but here, they're everywhere. You can hear them sometimes fighting during the night, screaming and growling at one another and biting each other on the face. Quite a ruckus they make! That's how they got their scary name. Farmers hate them! They eat their lambs and chooks." "Chook," I learned, was the Australian word for chicken.

When we arrived at Sue and Jack's house, I walked in nervously—but all seemed fine. Even the mattress was okay for me. In 32 hours of traveling, I'd had nary a problem. *The mold gods are truly smiling upon me.*

TASMANIA WAS A FAIRY-TALE kind of place. Jack and Sue's charming old cottage perched on a grassy hill that sloped down to a bay, with sparkling water on two sides. Sheep wandered through, keeping the grass trimmed. Jack spent his days digging in his garden, sipping gin and tonics on the porch with Sue at happy hour, dropping in on friends nearby.

Life moved slowly and amiably—which drove me mildly crazy. I wasn't interested in a relaxing holiday. I'd had quite enough not-working over the last couple of years—I wanted to work! So between games of horseshoes and strolls to the beach, I snuck off to my computer to do my reporting.

I'd arranged to do most of my interviews outside, but I didn't have that luxury for my first one with Menna Jones, a wildlife biologist at the University of Tasmania. She told me that her effort to save the devils now kept her mostly apart from them, supervising students and talking to state administrators rather than being in the field herself. I tried to imagine what I'd say if I couldn't tolerate her office, but I couldn't come up with anything that didn't sound crazy. So I decided to just hope for the best and deal with whatever happened when the time came.

I stepped into her office anxiously—and it was fine.

Jones smiled at me from across her desk, a warm but harried woman with a bush of hair so thick it wouldn't have surprised me if a bird had come flying out of it. She described how she'd spent a decade hiking through the Tasmanian bush, trapping devils, working out their mating patterns. Then in 2001, a devil showed up in her trap with a hideous tumor on its face. She showed me a picture of it: A mass obliterated his right eye and erupted into an oozing, red-and-black cauliflower across his cheek, and another swelling deformed his left cheek into a deceptive chipmunk-chubbiness. I gasped, but she said that she didn't think much of it at the time—scientists have to grow a thick skin regarding such horrors.

But then two more devils appeared with similar masses. Over the next months, she watched the disease march down the peninsula she was studying. When she returned to the initial spot a year later, she caught a quarter as many devils as she normally did, and a third of those had masses eating their faces.

Somehow, it seemed, cancer had become contagious.

Soon, another researcher figured out that the cancer cells from all these different devils were genetically identical. All the cancers in all the different devils had come from a single unlucky female devil who had died of the disease a couple of decades earlier. Somehow, her cancer cells had learned how to elude the immune systems in other devils. It had become a parasite.

Jones watched the devil population fall by 50 percent a year once the disease arrived in an area. And she realized that far more was at stake than just Tasmania's iconic animal: If devils vanished, other animals would fill their ecological niche—especially foxes and cats, which had been imported onto the island. And foxes and cats would wipe out a panoply of species found nowhere else, like the eastern barred bandicoot, the Tasmanian pademelon, the eastern quoll, the long-nosed potoroo, and the eastern bettong. The names of these species all sounded to me like they'd come from a children's fantasy novel.

When Jones described the state's effort to save the devils, I felt a pang of envy. Tasmania was spending many millions every year to fund microbiology research that might lead to a vaccine, field research to understand how the disease was spreading, captive breeding programs to preserve the genetic diversity of the species, on and on and on. If the CDC had responded as forcefully to the outbreak of ME/CFS in the '80s, would I be all alone in dealing with this damn illness? I wondered how much the Tasmanian devils were helped by the vulnerability of those potoroos and bandicoots and bettongs—no one outside the ME/CFS community seemed to feel much threatened by the disease, thanks in part to all the psychobabbling research suggesting we were just crazy people. Maybe what we needed was a Looney Toons character based on us, like the ferocious, whirling Taz. Taz might have few similarities to real devils, but he'd certainly created worldwide awareness of them.

A FEW DAYS LATER, John and I flew to the mainland to see one of the efforts to prevent this marsupial apocalypse: Devil Ark, a park where they were breeding devils in captivity to create an "insurance population" that would guarantee the species wouldn't go extinct. Someday, if wild devils were wiped out completely, the disease would vanish with them—and these captive animals could repopulate the island.

That night, the reprieve from the mold gods came to an end. We tried hotel room after hotel room, and I was forced to reject each one within seconds. We were prepared with camping gear as a backup option, and our GPS helpfully directed us to a campground nearby. But John was fighting a cold and was exhausted after driving and flying all day, and I could see that he was not thrilled about camping.

When the GPS told us we'd arrived, we were on a tiny dirt road with no sign of a campground anywhere. John gave a heartbreaking groan, and I froze. My illness seemed to be pushing him to his limits for the first time. *What if it pushes him too far?*

"We can just camp here!" I said brightly, and I moved to set up camp while John rested. But then I hesitated—we couldn't rinse the mold off our bodies. We'd contaminate our sleeping bags, and then we'd really be in trouble. So we'd have to sleep in the car, a minuscule two-door Hyundai. The only thing I could think of to make that less awful for John was to give him the passenger seat, free of the steering wheel. He accepted the offer without acknowledgment. *Boy, he really is fried.*

I slept, but poorly. I figured I was bound to be crippled in the morning, since I was sleeping with mold on me, but I couldn't figure out anything to do about it. I just hoped I'd be able to manage the day's reporting.

In the morning, everything was better than expected: I'd gotten off lightly, achy and miserable but ambulatory. John's cold, and mood, were much improved, and he even spontaneously thanked me for giving him the passenger seat. When we got up, we both goggled at where we were, with mist swirling around endless hills covered in eucalyptus and tree ferns. *I'm in Australia! I'm in Australia with my beloved, and I'm in the middle of reporting a story!*

As we toured Devil Ark, learning about all their efforts to create a safe haven for the devils from this terrible disease, I again felt a stab of envy. *I sure wish scientists were moving heaven and earth like this to create a safe place for me.* After the tour, the keeper brought out a baby devil he was hand-raising to take into schools. I leaned over to John and whispered, "Think that ME/CFS patients would be getting more help if we were this furry and cute?" John whispered back, "Not from me! You're plenty cute, and I wouldn't want you any furrier."

That night, our luck returned. We found a hotel room that worked for me that night, complete with a swooningly wonderful shower and bed. The next day, we flew back to Tasmania.

I had one last reporting trip, to Maria Island (pronounced mur-*eye*-er). The island had never had its own devil population, and researchers had just released devils there that had been certified disease-free, so that they could live truly wild lives while still being protected from the disease. We deliberated about whether John would join me—he wanted more time with his dad, plus this trip involved no buildings, so it seemed reasonably safe. Still, going alone felt daring given everything I didn't know. Could there be "ick" in the outdoor air somewhere here Down Under? I knew John would have sacrificed the time with his dad if I'd asked and that he had the emotional flexibility to get excited about joining me. But when I thought about asking him to change his plans, it felt as though it would put a small kink in the ever-thickening web of connections through which energy flowed between us.

Plus, I had a feeling as if I were caught up in a protective charm. It wasn't that I imagined that nothing bad could happen to me—after all, we'd had to sleep in the damn car, and I fully expected plenty more disasters to come—but those bad possibilities no longer turned my bowels to liquid. My fears in the past had concentrated themselves in the conviction that when it really mattered, those I loved would fail me and I'd be all alone. But Death Valley had plunged me into that fear and out the other side—and now, every day with John, I felt more met, more connected. Whatever happened, I could deal with it. So I drove off in our rental car in the early morning light, alone.

Maria Island felt like a fairy tale within a fairy tale. The water surrounding it was so clear that it gave the deceptive impression it must be as warm as a Hawaiian shore, though the island was actually one of the closest pieces of land to Antarctica. The bush was so thick that even a machete couldn't cut a trail. Flowers blossomed on bushes all around.

The researchers and I zoomed around the island on a Polaris, a sort of cross between a golf cart and a four-wheeler. Then we tromped through the woods to download pictures from the cameras they had sprinkled around the island, with stinking, fly-buzzing wallaby carcasses nearby to lure the newly released devils in (and to provide them some extra food, in case they didn't immediately catch on to finding it themselves). The devils had inspected the carcasses but barely eaten any, and the footage showed them sniffing around, sleek and fat and happy. I was struck by how historic those grainy images were. *Never in history has a Tasmanian devil been on this island before. And I'm getting to witness it!*

I FELT FAR MORE confident about flying home than I had coming, but sitting on the plane hopping from Hobart to Sydney, there was no denying that I was in trouble. I could barely breathe, barely move. It was too late to get off the flight.

"You okay?" John asked, and I shook my head almost imperceptibly. He pulled out my carbon mask, placing it over my mouth and nose. "Better?" he asked, and I managed another near-imperceptible shake.

Oh, jeez, I thought. *I may be in really, really big trouble here.* The flight was only an hour, but I found myself imagining going into convulsions.

John dug my respirator out, the big one that made me look like an insect, and placed it over my head. I breathed in once, twice, and my nervous system calmed. *Oh thank god, thank god.* I gave John a thumbs-up, and I saw a mirroring relief pass over his face.

A flight attendant came over, somewhat alarmed, to inquire about the respirator. I wondered if she imagined that I might be about to set off tear gas. When John explained, she transformed into helpfulness. They had oxygen on the flight, she said—would that help? I was tempted to try it, but I decided not to mess around. John asked the flight attendant to arrange for a wheelchair for me in Sydney, since I probably wouldn't be able to walk well. He also got her to arrange for me to be able to shower in the airport.

We also realized with some horror that we had only 45 minutes to make our connection—and that we had to change terminals. We explained this to the wheelchair pusher in Sydney, and he ran. He took us straight to the Qantas lounge (a revelation, complete with a gorgeous view, comfortable couches, free food, and booze), and I took the fastest shower in history. He called ahead so we wouldn't have to wait a moment for the bus that would take us to the next terminal. He shot us to the front of the security line, and then he turned the wheelchair over to John. John threw him a $50 tip and took off at a run, playing wheelchair derby around the shoppers in the duty-free area. We arrived at our gate 10 minutes after the plane was supposed to have left, but it was still there.

I walked onto the plane and apprehensively breathed in. It was okay.

I settled into my seat and rested my head on John's chest. He wrapped his arms around me. *It's really, really okay,* I thought.

CHAPTER 19

MOLDY SCIENCE

I couldn't seriously doubt the mold hypothesis anymore, but still, I kept longing for science. Good science, from respectable researchers, not crusading doctors with an agenda. I wanted papers in *Science* and *Nature*, conferences, uncontroversial findings, scientists quietly working away at their lab benches. And most of all, I wanted science to prove I wasn't simply crazy.

I started by taking matters into my own hands: I set out to prove I had a superpower. I wanted to demonstrate that I could reliably detect mold—or, well, whatever contaminants did me in, since I couldn't be sure it was mold, or mold alone.

To do it, I carried out the experiment I'd been pondering for months: I performed a double-blind, placebo-controlled, randomized trial, the kind often called the "gold standard of science." I bought two identical packages containing a dozen washcloths each. I sent one package to a friend in Berkeley, asking him to open it and place the washcloths around his house (which was also the only house I'd lived in that had visible mold). For two weeks, the washcloths absorbed whatever was in the air there, and then my friend returned them to me.

I kept the other package in my house in Santa Fe. These latter would act as a placebo control, since I had never experienced a mold reaction there.

After I got the washcloths back, I performed a preliminary test—not the official, double-blind one to come—to convince myself that the Berkeley washcloths were indeed detectably contaminated and that the Santa Fe washcloths were okay. Standing next to the shower, naked and ready to quickly rinse off, I held one of the Santa Fe washcloths to my nose first. No problem.

Then I breathed through a Berkeley washcloth. At first I thought, *Damn, it didn't work. This doesn't bother me at all!* But after about 10 seconds, I felt a sensation like someone toying with a dimmer switch on my consciousness. After another five seconds, the contamination slammed through my nervous system, scrambling the wiring inside my body so that the only signal it seemed capable of carrying was pain.

I threw the washcloth away from me and tried to get into the shower, but I couldn't even get over the rim of the tub. John helped me, and the water, as always, restored order.

The next day, we ran the experiment itself. My friend, Ondrej, a PhD physicist, manned the washcloths. Sitting alone at a table on the patio of my house, he flipped a coin, and if it came up heads, he chose a Berkeley washcloth; if tails, he chose a Santa Fe one. (That was the randomized part.) He then called John out and handed the selected washcloth to him. John carried the washcloth to me in the bathroom. (This was the "double-blind" part—neither I nor John knew whether the washcloth was from Santa Fe or Berkeley.)

Next, I held the washcloth to my nose until I made my determination. If I declared the washcloth contaminated, I showered before the next one. John took the washcloth back to Ondrej, washed his hands, and got the next randomly chosen washcloth.

We performed the same procedure on a friend who wasn't a moldie, as an extra control. After all, if the Berkeley washcloths simply smelled musty, my detecting them wouldn't be so impressive.

When John handed me the first washcloth, I had to steel myself. I felt like I was about to punch myself in the face—or worse, completely embarrass myself by showing that I couldn't distinguish the contaminated washcloths from the uncontaminated ones.

Bam! Within seconds, the strength seemed to pour out of my body into a puddle on the floor. I whimpered and let the washcloth fall. John helped me stagger into the shower, and the strength poured back into me.

John brought me the next washcloth. It was fine. The next one too, and the one after that.

Bam! The fifth one slammed into me. Again, the strength poured out of me, and again, the shower poured it back in.

By the eighth washcloth, a contaminated one, the reaction was notably stronger, my body curling, my nerves screaming. John struggled to get me into the shower because I couldn't lift my legs over the edge of the tub even with him supporting my torso. After that, I realized I was making this harder on myself than I had to, and I stayed inside the tub for the rest of the experiment.

The violence of my reaction to the 12th washcloth frightened me. *How much of this can my body take?* I wasn't recovering fully between the washcloths, and the image came to mind that I might go into convulsions. By then I'd determined that six washcloths were contaminated and six weren't. *Fuck this*, I decided. *I've obviously proven my point, so I don't need to torture myself further in the name of science. My reactions were so clear that there's no way could I have made a mistake.* I stopped.

Afterward, Ondrej reported the results: I had gotten 10 out of 12 correct, with one false positive and one false negative. My non-moldie friend, on the other hand, had done worse than chance and reported that he had absolutely no idea—the washcloths all seemed identical to him.

How on earth did I get any wrong? Truly assessing what the results meant would require doing some statistics, but immediately, all I could think about was whether a Santa Fe washcloth and a Berkeley washcloth could have gotten switched, or if the Santa Fe washcloth I declared bad somehow got contaminated despite our precautions, or if I had rushed when I called the Berkeley one okay. I started scheming about repeating the experiment to get more data and to see if I could figure out what happened with my mistakes.

But I spent the next day in a miserable miasma, and it took several days before I felt fully myself. The idea of inflicting that on myself again—*ugh*.

And when I recovered and did the calculations, the results looked pretty good. If I'd just been guessing, with no ability to detect contamination at all, I would have had less than a two percent chance of doing as well as I did. In statistical terms, my experiment had a p-value of 0.019. The threshold for a result to be considered "statistically significant" (and hence publishable) was far looser, a p-value of less than 0.05.

Woohoo! I could publish this! Scientific proof!

Well, not really. I knew that my little experiment couldn't really *prove* anything—all it could show was that I was unlikely to do as well as I did if I couldn't detect the contaminated washcloths at all. That suggested, but didn't prove, that I had my moldie superpower.

Additionally, this was what a scientist would call an "n of 2" experiment—there were only two subjects, me and my non-moldie friend. At most, its conclusions applied only to the two of us. It couldn't be generalized to say that other moldies truly detected mold, or that non-moldies couldn't.

Later, I asked statistician Philip Stark of the University of California, Berkeley to review my experiment. He declared it "pretty convincing" but pointed out that changing my study design by shortening the number of trials was a flaw that weakened the experiment a bit. My mind agreed; my body didn't care. I decided I'd sacrificed myself for science quite enough, and I left it at that.

MY PERSONAL WASHCLOTH TRIAL made me feel like I was on more scientifically solid ground, but it still left a zillion questions about what the hell was going on in my body. *Surely someone has studied this!* So over the next few years, I pored through the scientific literature and history about mold.

Even in Biblical times, I learned, people knew mold could be dangerous. The Old Testament gave explicit instructions for decontaminating a house with "defiling mold," and ordered that if the technique didn't work, the house "must be torn down—its stones, timbers and all the plaster—and taken out of the town to an unclean place."

And for centuries, scientists and doctors had also recognized that mold can cause illness. The very first textbook on asthma, in 1698, described how asthma could be triggered by visiting a moldy wine cellar. In the 1930s, mold got some of its first serious scientific attention after horses in the Ukraine started getting swollen lips, massive bruises, fevers, blindness, and tremors. Many of the horses died, and people who handled straw from the horses developed similar symptoms. Scientists traced the problem to a mold called *Stachybotrys chartarum* that had infested the straw.

This problem turned out to go far beyond the Ukraine: Moldy food was found to frequently make all manner of farm animals vomit, convulse, hemorrhage, become paralyzed, or die. In 2003, mold-related losses in agriculture totaled $1.4 billion per year.

These big losses had generated big money for science to understand the problem. As a result, most studies on health impacts of mold had focused on mold in food, not in the air. Scientists had traced the many ways ingested mold toxins poison the immune and nervous systems, cause inflammation, and damage cells.

The toxins are all part of mold's arsenal for defeating its microbial enemies: Since mold can't clunk other microbes on the head or run away from them, it instead engages in chemical warfare, oozing out nasty compounds that will poison bacteria or other fungi. Humans are just collateral damage in this nanoscale war. (And also, sometimes, we are beneficiaries of it. Penicillin, for example, is a mold toxin that doesn't poison us but whacks bacteria inside us.)

Mycotoxins are such good weapons for chemical warfare that humans may have used them in our own wars. The US Department of State has accused the Soviet Union of using mycotoxins as weapons in the 1970s in Laos, Cambodia, and Afghanistan, resulting in skin blistering, eye irritation, and then death within minutes. The United States itself studied the possibility of using mycotoxins as weapons. And Iraq stockpiled 2,200 liters of a mycotoxin in the late 1980s.

So there's no question that some mycotoxins are nasty substances indeed. But that isn't enough to establish that mycotoxins from moldy buildings can make people sick. A big question remains: Can we absorb enough of them from the air in water-damaged buildings to hurt us?

The possibility didn't receive serious scientific attention until the mid-1980s, not long after builders started more thoroughly sealing and insulating homes and office buildings in response to the energy crisis. Public health officials began getting reports of office buildings in which large percentages of workers complained they felt sick in their workplaces— and felt better when they left.

Scientists investigated, and they realized that the buildings had dangerous levels of toxins in their indoor air. Chemicals were leaking out of building supplies, outdoor pollution was accumulating in dust, mold was chomping through damp drywall and flinging its spores into the air— and with the buildings sealed up so tightly, all these nasties built up in the indoor air over time. Scientists patiently put together the clues and saw a clear signal that mold could cause or exacerbate serious allergies and asthma.

This was all part of the orderly, calm process of science—until the mid-1990s. Dorr Dearborn, a pediatric pulmonologist in Cleveland, Ohio, treated a string of babies with bleeding lungs in 1993. The condition is ordinarily very rare: Dearborn had seen only three cases in the previous 10 years. But within a year and a half, 10 cases came to his clinic, and three of the babies died. Some recovered in the hospital, only to relapse after they went home. All the babies were from a single, low-income area of Cleveland that had been flooded.

As the cases piled up, Dearborn grew alarmed and contacted the CDC. Ruth Etzel, the branch chief of air pollution and respiratory health, came to investigate. Together, Dearborn and Etzel compared the sick babies with healthy ones to examine possible explanations: Could the babies have been exposed to pesticides intended to treat cockroaches? Perhaps they were breathed fumes from crack cocaine, second hand? Cigarettes? Child abuse? None of these possibilities seemed like plausible explanations, but one thing stood out: All the babies lived in extremely moldy homes. The homes were contaminated with *Stachybotrys chartarum*, the particularly nasty strain of mold that had killed the Soviet horses long ago. Spore levels of *Stachybotrys* were 3,000 times higher in the homes of the sick babies than the healthy ones.

The media, naturally, freaked out. One AP headline read "Baby-Killing Fungus." An article in the *Plain Dealer* newspaper claimed that health officials were "99 percent certain" that *Stachybotrys* had killed the babies (though Dearborn and Etzel never made such a claim, only saying there was an association between the illness and the mold).

In 1999, even as Dearborn and Etzel were continuing to investigate the cases that kept appearing in Dearborn's clinic—close to 30 in seven years—the CDC launched a second investigation by an anonymous panel. It reported that Dearborn and Etzel's work had "serious shortcomings," criticized the methods of the CDC's own statisticians, and concluded that "the postulated associations should be considered, at best, not proven."

The CDC's decision to undermine its own ongoing investigation struck many as quite unusual, even bizarre. Nicholas Money, a highly regarded mycologist at Miami University, reviewed the controversy in his book *Carpet Monsters and Killer Spores: A Natural History of Toxic Mold*. Although Money agreed that Dearborn and Etzel's study had some shortcomings, he argued that most of the criticisms in the reevaluation were baseless. Money concluded, "I don't know if *Stachybotrys* is guilty of killing babies, but I think its presence in the homes of IPH [lung bleeding] patients is more than pure coincidence."

The Cleveland bleeding lung case alerted the world that mold could pose serious dangers, and lawyers perked up their ears.

In 2001, a court awarded a Texas homeowner, Melinda Ballard, $32 million for the cost of her mold-damaged 12,000-square foot mansion and the belongings inside, including punitive damages, emotional distress, and lawyers' fees. Ballard was an irresistible subject of news coverage: a Jaguar-driving, photogenic, loud-mouthed New Yorker-turned-Texan who described the deterioration of her house and family in frightening detail. The insurance company perfectly fit the villain's role with its refusal to pay for repairs, and the images of the mold in her house were viscerally revolting: The *New York Times* described it as "thick and black and gangrenous, with a dull, powdery sheen that makes it seem waiting and alive. Just looking at it makes you want to throw up."

On appeal, the judgment was reduced to $4 million, and then the parties settled for an undisclosed sum. The judge rejected arguments that Ballard's husband had suffered brain damage from the mold exposure on the grounds that science couldn't prove the link.

Nevertheless, the case marked the beginning of the Mold Wars. According to a buzz phrase at the time, "mold was gold." Insurance claims skyrocketed. The television celebrity Ed McMahon won $7.2 million from his insurance company, claiming that mold had spread through his Beverly Hills home, sickening both him and his wife and killing their dog, Muffin. Erin Brockovitch, the environmental toxicity activist, sued her contractor for more than $1 million over her moldy home. Mold litigation became a legal specialty, with one lawyer handling 1,000 cases, according to the *New York Times*. In 1999, before the Ballard verdict, Farmers Insurance handled only 12 cases in Texas. In 2001, it handled 15,000. Expert witnesses could sometimes charge $1,000 an hour, arguing that science did or did not support litigants' claims.

The insurance industry was reeling from the asbestos disaster, which industry analysts projected could cost $275 billion, and it feared that mold could be a second calamity. So it acted fast to protect itself. Companies added riders to essentially every insurance policy refusing to cover mold. They also lobbied to pass legislation in many areas protecting industry from mold claims.

The insurance companies also gained a huge legal tool from an official statement by the American College of Occupational and Environmental Medicine (ACOEM), a professional organization of nearly 5,000 doctors and other health care professionals. "Molds growing indoors are believed by some to cause building-related symptoms," the statement said. "Despite voluminous literature on the subject, the causal association remains weak and unproven." This proved invaluable to insurance companies in subsequent litigation.

The statement acknowledged that mold was involved for some people with allergies or asthma, but granted it only "an important but minor overall role." It conceded that it was a good idea to remove mold in buildings, but only because it was ugly, smelly, and damaging to building materials, along with being allergenic to those susceptible.

The three authors of the ACOEM statement were all physicians who had earned money as expert witnesses for insurance companies defending themselves in mold cases, none of whom had significant experience in indoor air-quality research. Two of them, Bryan Hardin and Bruce Kelman, worked for GlobalTox, Inc., a firm that regularly testified for the defense in mold cases. Kelman was a seasoned player in the toxin-denialism drama, having participated in the organized effort to sow doubt that cigarettes cause health problems. The third author, Andrew

Saxon, went on to earn more than a million dollars over three years as a private expert witness in mold-related trials.

Even before the statement was published, scientists objected. They argued that the statement was at odds with the science of the time, which had found strong links with allergies and asthma and identified the allergens, irritants, and toxins that can inflame our lungs. And asthma was no small matter—it could be deadly, and its rates were dramatically rising without explanation. Several ACOEM members called the statement "a defense argument" to protect insurance companies in mold litigation, rather than a dispassionate scientific evaluation. Some pointed out that the authors' conflicts of interest weren't disclosed and needed to be.

Nevertheless, ACOEM published the statement with few revisions and without a disclosure of conflict of interest.

The statement immediately became a tool for the insurance industry in litigation. Within months of its publication, the US Chamber of Commerce, the largest business advocacy group in the United States, sent an adapted version of the statement to judges around the country. "The notion that 'toxic mold' is an insidious, secret 'killer,' as so many media reports and trial lawyers would claim," it argued, "is 'junk science' unsupported by actual scientific study."

One of the authors of the ACOEM statement, Saxon, went on to coauthor a similar report in 2006 for the American Academy of Allergy, Asthma, and Immunology (AAAAI), an association of more than 6,000 allergists and immunologists. He bolstered the credibility of the new report by adding an author with a strong reputation in indoor air-quality research—Jay Portnoy, chief of allergy, asthma and immunology at the Children's Mercy Hospital in Kansas City. But Portnoy never approved the paper for publication. He discovered only after the paper was in print that his coauthors dramatically weakened his section of the article so that it denied the evidence that mold causes even hay fever. When he read the revision, he was so incensed that he asked to have his name removed.

Other scientists continued to work to get the statements retracted, and in 2007, the *Wall Street Journal* published an exposé revealing the insurance industry's influence on these statements. But such rebuttals had little apparent effect. ACOEM reissued its statement with only minor changes in

2011—even though by then, studies had shown that more than 20 percent of asthma cases were attributable to water-damaged buildings.

When I realized that special interests were powerful enough to override science in official statements from professional organizations, I saw the CDC's reversal on the Cleveland bleeding lung cases in a different light. In an argument I found persuasive, Nicholas Money, the mycologist and book author, speculated on the reasons the CDC might have chosen to take on a second, highly skeptical investigation:

> The potential for insurance claims by homeowners maintaining that they were sickened by mold exposure is astronomical. The prospect of a peer-reviewed scientific article demonstrating a clear association between *Stachybotrys* and human illness must have kept plenty of insurance agents awake at night, and also made attorneys salivate. Also, everyone is aware that the insurance industry donates a great deal of money to finance political campaigns. The CDC is a government agency. I presume, then, that somebody made a phone call from Washington, DC, to Atlanta [the location of CDC headquarters] and told the CDC to shut those meddling scientists down in Ohio.

This possibility seemed even more plausible when I learned that a few months before the CDC initiated its 1999 reinvestigation of the Cleveland babies, the agency got a new director: Jeffrey Koplan, who came to the agency from the research arm of Prudential, a large insurance company.

Very slowly, scientists have prevailed in bringing down the ACOEM and AAAAI statements. In 2015, ACOEM removed the statement from its Web site, largely due to the efforts of Michael Hodgson, former head of occupational health at the US Veterans Health Administration, who had joined the organization's board. He told me that he argued, "We can't do this. We're making ourselves a laughingstock. The science simply doesn't support it." The AAAAI statement expired as official policy in 2011 but was not retracted. It was only replaced with a new statement affirming the respiratory dangers of mold in 2016. The US Chamber of Commerce has never sent a revised paper to judges. No one from ACOEM, AAAAI, or the Chamber of Commerce answered my e-mails asking for comment.

The ACOEM statement and its progeny shut down one mold-related court case after another. And in the long run, the cases stopped being filed at all because of the riders insurance companies added to their policies that excluded mold from coverage.

Learning all this, I felt as if my brain were quietly exploding. A scientific organization put out a statement that was contrary to science, and scientists couldn't get it removed for *12 years!* How could that happen?

And if respected organizations could sow doubt about whether mold is a significant risk factor for asthma—a link that had been observed in the very first textbook on asthma ever written, in 1698—what hope did I have that science would come to understand my weird illness?

CHAPTER 20

CRAZY NEUROLOGICAL PEOPLE

None of my research so far had shed much light on what I really wanted to know—what was going on in my body. The question burned for me: What was the mechanism?

I had learned enough to understand the mechanism for ordinary respiratory effects. Compounds in mold itself could trigger both allergies and inflammation.

But for neurological effects like mine, the mechanism wasn't so clear. There was an obvious suspect, though: mycotoxins. After all, these mold toxins were known to kill brain cells. There were other plausible culprits in the great airborne stew floating around in moldy buildings—volatile organic compounds, bacteria, bacterial toxins, particulates, manufactured chemicals, some combination thereof—but none of those were known to be powerful neurotoxins, as some mycotoxins are. So everyone seemed to focus on mycotoxins as the most likely culprit.

The 2004 National Academy of Medicine (NAM) report gave good reasons for worry about the impact of airborne mycotoxins on our health. Humans absorb mycotoxins through their lungs and skin as well as through their guts, and for some mycotoxins, breathing them is as toxic as mainlining them straight into a vein—and 20 times as toxic as eating them. Mycotoxins had been found in human blood, tissue, and breast milk. (Breast milk was especially alarming since babies are more vulnerable.) In animals, mycotoxins had been shown to be toxic to the lungs, the skin, the gut, the liver, the kidneys, and the brain, and even low-level exposure to mycotoxins depressed animals' immune systems, leaving them susceptible to infection. The report said that research on mycotoxins from *Stachybotrys chartarum* in particular "suggests that effects in humans may be biologically plausible."

But the report sounded aggravated with the insufficiency of the science. Over and over, it called for more research on the toxic effects of mold. By the umpteenth call, the statement had come to take on a pleading tone to my ear.

It had been a decade since the NAM report was issued, though, so I wondered if the report's call for more research on mycotoxins had been heeded. To find out, I asked the author of the toxicity chapter of the NAM report, Harriet Ammann, a former senior toxicologist with the Washington State Department of Health. Overall, how strong was the evidence that mycotoxins caused non-respiratory problems now?

"I think the evidence is quite strong," Ammann told me, "much stronger than in 2003." My heart leapt.

Ammann explained that one of the biggest arguments against problems from mycotoxins had been that many researchers didn't think you could breathe enough of them in to poison you. But recently, they'd realized they'd been calculating exposure levels the wrong way. They'd been collecting air from moldy buildings and then counted the number of intact spores, which, like plant seeds, can germinate into new mold colonies. They then calculated the amount of mycotoxin each spore could carry, and the total quantity of mycotoxins seemed awfully low. Admittedly, nobody really knew how much mycotoxin it took to poison people, especially people who were exposed day after day and month after month. But still, this had made many researchers skeptical.

It turned out, though, that whole spores weren't the only things that mattered. Mycotoxins also oozed onto broken spores and tiny fragments of the mold itself and surrounding dust, all of which could float in the air. When environmental health researcher Tiina Reponen of the University of Cincinnati looked for these fragments, she found between 1,000 and 1,000,000 times more of them than intact spores.

So our potential exposure to mycotoxins was vastly greater than previously thought. Furthermore, these fragments were far more dangerous. These smaller particles have more surface area to soak up the toxins and can penetrate deeper into our lungs, delivering their loads of mycotoxins, irritants, and allergens into the bloodstream more efficiently.

Reponen's work solved another puzzle too: Buildings that made people sick hadn't seemed to be consistently moldier than buildings that didn't. But that was when researchers were only counting spores—once Reponen counted the fragments and dust, she found that the more of it present in a building, the sicker people got.

Another major advance was that we now had objective evidence for neurological impacts from mold. People who had lived in moldy buildings had poorer balance, slower reaction times, slower reflexes, weaker memories, and other problems, compared with those without known mold exposure. In addition, a Polish study had shown a 10 percent drop in IQ among children who lived in moldy homes for two or more years, after controlling for other factors.

Furthermore, researchers had begun to realize that air pollution as a whole could cause systemic effects, not just the respiratory ones they'd long recognized. It had recently been linked to diabetes, heart disease, and dementia. The mechanisms for these associations were unclear, but many researchers fingered inflammation as a likely culprit.

For my own symptoms, inflammation always struck me as a plausible culprit, at least in part. When I woke up in the morning, before my coffee enema or sauna, my face was usually swollen, sometimes so much so that I could barely see. It also seemed plausible that inflammation of the brain and spinal cord played a role in my walking problems. Neuroinflammation was known or suspected to be integral to Alzheimer's, Parkinson's, and multiple sclerosis. I knew that inflammation could happen fast, since severely allergic people can go into anaphylactic shock, with its massive inflammation, within seconds of an exposure. But could it really resolve as quickly as my symptoms could, vanishing when I stepped into a shower?

Ammann pointed me to another key discovery that, I thought, might possibly explain the shower phenomenon, at least better than anything else I'd come up with. Mycotoxins can travel from our noses, along our olfactory nerves, and straight into the brain, James Pestka of Michigan State University and his colleagues had found.* This route acts as a molecular version of TSA PreCheck, speeding mycotoxins past the blood-brain barrier that ordinarily would flag them as potential terrorists. When monkeys breathed mycotoxins from *Stachybotrys chartarum,* they lost their sense of smell, neurons in their olfactory bulbs died, and their brains grew inflamed. Similar particles, studies had shown, could travel past the olfactory bulbs to the rest of the brain.

Whether this happens in humans from quantities of mycotoxins they absorb in moldy buildings wasn't clear—the monkeys received very large doses. But repeated exposures had a vicious cumulative effect: Monkeys who received five micrograms of the toxin each day for four days showed even more damage than ones who received 20 micrograms once. It may be, then, that breathing still smaller quantities day after day could be similarly harmful.

I doubted that mycotoxins were killing neurons in my brain, since I hadn't lost my sense of smell and most of my symptoms could be swiftly reversed.† But neuroinflammation fit. I also thought this mechanism might apply to me in another way: Perhaps the mycotoxins were traveling up my olfactory nerve and causing some of my neurons to fire in some pathological way, and that was producing my semi-paralysis. Some mycotoxins could cause neurons to fire, I'd learned, so that didn't seem like too big a stretch.

That might explain both the quickness of my reactions and the quickness of their resolution. Research suggested that molecules might be able to travel along the olfactory pathway very quickly—certainly within minutes, possibly within seconds. And perhaps when a shower

---

* Somehow, the notion of molecules traveling along a nerve sounded immensely implausible to me—I was convinced that only electrical signals could travel along nerves. I checked references Ammann gave me, and indeed, this is an established fact. This is one of the ways that air pollution may increase dementia risk. And pharmaceutical companies are eyeing this pathway as a route to deliver drugs. Intranasal insulin, for example, may provide a treatment for Alzheimer's disease, since insulin levels in the brains of Alzheimer's patients are thought to be low. Using the olfactory nerve to deliver the drug would, potentially, raise insulin levels in the brain without affecting the rest of the body.

† I did have some fairly mild cognitive effects that were lasting. Interviewing sources on the phone for more than about 45 minutes often left me feeling concussed, and it took hours to get functional again. I took some solace in learning that over months, the monkeys' neurons regenerated.

rinsed the mycotoxins away, the abnormal firing of my neurons stopped too.

I learned of another mechanism that might result in neuroinflammation: Our immune systems come preprogrammed by evolution to detect some pathogens people have been exposed to for millions of years—including bits of the cell walls of mold spores. That means that when we breathe in mold, our immune systems may become convinced that they're under attack, triggering inflammation and flulike symptoms. Cheryl Harding of Hunter College developed the hypothesis that this immune response could be driving inflammation in the brain as well, causing the neurological problems people report. She exposed mice to the cell walls of mold spores and found that they grew more anxious and forgetful, and they also had signs of inflammation in their brains. When the mice were exposed to intact *Stachybotrys* spores, complete with their mycotoxins, many of the effects were even stronger.

I was astonished to read of a third, entirely new mechanism that had been discovered as well: The gases that give mold its characteristic smell may damage us. Joan Bennett of Rutgers University pumped a volatile organic compound (which, roughly speaking, is the type of gas we smell, commonly abbreviated VOC) from mold into a chamber filled with fruit flies, and the flies staggered and shook like Parkinson's patients. When Bennett treated them with L-dopa, a standard Parkinson's drug, they recovered. She also found that the mold VOCs killed human cells in a petri dish.

I didn't have Parkinson's of course, but there are many mold VOCs, and perhaps one of them caused my particular flavor of nervous system problem. Buildings didn't have to smell of mold to do me in, but our noses can't detect every VOC out there. And thinking of the compound as a kind of scentless smell made some sense. I thought about how it could be nearly impossible to get rid of the reek in the house of a heavy smoker, how the smell could follow them around like a cloud. Perhaps that explained how difficult it was to decontaminate objects that had been in a moldy house for a long time.

Of course, these theories about my reactions were all only possibilities, probably far more likely to be wrong than right. My theories were particularly tenuous because it was unclear whether people living or working in moldy buildings were actually harmed via any of these mechanisms—the work was preliminary, and the doses were unrealistically high. But I found it pretty incredible that we were finding entirely new mechanisms mold could use to hurt us.

Especially because we were finding them even when we were barely looking. When I talked to Pestka, Harding, and Bennett, the researchers who had uncovered these new mechanisms, all reported they had given up their research because they couldn't get funding to continue it. They had each repeatedly sent grant applications to the NIH that had been denied, and they'd concluded that the NIH was simply not interested in research into non-respiratory effects of mold. Pestka had returned to studying ingested mycotoxins. Harding had retired but was continuing work to finish and publish her research. Bennett had turned to studying the positive effects of mold VOCs (including a promising treatment for white nose syndrome in bats).

Some mold researchers were getting funded, though—the ones studying respiratory effects. So I turned to them, figuring they must have some perspective on the range of possible impacts of mold. I often found, though, that as soon as the words "mycotoxin" or "neurological" passed through my mouth, I felt as though I could hear their eyes rolling through the telephone. Many adamantly argued that there weren't enough mycotoxins in the air in moldy buildings to make people sick.

"They're just not there!" barked Jay Portnoy, the researcher whose name was falsely put on the AAAAI report. "We looked, and they're not there!" Despite asking repeatedly, I couldn't get him to cite a single study to back up his claim. I asked him about the study showing that airborne dust and mold fragments could carry vastly great loads of mycotoxins than spores alone, but he simply repeated his irritated dismissals. And when I asked him about the AAAAI report, he sighed, said it happened so long ago he could barely remember the details, and said it was "just a snafu." He seemed angrier at the activists who had complained about the report than he was at his colleagues who had hijacked his name to prop up a statement he disagreed with.

What the hell? I thought. *Maybe he's just having a bad day.*

Next I turned to David Miller of Carleton University in Ottawa, perhaps the foremost researcher on indoor air quality. In the mid-1980s, when workers in entire office buildings suddenly complained of feeling ill at work, Miller had been called in to investigate. He had patiently put together the clues linking the complaints to toxins trapped in the air of tightly sealed buildings, including VOCs, concentrated outdoor pollutants, and mold. He and his colleagues had raised the alarm, helping to change building practices around the world. This guy, I figured, must have a broad perspective on what's going on.

Miller was no less dubious about mycotoxins than Portnoy, though he was far friendlier. To get sick from mycotoxins, he said, you'd have to do "something stupid," like carrying badly moldy boxes right up to your chest, so the mycotoxins would get shaken loose and breathed right in (though, as with Portnoy, I couldn't get him to give me any citations to back up this claim*). Yes, he said, mycotoxins[†] could contribute to asthma—he himself had shown that—but their role was minor. The more significant danger, he argued, was the mold itself, rather than the toxins

---

* I worked really hard to sort out this controversy, asking Miller for references so many times that I strained his patience. He never gave an argument that long-term exposure to mycotoxins in moldy buildings couldn't plausibly have neurological effects, at least not one that I could understand even with great effort.

Instead, he made a blanket claim that 25 years of good epidemiology had proven his claims; he asserted that he didn't make things up; he sent me a dozen highly technical papers at once with no explanation of how they addressed my questions (I read them all, and so far as I could tell, they didn't); and he argued that the health effects could be satisfactorily explained without a significant role for mycotoxins (though, when pushed, he acknowledged this applied to respiratory effects only, not neurological ones).

In particular, he never addressed the three studies that, it seemed to me, made such effects plausible:

1. Reponen's study showing the vastly greater levels of mycotoxins in dust and mold fragments than in intact spores.
2. The greater toxicity of airborne mycotoxins, compared to ingested ones.
3. The complete lack of studies of long-term, low-dose effects.

I also found it odd that, according to him, carrying moldy boxes could make you so sick that you would land in the hospital—but no lower dosage, even over a long time, could have any significant effect. Again, I couldn't get a response from him about this.

† Miller reserved the term "mycotoxin" for the toxins that occur in agricultural settings, and he described the toxins molds emit in indoor air as "low molecular-weight compounds." I chose not to follow his convention because as far as I could tell, it was idiosyncratic to him. Furthermore, it seemed to me that the term "low molecular-weight compounds" failed to capture the essence of what we were talking about, since many small compounds aren't emitted by molds and don't poison people. "Mycotoxin," on the other hand, literally means "mold toxin," which seemed quite appropriate.

it produced. Proteins in mold could both irritate the lungs and cause an immune response.

"What about neurological effects?" I asked. "Can mold, rather than mycotoxins, explain them?" Then Miller grew hesitant. He said that mold can cause allergies, and allergies can wind up the immune system and leave people feeling muddle-headed, but beyond that, he couldn't identify a plausible mechanism through which ordinary moldy buildings could cause neurological effects.

Still, Miller didn't deny that neurological problems might occur in mold-exposed patients. He'd certainly heard people complain about it. Whenever he oversaw the remediation of a moldy building, he said, at the end, a couple of people continued to complain they were sickened by the building even when everyone else felt fine in it. Some of those outliers even reported that if they handled a single piece of paper that had been in the building before its remediation, their symptoms would flare up again.*

Now that *sounds familiar,* I thought. And suddenly I confronted a decision: Was I going to fess up to being one of those folks?

I'd been through this with other researchers. Once I divulged my secret, our nice, easy, relaxed conversations about their research suddenly became stiff and awkward. They'd started to measure their words carefully and then quickly tried to get off the phone. *But,* I reminded myself, *data is data.* I'd had the experiences I'd had, whether they fit into a tidy theory or not. If I stayed silent about them, it felt like I'd be turning them into something shameful.

So I came out: I was one of those crazy neurological people. Then I told Miller about my washcloth experiment, partly to salvage my scientific creds. I described the placebo control and double-blinding and how just breathing through a contaminated washcloth crippled me. What did he make of that? If he didn't think mycotoxins could do that, what could?

Miller's affable voice stayed even but became more careful. Perhaps, he suggested, I had at some point been exposed to multiple chemicals in

---

* I later heard this same story from several indoor air-quality researchers. One reported it with incredulity ("I wouldn't say she needs a psychiatrist," he said, "but she needs something that isn't medical") and another with a kind of wondering sympathy. Miller told the story in a neutral tone.

a building at once, not just mold, and it was the combination of chemicals that had done me in. I was excited—I'd read that some evidence suggested that these combined exposures could be worse than the sum of their parts. *Maybe he can point to other chemicals that can produce my symptoms!* But when I asked, he said no. He just thought a combined effect was more biologically plausible than mold alone.

Then he delicately suggested another explanation: "conditioned immunity." If you give a mouse an allergen mixed with almond extract (with its distinctive smell), the mouse will of course react to the allergen. But if you do this again and again, slowly reducing the level of the allergen to nothing while maintaining the almond scent, the mouse will end up having an allergic reaction to the almond extract alone. That's conditioned immunity, he explained.

But what then, I asked, was the equivalent of the allergen for me? In this analogy, there had to be something—mold or some other compound—that set off my neurological response in the first place. Only then could that reaction be transferred to the almond extract alone. And for that matter, what was the equivalent of the almond extract's scent? In my washcloth experiment, neither I nor my non-moldie friend could smell the mold or detect any other difference between the washcloths, other than that some crippled me and some didn't.*

"Fair enough," Miller said—but then he kept raising that possibility. He called conditioned immunity "the mirror of the placebo effect," in other words, the nocebo effect. He was considering, in more polite language and more specific form, whether my reaction was all in my head.

Then he jumped, saying, "From my perspective, it can seem like more of a mystery than it really is." The problem wasn't the science, he said. It was the politics, particularly the Mold Wars and the ACOEM statement. "Because there was such aggressive marketing on both sides—one side saying mold is doing everything, the other saying mold is doing nothing—it really was difficult to find the center of opinion," he said. But by now,

---

* Later, I experimented a bit in an attempt to use the phenomenon of conditioning in my favor. I put lavender from our garden in my sauna, to build an association in my brain between the smell and the physiological processes I underwent in the sauna. I carried lavender with me, and at times I was feeling lousy but couldn't use my sauna, I'd sniff the lavender. Plus, some evidence suggested lavender on its own had a calming effect. I found it quite pleasant and possibly helpful, though I couldn't know what the mechanism was.

it had all come clear. He'd even just published a series of papers for AAAAI, superceding its earlier, flawed statement, describing the respiratory risks from mold. The science was pretty well settled.

Even though it didn't explain people like me.

When I got off the phone, I felt like a refugee, my citizenship in the land of science having been unceremoniously revoked. I felt like I was as trapped as the snake eating its tail: The way to reclaim my citizenship was to agree to the perspective that Miller had presented with such genial authority. But Miller's claim was that the science was clear—even though it couldn't explain experiences like mine, which he acknowledged occur regularly. So accepting that thrust me and my kind back into exile.

But why, I wondered, didn't he seem to care about folks like me? He seemed like an open-minded, engaged, thoughtful, caring guy. Plus, the problem might well go way beyond a few freakish people like me. Around the world, mold problems occur in 20 to 50 percent of buildings, including schools. Given the huge number of people exposed, especially children, it was imaginable that many people were being affected in lower-level ways. The study that showed a 10-point IQ reduction in Polish children who lived in moldy houses strongly suggested this. Miller was a public health guy. This was potentially a huge public health problem. What gave?

Thinking back on his comments about the Mold Wars and the ACOEM statement, I felt like I had a clue. I imagined him as a young researcher, steadily accumulating solid scientific evidence to prove the respiratory dangers of mold—only to be ignored in the legal clashes, with unscientific claims made on both sides and his own careful evidence getting disregarded. In his shoes, I might want to scream, "Ignore those crazy insurance people! Ignore those crazy neurological people! Listen to me! I'm the one with the science!"

Miller and his researcher comrades had finally won the war against the crazy insurance people. But I could imagine it being very hard to then open the door to the crazy neurological people in order to see how science could be used to investigate their claims. Much safer to keep the focus on the core issues, the ones where we already had solid results, the ones that seemed to affect vastly greater numbers of people. Especially when the mechanism for neurological problems was unclear, and when it was so easy to imagine that they were just a nocebo effect.

Plus, from Miller's point of view, he'd succeeded. He'd established that mold in buildings was a human health threat and that mold levels needed to be as low as possible. He was done.

I, HOWEVER, didn't have the luxury of dismissing crazy neurological people like me. So I contemplated what to conclude about what was going on in my own body.

As much as Miller's lack of interest in neurological issues frustrated me, I also agreed with him that whatever was debilitating me in water-damaged buildings, it was unlikely to be an ordinary toxic effect from a mycotoxin alone. I reacted too quickly and recovered too quickly. If toxins were damaging my cells, I couldn't imagine how the cells could immediately undamage themselves during a shower.

The other problem was that I reacted to such unbelievably tiny quantities. How much mycotoxin could possibly be reaching my body from the sheets of a bed on which a backpack had been set for a couple of minutes, hours earlier? Doctors who treated mold patients universally reported such hypersensitivity, and certainly it was true of all my moldie friends. But that didn't provide a mechanistic explanation.

The only medical condition I knew of that involved that degree of reactivity, other than extreme allergies, was multiple chemical sensitivities,* so I researched the current understanding of its mechanism. Not surprisingly, nobody knew, but the hypothesis that seemed most relevant to me was called "kindling": Neurons that are given a strong or repetitive electrical or chemical stimulus can become trigger-happy, requiring only a tiny spark of stimulation to kindle an enormous fire of a response. That phenomenon was thought to play a role in epilepsy and alcohol withdrawal as well as, perhaps, chemical sensitivities. That fit with my idea that my neurons were pathologically firing in a way that paralyzed my legs.

It was an intriguing idea, but for cases like mine, kindling was no more than an unstudied hypothesis.

---

* The foremost researcher on multiple chemical sensitivities was Claudia Miller (no relation to David), and she had introduced a new term for the illness, toxicant-induced loss of tolerance (TILT), which she argues is more precise and accurate. Since my discussion of it here is so brief, I've stuck with the more familiar term.

So ultimately, after all my research, I still had little idea what was going on inside my body when I reacted to mold. My theories about my reactions were all only possibilities. To really know would take serious research—which would take serious money.

The science did show, however, that moldy buildings were probably harming people in many different ways and that we'd only just begun to scratch the surface of understanding mold's impact on human health.

I felt even more discouraged about the prospects for scientific progress on non-respiratory effects of mold than I did about ME/CFS. ME/CFS was at least an official illness, with a cadre of determined researchers trying to understand it scientifically. They were facing quite a battle given the very limited research funding, but still, they'd accumulated lots of evidence that ME/CFS caused physiological abnormalities, which was an important first step. For non-respiratory effects of mold, the research budget was pretty much nothing. With no money, even the most committed researchers couldn't do their work. And, of course, almost none of the researchers on mold were committed to understanding neurological effects anyway.

So, I felt as though I was taking one more step away from the naïve assumption that, given time, science would save me. At this rate, the universe would come to an end first.

Still, it hardly made me abandon science. I held on to the knowledge that my illness could and should be understood scientifically. I continued to use my scientific skills and mindset to try to understand and treat it. And most of all, I continued to claim my citizenship in the land of science.

CHAPTER 21

TIMMY THE WOOD ELF

One day a couple of months after we got back from Tasmania, John excitedly told me that he'd been shuffling through tunes on his iPod and had come upon a recording of a session he'd had with a psychic a year before. He wanted me to hear the recording.

A psychic? I thought. *Really?*

Few things aroused my skepticism more than the idea of a psychic. Not long before my mother died, she went to see one, on a friend's insistent recommendation. The psychic told her she would get married and go live in a Mediterranean country—a vision that fit well with her fantasies, but not, as it turned out, with reality. My mother's experience fit with my expectations: I had always figured that either psychics said things that were so general that they could apply to anyone in any situation, or they were observant and attuned what they said to people's images or fantasies. Some might be well intentioned but self-deceiving, I figured, but most were probably just con artists.

John's comment about the psychic hit on one of my few anxieties about our relationship: He was not particularly science-minded, or even inclined toward careful, rational analysis. When he drove down from Boulder to see me for the first time, he called me from the New Mexico border and said he'd be there in an hour, when the drive ordinarily takes two—a case of wishful thinking he was quite prone to. He enthusiastically took a homeopathic cold treatment that I figured *had* to be nothing more than a placebo whose primary efficacy lay in its fancy-sounding name, Oscillococcinum. He described a form of alternative medicine linking symptoms to organs and thence to emotions as though it were plausible. And he certainly wasn't the kind of person I could ever talk math with.

A small voice in my head said that perhaps that was why he was so willing to accept all my strange moldie rituals. *Maybe he's just not savvy enough to recognize how ridiculous I'm being.* I immediately rejected that—*Hey! It's working! Nothing branded "scientific" has. Give him and yourself a break.*

I also recognized that in some way, I *liked* his nonscientific orientation. More primary for him than careful, rational, scientific analysis were intuition and feeling. His strengths lay in his acute understanding of human nature, his awareness of his own psychological underpinnings, and a kind of attunement to the underlying patterns of the world that fit in very much with my own. When I described my childhood experiences with my mother and my own intuitive, mystical orientation to him, I didn't feel sheepish, as I so often did. He seemed to know just what I was talking about when I described my time in Death Valley and how I felt hollowed out, like I didn't really matter anymore, even to myself. He quoted his Sufi teacher: "It's not about finding yourself. It's about losing yourself."

At the same time, my scientific side felt just as central to me. I felt enormous power in holding both these perspectives at once, rubbing them against each other while betraying neither, withstanding the tensions between them. Science without mysticism struck me as narrow and misleading, but mysticism without science could veer off into insanity, as it sometimes did in my mother.

I reminded myself that John was very different from my mother. And if my science-writer friends might sneer at some of the things he said? Well, fuck 'em.

But now he was talking about a psychic.

As he described the recording, he reminded me of a little boy who wanted to show me the lizard he'd caught. His face was alight, and he was nearly bouncing. I couldn't help but smile. "Sure, I'll listen," I said.

And I *was* pretty curious. Despite my discomfort, I figured that if

John was so excited about this, it had to be interesting.

That evening, we snuggled on the couch together and he gave me the context for his session: He had gone to see the psychic, Timmy Wood, a few months before he met me, primarily because he wanted advice about a recent breakup that he had belatedly regretted. During his first visit, Timmy had been encouraging about his prospects for a reunion. But since then, John had been feeling ever more disheartened. He went again, looking for a fill-up on hope, and it was the recording of this second session that had come up on his iPod.

John pressed play, and a deep voice spoke: "Let's invite in your guides. Let's ask for the highest, clearest messages. I'm going to channel your higher self. Do I have your permission?" John agreed. "We give thanks for the messages for the good of yourself and others. Amen."

Then the voice shifted and became artificially high-pitched and staccato, as if a lumberjack in ballet shoes were dictating to voice recognition software. Timmy began a high-speed riff: "As we look into your soul vibration we want to remind you and be perfectly clear that you have a lot of red in your soul, you have a lot of yellow in your soul." *Oh, god,* I thought. *Soul vibration, yeah right.*

But as he continued on, he painted a portrait of John that I recognized. John's "yellow vibration" was his optimistic outlook, his sunniness, his enjoyment of life and its physical pleasures. His "red vibration" was his sexuality and sensuality—which I was happy to attest to.

Timmy described the importance of John's soft, feminine side, one of the things that had drawn me to him in the first place. He encouraged John to trust that aspect of himself more. He told him it was time for him to do the work that he loves (advice John hadn't yet taken—he was writing technical manuals for a living, but longed to do his own creative writing and to help people write books).

Then Timmy said something that really caught my attention: John was going to meet someone wonderful in June and have lots of great sex, a prediction that happily had turned out to be precisely true.

Timmy hadn't seemed to take a breath for several minutes during that barrage of words. "First question?" he asked, finally inhaling.

John edged toward the real issue, starting with less intense questions about work. Then finally he came out with it: He wanted advice about his old girlfriend, Karla.

"That's still stuck in you. Let's clear that up and release that and move on," Timmy declared briskly. "Go out and meet some ladies."

John didn't want to hear that. "If I date other women, does it have a bad effect on the friendship I have with my last partner and the potential that's there for that to become more?"

"Why do you think there's potential to develop more with her?"

"After I broke up with her, I realized how strongly I cared about her."

Timmy's voice grew sharper. "Yes, but what are you currently doing about that?"

"Being friends," John said in a puppy-dog tone.

Timmy was having none of it, and John's voice rose into a slight whine: "This is something we talked about a lot last time, but it was different. You said there was still hope."

"Well, it's changed," Timmy pronounced. "It's time to release her and move on. That's what we're picking up now."

Hearing this, I laughed, my head bouncing against John's chest where it was snuggled. Timmy kept trying to lure him toward interest in moving forward—*Great sex ahead! Wonderful new partner! This summer! All you have to do is release the past!*—but John kept turning back to Karla.

"What about affection?" John asked.

"No!" Timmy ruled instantly.

"But yesterday, I asked her to hold me, and she did," John said. "It felt good. It didn't feel sexual."

"Did you feel like it was allowing you to move on?"

Long pause, and then a small voice: "No."

My head rocked against John's chest as we both guffawed.

At one point, Timmy's voice shifted back to its deeper cadence: "This is Timmy now. I can totally relate to this. I've been there. This is for both of us together, because I can identify completely."

By the end of the recording, I was impressed. It was like a really good therapy session, but without the extended getting-to-know-you. By the end of the session, John was able to discuss the possibility of dating, and he reported to me that it had indeed been very helpful, even a turning point. A few months after that psychic-therapy session, on the very night he finally fully accepted that Karla wasn't the woman for him, he'd checked his OkCupid online dating account, seen my profile, and written to me.

Whether Timmy had any powers of clairvoyance or not, he had clearly done John a service. Maybe he was just a wise and perceptive fellow, with no supernatural powers—*but hey, that sounds good.* Maybe he could offer me insight about my life and my illness that would help me move forward too. My reactivity to moldy buildings was a big fucking drag and only seemed to be getting more extreme, and I had little idea what to do about that other than hope it would resolve over time. Maybe Timmy would stir up some idea for me. *Plus, why not? I've got nothing to lose except a modest amount of money. It'll be fun!*

TIMMY WOOD WELCOMED ME with a huge "Hey!" Beaming, he asked me to remove my shoes and then padded toward the back of his dimly lit house. His round belly, short legs, and curly hair made me think of a hobbit. Pointed ears would have suited his face perfectly. John and I later dubbed him "Timmy the Wood Elf."

No bad reactions so far, I thought, though the cluttered, dusty house didn't inspire confidence. We passed through his kitchen and sat in his office, at a card table covered with piles of bric-a-brac: gems, rocks, little carvings.

As I listened to him intone the same invocation he'd used with John, I reminded myself of a resolution I'd made before I came: My job, for the duration of the session, was to set my skeptical mind aside and just let the experience move me. I was not to let myself be an asshole, ripping everything he said to shreds as the words left his mouth—if I did that, what was the point in coming? Instead, I'd imagine, to the best of my ability, that all this was real, and I'd give Timmy the full chance to move me to a different place emotionally, just as he had with John. Later, I could analyze and dissect it all I wanted.

After the invocation, Timmy barreled off, painting a portrait of my character. Red was my soul's color, he said, the color of passion and fire. I was very connected to the earth.

My sensitivity, including to mold, was a gift, and now I just needed to learn to master it. (I had mentioned mold when I first called him, and I now regretted that—would he have figured that out on his own?)

"Be careful that you're not questioning yourself, that you're refining your awareness of your own sensitivities," he said. *Hmm, well, that's pretty astute,* I thought. *I certainly do question myself about mold more than I think is truly helpful.*

He riffed a bit more and then invited my first question. I asked, "What does my body need from me?"

To listen to it, he said, and to learn its language. It's when I failed to do so that my body got "a little off." *I guess that's one way to describe it.* He emphasized that the sensitivity was "an advancement of the soul," not a brokenness. "As you refine this really well, you're going to live a long time," he said, explaining that being forced to avoid mold and pay attention to my body's needs would keep me in good health.

Then he laid out his theory about any sensitivity or allergy. During childhood, he said, something traumatic happened to me while I was in the presence of mold, and my body had falsely associated the trauma with the mold. It was when I was between four and six, he felt. Had my family moved when I was that age, he asked, or had some other dysfunctionality?

Why yes—we moved from Houston to San Diego. *Lots of families move with young children,* I thought. *Big whoop.*

But there was a far bigger dysfunctionality around that time: When I was seven, my mother sent my brother and sister away. My sister, who was eight years older than me, went to boarding school and to my uncle's for holidays; my brother, who was three years older than me and had been adopted, went to foster care and then eventually to his adoptive father (my mother's ex-husband).

I told Timmy about this briefly, though I also thought, *Gee, my siblings left when I was seven, not when I was between four and six. Yeah, it's close, and my family wasn't doing well leading up to that point, but isn't this exactly the kind of wiggle room psychics rely on? Plus, how many people have had nothing at all traumatic happen when they were young, not even a move?* Then I reminded myself, *Don't be an asshole. You can worry about that later.*

"You haven't dealt with all that," he declared. "That was also associated with mold."

I felt my body stiffen, thinking of PACE and all the ME/CFS patients who had been horribly mistreated because people believed their disease was psychological. It was one thing to consider myself that psychological trauma might be affecting my body, and quite another to have some know-nothing psychic push it on me. But again, I set aside those thoughts to consider later.

Then something else occurred to me: *Hmm, my bedroom when I was that age was in the basement. It could easily have been moldy. Who knows?*

He riffed on about this a bit, describing my wounded inner child who had been frightened and unable to understand what was going on. In passing, he commented, "Mom was off the charts a little bit." I hadn't told him anything about my mother. She was definitely "off the charts a little bit" in those days, just like my body could get "a little off."

He pointed out that because I was dependent on my mother then, I had needed an explanation for the turmoil that allowed me to continue believing I was safe with her. I had unconsciously blamed mold, he said, and now, 30-some years later, exposure to mold reactivated that bodily sense of trauma, leading to my body's freak-outs. "The mold is the symbol of your inner child not getting nurtured."

The way to deal with this, he advised, was to go back and reexperience the trauma and bring my adult self to my frightened inner child. I needed to hold her, listen to her, comfort her—and then to break the association between the trauma and the mold. "Timmy will work with you," he (or my guides, or whoever) said, by doing "energy work" (whatever that was). Or I could work with a therapist.

He asked what was happening in my life when I first got sick, and I quickly described building the house, Geoff's dissolution from his bipolar disorder, the moldy trailers. Timmy was delighted by the grim tale: That experience of extreme stress and mold together had reactivated the childhood trauma, he declared. My response to the difficulty had been to become very strong and masculine, to hold everything together, and now I had to learn how to be soft.

"Once you release all that trauma and forgive your ex-husband," he said, "then the presence of mold won't affect you."

But I forgave Geoff long ago! I thought. *It's not his fault that he got sick. Plus, that sounds like just the kind of ridiculous thing a psychic would say.* Then I reminded myself, *Later. Don't be an asshole.*

Timmy also said that I was feeling somewhat scared. That was certainly true: My relationship with John felt swooningly dreamy after so many years of aloneness and struggle, and while I felt myself coming to trust in the relationship, I was also frightened that it would all fall apart. And it wasn't just John—for so long, things that had seemed like they should work just didn't. I'd almost felt cursed, and suddenly, that curse had vaporized. But I didn't fully understand why life had been so hard in the first place, or why it had turned wonderful—or if it could start being that hard again.

I asked Timmy whether it was possible for me to have a baby, which would feel like a kind of ultimate lifting of the curse. He had me close my eyes and pick six objects from his pile of knickknacks. One of them was a skull, and Timmy told me that it showed that there was a block in my sexual energy that was impeding having a baby.

Initially, he suggested that this was a problem in my relationship with John. When I said I was having the best sex of my life, he looked for other explanations. He asked about my sexual relationship with my ex-husband, and I told him about how it had been powerfully sexual early on, but by the end, not at all. He said that I still carried wounds from that, and I should ask John for support, through "making love to God." I tried to imagine what that meant, visualizing us in the lotus position, hands folded in prayer, looking upward as we thrusted. I suppressed a giggle and then remembered, *Don't be an asshole, Julie.*

But he also told me it wasn't too late to have a baby, and that there was the spirit of a boy waiting to come through. "As this gets corrected, you can bring a child forth. Do that work in the next several months, and by August you could be pregnant." *That's way too soon,* I thought, but I kept quiet.

He began to wrap the session up with another high-speed riff. He enthused about my relationship with John, calling it "good good good stuff." He reassured me once more about my health: "It may be a little bit of an issue for you your whole life, but it doesn't have to knock you down like you're afraid it will." He told me that I'd have a "spiritual awakening" the coming summer, that I'd express myself creatively through my writing, that my forties would be very active and successful and playful. I would "manifest my reality."

"We love you and bless you. Amen."

As I DROVE HOME AFTERWARD, I let my skepticism pour back in. Certainly, the idea that my extreme sensitivity to mold was *purely* psychological (if that's what he was saying) was absurd. I thought of the fruit flies staggering about with Parkinson's after their encounters with gases from mold—had they reexperienced some childhood insectile trauma while the mold gas had been pumped into their chamber?

Timmy also had claimed that this psychological explanation applied even to allergies. But the physiology of allergies was well understood, and I'd never heard any scientific support for the idea that it had a psychological basis. Science could, of course, have not caught up to the idea, but even so, the theory didn't make much sense to me. I had never had any allergies as a kid, but a few years after I moved to Santa Fe, the springtime juniper pollen had me sneezing. That pattern was typical for transplants to Santa Fe. Was spring a particularly traumatic time of year for new Santa Fe residents?

Plus, I'd put so much effort into psychological explanations for my illness that hadn't led to anything. Early on, psychology seemed so compelling: The problem was obviously just too much stress and overwork. *Finish the house, get divorced, do some therapy, and I'll be fine*, I figured. I wasn't. Then when I lost my job at St. John's and was miserable even after I got my job back, I figured, *Find a new career path, get my life growing in new directions, do some more therapy, and I'll be fine*. I got worse. Then my relationship with William wasn't working and I was desperately missing my home in Santa Fe. *Leave William, go home, keep working on my own psychology, and I'll be fine*. It didn't help.

Of course, Death Valley had led to a profound psychological shift for me, and it's true that I got dramatically better just after that. But what if I hadn't had such a profound experience? Would mold avoidance alone have led to my improvement? I couldn't know for sure, but I was inclined to give mold avoidance most of the credit. And the fact was, I was always focused on personal growth, so if I'd gotten better at a different moment,

I could almost certainly have linked it to some other psychological shift.

But while I had grave doubts about drawing a simple causative line between psychological growth and physical improvement (or between psychological issues and illness), I certainly didn't see the two as disconnected. It seemed obvious to me that anyone is likely to deal with any life circumstances better if they're functioning well psychologically. And if someone happens to be sick, that better functioning will help them get better, in straightforward ways: They'll be under less stress, they'll think more clearly about their options, they'll waste less energy on fruitless worrying and hence have more available for productive thinking, on and on and on. There's nothing surprising or mysterious there.

At a deeper level, I saw our minds and bodies as so inextricably linked that there aren't really even two things to connect. Something profound happened to me on all levels in Death Valley, and asking how much of the shift was physical and how much was psychological struck me as ultimately nonsensical. My being as a whole changed. The hidden threads that I had been following led me to that spot, alone in the desert, and they carried me out of it into a transformed life.

But Timmy was making a very specific claim far beyond these generalities that I strongly believed: He was connecting a specific traumatic event in my life to my illness and claiming that working on it would directly make me feel better. Figuring out whether that made sense to me was far more difficult.

There was no question that I'd experienced trauma and that it had affected me profoundly. In the period leading up to my family's dissolution, my mother's craziness had spun out of control. The worst of it was that she had beaten and humiliated my brother. I loved them both desperately and had tried, impossibly, to mediate between them.

Most of my memories of that time were hazy, filtered through stories I'd heard about it from my siblings, blanked out by my confusion and pain. My clearest memory was ironic for its seeming triviality: My mother cut up my brother's *Star Wars* T-shirt and used the shreds as rags. That T-shirt was a talisman for my brother, perhaps the most sacred object in his young life, and defiling it struck me as an unambiguous and unforgivable offense. Spanking him with a belt and leaving welts on his butt, or hitting him on the head with a hairbrush until he got a black eye—maybe there was some explanation for those things that my six-year-old mind couldn't grasp. But cutting up his *Star Wars* T-shirt—*that's wrong!*

Still, I hadn't simply condemned my mother. For one thing, I knew as a child that if I did, I'd lose whatever power I had. If my mother was hitting my brother and I told her to stop, she did—but I was sure it was a privilege that would vanish if I overused it. It was my connection to my mother that allowed me to influence her.

Plus, I simply couldn't bear being disconnected from my mother. Occasionally, she would get so angry that she would simply drive away, leaving us three kids behind. I'd see her lime-green Cutlass Ciera convertible starting to pull away and I'd tear away from my siblings, running after her, crying for her to take me with her. I was the golden child, my mother's unambiguous favorite, and she would stop the car and let me climb in. Then she'd take me to Toys "R" Us and let me pick out whatever toy I wanted. We'd go home, and I'd slink past my siblings with my Barbie doll, amazed that they didn't seem to hate me when I was so obviously a traitor.

One day when I was seven, my mother called my 10-year-old brother into her room. I sat on the porch swing outside her bedroom window, trying to eavesdrop. Ominously, I didn't hear the sounds I expected, of her spanking him and him crying.

Ty finally emerged, dry-eyed and quiet. He sat next to me on the porch swing.

"She said I have to leave," he told me. "She's sending me to foster care."

I had no idea how to respond, what to say, what to feel. We sat together on the porch swing, holding hands in silence.

I didn't see my brother again until I was 18.

Around the time Ty left, my mother sent my sister away too, to boarding school and to my uncle Steve's for holidays.

After my siblings left, my mother told me, "Now I have all my energy for you!" and I wriggled like a puppy, despite a frisson of guilt. A few months later, I looked back at my response with all the cynical disgust a seven-year-old can muster. I'd discovered that all my mother's energy included all my mother's *negative* energy too, which my siblings had previously taken the brunt of. Before, when my mother's mood mysteriously shifted dark, she'd spank my brother or yell at my sister while I got off scot-free. Afterward, my own fanny was on the line, though I never got it nearly as bad as my brother had.

These experiences must have bathed my body and brain in stress hormones for years on end when I was a child, and that couldn't have done good things to me. Although I hadn't been through a war, it was easy to imagine that my brain and body had been affected by a sort of post-traumatic stress disorder. Mold might be a trigger, like a car back-fire that sends a veteran flying to the ground.

That idea has some scientific backing too, given that research has linked adverse childhood experiences like mine to ailments including chronic obstructive pulmonary disease and ischemic heart disease. Studies also claimed to link ME/CFS with childhood trauma, though they held little weight for me since such research rivaled the PACE trial's psychotherapy and exercise advice for quality and scientific care. I had my scientific doubts about other similar studies as well—mind-body science seemed to be a field that attracted low-quality research. But still, maybe some of it was solid.

It was one thing, though, to consider such possibilities in my own mind and quite another to have some psychic assert it. It struck me as a cheap and easy explanation, so appealing that who could resist? All Timmy had to do was guess I'd had some childhood trauma, and then he had a tidy explanation to offer. And really, who hasn't had some childhood trauma? Though, admittedly, mine was probably more extreme than most.

Adding it all up, I certainly wasn't persuaded that Timmy had truly shown any clairvoyance. At one moment, for example, Timmy had started free-associating about mold, asking me if I had a fear of wetness. Was I afraid of drowning? Did I dislike gooey things? When I said no, he'd eventually made his way to this connection: Mold is growth occurring where we don't want it. Since that's what my body was freaking out about, I needed to give myself permission to flip out and be out of control from time to time, to grow in ways I didn't intend. Finally, he'd found an explanation that resonated with me a bit—but after an awful lot of fishing. He also recommended that I wear a ruby for my "red energy." *Seriously? Start wearing crystals?*

But ultimately, all that second-guessing just wasn't the point. The question was whether I could use his comments and suggestions to improve my health or my life as a whole. If so, it was worthwhile, and if not, it wasn't. Nothing else mattered. And I wasn't going to let prideful skepticism get in the way of anything that might help.

Then the question became how I might be able to make use of it. *Jeez, I've done so much therapy already!* I had talked over and over again about my childhood, my mother, my brother, my sister. Those events couldn't be undone. How could I fix them now?

Still, it had been a while since I'd revisited all that, and I'd experienced big internal shifts in the meantime. Perhaps working through it all once more would be useful.

The idea of doing "energy work" (whatever that was, anyway) with a psychic was a stretch, though. Maybe I could work on the trauma with a therapist, I thought. Someone licensed, credible, not so embarrassing. Someone who would put me back on firm scientific ground.

CHAPTER 22

REBIRTHDAY

The morning after my session with Timmy, John and I headed off to Death Valley to celebrate my one-year "rebirthday," the anniversary of my trip there. I wanted to take John to the desert from which I had emerged, reborn.

We were driving a 1984 Vanagon camper that we'd found after months of looking for a car. Each time I'd sat in a car for sale, I'd gotten crippled within seconds to minutes. John would then make apologies to the astonished owner as I staggered away. The more cars we tried, the more miraculous it seemed that I'd never had a problem with John's car or with Gary's little Impreza that I'd been driving for months. We got desperate enough that I tried a new car. I felt fine in it, but I couldn't see dropping 20 grand for one.

One day I mentioned to John the fantasy I'd had in Death Valley of living with Frances in a Vanagon in the desert. "A Vanagon!" John cried. "Let's buy a Vanagon!" He began spinning fantasies about road trips through the Southwest together, pointing out that it would allow us to travel without risking hotel rooms. Maybe we could even rig up a shower inside a Vanagon, he said, so that if I went into a building and "got molded," I could rinse off right away.

I was doubtful that we'd be able to find one I could tolerate, since they were all more than 20 years old, but I was willing to look—and astonishingly, we succeeded. We bought a 1984, chocolate-brown camper van that we named Maxine, and she became my mold-free home on wheels, complete with bead-bedangled curtains that radiated good hippie juju.

On our way to Death Valley just after my session with Timmy, we camped in Maxine at the base of great red cliffs in Capitol Reef. We drove through country so fantastically beautiful, dry, and difficult that I had to laugh at the perfection of the metaphor for my life over the last few years. We stood together at a pull-off on Boulder Mountain, with Rachmaninoff's Vespers playing on the stereo. We were overlooking what must have been many thousands of square miles of land, with snow-capped mountains shining in the background and canyons and cliffs and red rock in the foreground, so much that you could have looked forever and kept seeing new things. I had the same feeling I'd had in Death Valley, that my soul was expanding across all that space, growing out into the great nothingness over the land—but this time, I had John's hand in mine. Tears sprang to my eyes, and when I looked at him, I saw matching tears in his.

We stopped in St. George, Utah, and John did the shopping while I waited in the van, not wanting to risk an unfamiliar building. When he returned, the van's starter turned over slowly, then more slowly, then not at all. Maxine was dead.

"Hey!" I said. "We can jump her ourselves!" We'd brought the marine battery that I'd gotten for my first Death Valley trip to provide power, along with a solar panel. We wired the batteries together, turned the ignition, and heard Maxine rev to life.

We were proud of our ingenuity—but also rattled. We'd just been driving for hours, so why had Maxine's battery died? What if Maxine wouldn't start when we were camping miles up a jeep trail?

As I drove through Las Vegas and out toward Death Valley, a shifting wind battered Maxine's sides. She was struggling to maintain 50 miles an hour against the blasts. John looked stiffly out the window. He seemed lost in misery, and I couldn't catch his eye to smile at him. When I asked what was up, he said he wasn't feeling very well, and the wind was bugging him. My hands were tight on the steering wheel, working to compensate for the wind's blows. I reached out to touch his arm, but I got little response, and I needed both hands to steady us.

I couldn't help but remember Geoff dissolving into bipolar disorder.

Could this be the first step in something similar happening? Could the wonderfulness of the past eight months be an illusion beginning to crack? People do commonly get blinded in the early stages of relationships, I thought, so perhaps I'd missed incipient signs of trouble.

Don't be ridiculous, I told myself. *So what if John has a moment of being distant? He's amazingly good-natured nearly all the time. He does so much to support me, and I should return the favor and be strong for him when he needs it. Happily, I'm well enough to do so right now.* We drove on in silence.

Suddenly, Maxine banged so loudly it sounded like she was being ripped in half. Then she clattered and died.

I pulled to the side of the highway and we emerged from the van into the wind. We quickly determined that this problem outclassed our meager mechanical skills, despite our earlier triumph. Time for AAA.

Hours later, the tow truck driver arrived, and we begged him to let me ride in the van on the flatbed, explaining that I had an environmental illness. "Not in this wind," he said, face closed, continuing to load up the van.

I put on my respirator and climbed in, hoping for the best. But within a few minutes, I could barely breathe, even with the respirator on. John rolled down the window for fresh air and wiped my face off with his dampened sleeve. *In, out,* I thought. *You can do it, Julie.*

Then a sudden certainty came over me: I was going to have a seizure.

It hit me like a train, contorting my body and wrenching out a scream that surged from my chest uncontrollably, on and on and on. I wasn't in pain; the scream felt as involuntary as the convulsing, a direct product of my disordered nervous system.

Some small part of me was coolly observing this, thinking, *Geez, Julie, you sure are screaming. You should figure out how to stop, because this is thoroughly socially unacceptable. And how odd—people don't ordinarily scream during seizures, do they? Are you really sure you're not somehow faking this?* But the screams continued ripping through me.

I distantly heard John hollering, "Pull over! Pull over!" As soon as the truck stopped, he climbed over me and carried me to the side of the road. The icy wind whipped around us as I screamed on.

John said something about pouring water on my head, a reasonable thought given the usefulness of showers. But the idea of being wet as well as cold and convulsing sounded awful to me. I shook my head and pulled at the mask, and John took it off for me. The screams muffled into sobs. John held me, saying over and over, "Ah, sweetie," in a tone so soaked with love that I hung on to his words like a life preserver.

My body gradually calmed down. The tow truck driver babbled incoherently. I worked out that he was saying that he'd let me ride in Maxine to the end of his zone, but after that, we had to transfer to another truck, and once we switched trucks, I couldn't stay in the van.

I was finally able to get up and walk, with John's help, over to Maxine. I lay down a towel, climbed in, covered myself with another, and pulled Frances into my lap. I held her tight as she nuzzled her nose along my neck, and I drew strength and calmness from her solid little body.

Meanwhile, John was in the tow truck, begging the dispatcher to let me stay in the van for the rest of the trip. It was a no-go; the dispatcher was sympathetic but said that it was against the law.

When we reached the next town—really just a couple of gas stations and casinos—John walked back to the van and asked, tentatively, if I was up for trying the tow truck that was waiting for us.

"No," I whimpered.

"We could stay in Maxine here," John said, his voice gentle.

I closed my eyes, took a deep breath, and forced myself to focus. Most likely, no tow truck would let me ride in Maxine in the morning either. Somehow, then, I had to get to Las Vegas outside the van. And a taxi was as likely to be as bad as a tow truck, maybe more so. *Jesus*, I thought. *The world is not designed for people like me. There is no safe way to deal with this.*

John stroked my hand as we talked about our options. Staying in this gas station parking lot sounded awful. Plus, I told John about a hypothesis I'd come up with: Maybe I'd reacted so violently because the mask itself had gotten saturated with contaminants from previous use and had actually made things worse. If so, I might be okay if I didn't wear the mask.

So I decided to try it: I climbed in the next tow truck, mask-free. Almost immediately I could tell that it would be okay. *Thank god, thank god, thank god*, I thought, almost in tears. I could see the relief etched in John's face too.

As we drove, John told me that when I was convulsing, he'd assumed I was dying and in horrendous pain. The thought that went through his mind was, "Well, we sure had an unbelievable eight months together. Too bad it couldn't be longer." Tears sprang to my eyes and I squeezed his hand. At one o'clock in the morning, the tow truck pulled up to the garage. Even at that hour, traffic whizzed past and street lamps blared. Still, we gratefully climbed into the van and popped the top up. We stripped off our clothes, put it all in giant Ziploc bags to try to keep the contamination from spreading around the van, gave ourselves sponge baths, and poured water over our heads before collapsing into bed. We just had to hope our efforts were enough to keep Maxine contamination-free.

Just before eight a.m., the garage owner arrived. He seemed unsurprised to see marooned Vanagon owners sleeping in his parking lot, and as he opened his shop, he called out cheerily, "Be with you in a moment!" His mechanics found a huge metal plate at the transition between the transmission and the engine that had ripped in half. Seven hundred dollars and a day later, we were heading to Death Valley once more.

We listened to the recording of my session with Timmy as we drove. Hearing Timmy's advice, I rethought my response the day before in Las Vegas, when John had been distant and I had been frightened. Timmy had advised me to be soft, to allow my emotions to swing, to not always keep myself together—all the opposite of how I'd responded.

"Yesterday, when you were so distant," I asked John, "what if I'd told you I was feeling scared and needed to connect, instead of trying to be strong for you? How would you have responded to that?"

"Oh yeah, absolutely!" he said. "That would have been easy for me to be open to."

I felt a band loosen from around my chest, the same feeling I'd had when I'd been feeling anxious as I drove into Santa Fe after Death Valley and the thought had fallen into my mind, *I died out there in the desert.* I wasn't responsible to make things work out. I could just be where I was, feel what I felt, inhabit my poor, beaten-up body free of burden and duty. I could live that way by myself, and I could do so with John too.

Huh, I thought. *Well, that's something that's come out of that session with Timmy. I still don't know if he had any special insight, but hey, he managed to spur something in me!*

JOHN WAS DRIVING when we got to the jeep trail snaking up the rocky moonscape of Trail Canyon. At one point, I warned him the next bit was a little tricky, and he should speed up and stay to the right. But instead, he stopped and inched forward—and then got stuck.

"Can I drive?" I asked, fighting back my irritation. John got out and gave the van the slight push it needed to get unstuck, and then I gunned it up the hill, dodging the potholes.

When John got back in the car, he said, "All right then!" He also reported that a fellow camping down the road had walked up to see if we needed help, and after I got up the hill, he'd asked, "Got a four-wheel-drive van there?" John had laughed and said, "Nope! Just a very determined woman."

My breath caught as we pulled up to my campsite from a year earlier. It had come to feel mythical to me. It looked unchanged, and I wondered if anyone had camped there since me. I felt an odd nervousness, like I was bringing my boyfriend home to meet the family.

I looked out at the familiar view and thought back to the woman a year before, sitting in this spot, facing a cavernous darkness, with no idea of the transformation that lay ahead. I'd focused my hope on the fantasy of living alone in the desert with my dog in a Vanagon, and now here I was, in my Vanagon with my dog. I couldn't have imagined then, though, that I'd also be here with my beloved, and that I'd have a safe home and my health (well, mostly, albeit with some frightening reactions). I felt my gratitude spilling beyond my body, reaching toward the Amargosa Mountains on the other side of the valley.

Then I heard John say "Julie!" Portent dripped from his voice. As soon as I jumped out of the car, I heard a hissing sound. John pointed underneath the engine. Drops of green fluid sizzled against the radiator.

"This has to be from bumping up that bad spot," John said, with an accusatory tone I'd never heard from him before. "I saw the exhaust pipe scrape on the ground. The car is almost thirty years old. It's just too delicate for that."

I froze. *He could be right.*

The engine was so hot that we had to wait before we could figure anything out, so we sat quietly next to each other in Maxine, thigh to thigh on her bench seat, retreating into her tiny protected space. We didn't say it, but we both knew we might be in really big trouble. Would a tow truck even come up here? If it didn't, what could we do?

Defensive thoughts swirled in my brain. *Gary's low-slung Subaru had no problem with that. And coming here in Maxine was part of my original image in getting her. If she's too delicate to bring to places like this, I'm not sure I want her.* I thought I could almost hear the reversed mirror image of these thoughts swirling in John's brain, a cacophony of blame.

I looked out the window at that enormous view, breathing it in, absorbing the hugeness of this place, its stillness, its ancientness. These mountains didn't care a whit about whether I'd screwed up, or whether we'd get Maxine out of there, or whether we'd have a big fight. I felt the part of me that didn't care much about any of those things either, the part of me that was as ancient and enormous and calm as this valley. If we were going to have a fight, well, okay. Worse things had happened.

I leaned against him, feeling his solidity. John wrapped his arm around me. "I'm really glad to be here with you," he said. "If we can never come here again in Maxine, at least we're here now."

I put my head against his shoulder, the divisive thoughts swirling past me and away. *I'm safe,* I thought. *Even if I really screwed up, I'm still safe.*

We decided to enjoy ourselves and deal with Maxine later.

WE QUICKLY FELL into the rhythms of the place. John rode his bike way up the canyon, and on the way up, Frances stopped to sniff and then caught up with him. On the way down, she ran full-out, delighted to at last have her speed tested. We prepared gourmet dinners on Maxine's two-burner stove and ate them by candlelight. We spent hours making love in her pop-top, feeling the van rocking beneath us. Unlike a year earlier, I spent no time as a zombie in bed.

A couple of days before we left, John called our mechanic in Boulder to ask for advice. "John," he said, "you're a smart man, and Julie's a smart woman. You've just got to get inventive. Got any duct tape? Got any electrical tape?"

We managed to trace the leak to a crack close to the end of a hose. When we reported our findings to our mechanic, he said that the hose was old and poised to break. At worst, my bouncing up the road sped it up slightly. We found that there was enough slack in the hose for us to trim the end and reattach it. Maxine was ready to roll.

I CALLED TIMMY when we got back to Boulder. The convulsions had scared the hell out of me—I had to find some way to calm down my reactivity. Plus, I'd found the reading helpful. It seemed dumb not to give his "energy work" a try, no matter how ridiculous I felt.

A few days later, I returned to Timmy's dark hobbit house, walked through the kitchen, and returned to the room with the table covered in tchotchkes. He asked me to lie down on a single bed. I eyed it nervously: Beds were dangerous objects for me. But I cooperated, and he put pillows under my legs and asked if I was comfortable. I was—so far, the bed didn't seem intent on killing me.

He started with fairly conventional relaxation exercises, having me progressively tense and relax different parts of my body, breathing deeply. *Okay,* I thought. *So far, I can handle this.*

Then he asked me to think back to when I was seven and my mother had made my siblings leave. Was there a specific moment that I remembered?

I described the day my brother came out of my mother's bedroom and told me she'd said he had to leave. I recalled the porch swing, my unsuccessful attempt to eavesdrop on their conversation, my brother's body next to me on the swing, the feeling of not knowing what to say, my confusion about what it meant that he had to leave, the impossible effort to hold on to my mother and my brother both.

I could feel the fear in my body: There were terrible possibilities in the world that I had never imagined—and now one was happening to me. Not only was the loss of my brother unfathomably awful, I had no idea what the next unimaginable calamity might be. I felt my love for my big brother, the shock of having him just gone. I felt the extremity of my effort to make my mother happy, the exhausting, grinding, depleting work, the feeling that everything depended on my doing it right.

"Breathe that out!" Timmy said, as enthusiastically as a track coach. "Hoo-hoo-hoo!" He panted like a woman in childbirth, and I followed his example.

"And where was your father in all this?" Timmy asked. I suppressed the urge to give the answer I'd given as a child: "I don't have one." I'd always been irritated when people didn't accept that answer, which had struck me as quite sufficient. Instead, I told Timmy the history: My parents had been married to other people when I'd been born; my mother left her husband but my father stayed with his wife, and I had never known him. "Hmm," Timmy mused. "So you were all alone in dealing with your mother after that, with no one to protect you?" I nodded mutely.

We talked about how terrified I had been after my siblings left that I'd be sent away too. When I was 10, a few months after my mother rescued me when I'd walked out of class, I was sitting on her bed talking to her as I so often did, trying to figure out how to make her happy. And, as often was the case, she was mad at me for not doing it well enough. She repeated a common statement of hers: "You don't have to do it"—where "it" was completely undefined and the object of my desperate efforts at ascertainment—"but if you don't want to, you have to tell me. It's only fair." She paused, and then added, "Then I'll know what I need to know about you."

I was quite certain I knew what she'd do if she "knew what she needed to know about me."

She sent me off to think about all this. My thoughts scrabbled: *What do I need to do? What is going to make her happy?*

Then something broke in me. *I don't want to do this. I don't want to work so hard to make her happy, only to be told I'm failing. This is wrong.*

I imagined packing my stuff up and going off to Houston to live with my uncle Steve. I'd heard a bit about life there from Robin: The children's schedules were very regimented, with school performance valued above all, and I got the sense that Robin felt like an eternal guest, obliged to be on her best behavior. Though I did very well in school, performing wasn't on my agenda, and all the rest sounded bad too. Much more appealing to stay with my mother, who loved me and whom I loved.

But this wasn't right.

I went back into my mother's bedroom. "Send me away," I said. "I don't want to do it."

As I told Timmy the story, I could feel the rigidity in my back, my muscles offering all their strength to support me. I described seeing the shock spread over my mother's face. She was nowhere close to sending me away, I realized. I had called her bluff.

She never said anything like that again.

"Hoo-hoo-hoo!" Timmy panted. "Hoo-hoo-hoo!" I huffed in return.

Timmy asked what I would say to that little girl now, if I could, and I came up with this: "You are so radiant, and you do so much for your mother simply by being who you are. It's not your job to make her happy or meet her needs, even if she thinks it is. Nor is it your job to save your brother. Your only job is to be your own beautiful little self, and in so doing, you *are* helping your mother and your brother, tremendously. And, my god, you are brave. You are so, so brave. It's going to take a while, but someday, you won't have to be quite so brave."

I imagined me now, or my "higher self," going back in time and holding the child me, dissolving time and telling her that whenever she needs me, she can call on me and I'll be there for her. I could feel her wiry body melting in my lap, snuggling against me like Frances did. I told her that yes, there were terrible things that would inevitably happen, but even so, she was safe. She would hurt, but still, she'd be okay. Profoundly okay.

After a few more minutes of breathing, Timmy led me to another event that I had mentioned to him only briefly: When I was six, a stranger had picked me out from among my friends in a park and asked me if I'd like some honey. "I don't like honey," I'd said guilelessly. He offered me chocolate next, but I told him I didn't like that either (I was a strawberry ice cream kind of girl). Then he'd said with some frustration that he had lots of candy, and I should come check it out. That got me: *Lots of candy? I want to see that! Anyway, I don't have to eat any.*

The man led me to a protected portal around the side of the rec center, pulled his penis out of his pants, and forced me to put my mouth on it. I gagged, but he pushed my head down, over and over, as he stroked his penis and grunted. Then a vile taste filled my mouth. (Timmy suggested that this was the "wetness" I was afraid of, though I was doubtful.)

The man let me go afterward, and as I walked away, I threw up. He yelled something mean sounding at me, but I kept walking. When I came around the corner, my mother came toward me. I was convinced I was going to be in trouble and panicked, running crying to the car.

Although that strategy was spectacularly unsuccessful at hiding the situation from my mother, it was excellent for getting the help I needed: My mother quickly made the brilliant deduction that something was wrong and got me to tell her what happened.

Then she handled it beautifully. She not only reassured me that it wasn't my fault, she called the police. Black-uniformed police officers drove up to our house in their white police cars, and then they gently asked me questions.

"That was a very bad man," they told me. "If we find him, we'll put him in jail." I believed them, and I believed that it wasn't my fault. I'd always thought that the quick intervention had spared me from most of the trauma, and I'd never felt like it had a major, lasting impact.

Timmy had me holler "No!" to the man over and over, encouraging me to say it deep from my belly. "No, you can't touch me! No, you can't hurt me!"

Then I thought about the poor guy who molested me, who had to have been a desperately tortured soul. I imagined my higher self in the park that day, talking to that sad, twisted man. In my mind, the two of us watched my child-self together, and I told him that he wasn't allowed to touch her but he could draw strength and hope just by watching her. He could know that within him was a child as blameless and beautiful as the one he was watching, as deserving of protection and love. My child-self continued to play obliviously with her friends, swinging on the monkey bars, her luminousness undimmed, as if in a bubble of protection.

AS WE WERE ENDING the session, I wasn't sure what had come from it. What does it mean to process trauma anyway? Was I in any way different after this than I was before—and what difference could I hope for? I didn't feel any different.

But it also struck me as a reasonable-enough approach, and something that was generally useful, not so different from what a therapist might do. I'd talked about these events with therapists in the past, but it hadn't included the breathing exercises or the visualizations about my "higher self." I'd liked those aspects of the session, and maybe they'd been helpful.

Just before I left, Timmy said something that shocked me: "The association with mold is entirely broken." I would never be bothered by mold again, he claimed.

I almost laughed. *Yeah, right,* I thought. *Fat chance.* But then I caught myself. *Hey, I am not too proud to have the power of suggestion work on me! Let's not channel too much energy into skepticism.*

John and I met for dinner that night at a restaurant in a hotel, and I told him about the session. After John heard the story, he said, "Let's test it!"

The restaurant was fine for me, but we knew from previous experience that the lobby of the hotel wasn't. So after dinner, I walked into the lobby.

Instantly, I felt the mold hit me: My legs weakened, my consciousness dimmed. *Ah, shit. Well, what did I really expect? One session doing woo-woo stuff with a psychic couldn't possibly fix me.*

I was going to turn around to leave, but then I realized I could cross the lobby and get to the outside nearly as fast as I could return to the restaurant. So I kept going, rushing to get out before I collapsed.

But when I reached the exit, I realized that I didn't feel so bad. I stood with my hand on the handle, ready to flee, monitoring my body. *I feel kind of okay.* I decided to try walking around the lobby, returning to the spot that had felt so bad.

I was definitely aware of the mold—it felt a bit like a swarm of gnats inside my head, buzzing away—but the weakness and dimming-of-consciousness was gone. The mold wasn't felling me. It was nothing more than an irritation.

Oh my god. I think it worked. I may have been healed by a psychic.

CHAPTER 23

PSYCHIC SCIENCE

Over the following weeks, I tested Timmy's bewitchment further, going into places that were previously forbidden to me. I could go to Trader Joe's! I could wait hours to take a shower after an exposure, letting laziness reign! I could venture down into the dank basement at John's house in Boulder! John was even more pleased about the basement than I was—the washing machine was down there, so he had been forced to do the endless laundry himself.

I still felt mold very strongly, and I still got the hell out when I did. But I didn't get paralyzed, didn't collapse, didn't go into screaming convulsions.

I also wouldn't have said I felt cured. I woke up every morning feeling crappy, and getting functional required a couple of hours of detox (primarily saunas and coffee enemas, which continued to be amazingly effective). But I felt vastly safer in the world.

The whole thing was rather intellectually embarrassing. I forced myself to be open about it, even reporting the experience to my science-writer friends. After all, I figured, the first step in the scientific method is to gather data—even data that doesn't fit your preferred theory, even data that seems kooky, even data that might make you look crazy. And certainly, my preferred theory was *not* that my illness was caused by psychological trauma or that the appropriate cure was a healing by a psychic.

When I thought about the situation carefully, I didn't think those conclusions explained my experiences all that well. To say that psychological trauma was the sole cause, I would have had to know that without the trauma, I wouldn't have gotten sick no matter what my mold exposures were. That was a huge leap beyond the evidence at hand.

Furthermore, my Berkeley washcloth experiment gave strong evidence that contamination was doing something directly to my body, independent of my awareness. So to explain the whole phenomenon on a psychological level, my brain would have to be reacting to a stimulus that I was unconscious of. That would be extraordinary—like a vet flying to the ground when a car silently backfired.

And finally, if psychology was the sole cause, then presumably addressing psychology would be the sole cure. But as big a difference as Timmy's treatment made and as much as I hoped it would cure me, I couldn't get that far. I still suffered if I spent too much time in a moldy building, or if I failed to decontaminate within a few hours. Moving into a moldy house would almost certainly send me back into terrible illness. Perhaps that meant I just needed to do more psychological work, but if so, I couldn't figure out how.

Still, it was clear that somehow, Timmy had dramatically reduced my reactivity. But how? "Psychology," after all, isn't a magic wand that can accomplish anything, good or bad. Whatever Timmy had done for me, it had to have operated through some mechanism.

I developed a theory: In learning to avoid mold, I had focused on the tiniest indications that I was exposed, and then I'd made a very big deal out of them, getting the hell out of wherever I was and going through elaborate rituals to decontaminate myself. I was essentially teaching my brain that certain sensations were really alarming and important. And subsequently, those responses became stronger. I had trained my body to react.

That training was very useful: Without it, I couldn't keep myself from getting poisoned. And I had little question that I *had* been poisoned—I couldn't explain the whole thing as a trained response. After all, I was terribly ill long before I suspected that mold could be a cause, and avoiding mold had brought me a dramatic and lasting improvement (at the cost of some terrible reactions).

The problem was that I had gotten into an upward spiral, with each reaction digging a kind of groove into my brain that made the next reaction stronger. Somehow, I figured, Timmy had broken this spiral. That narrowed things down, but it still left the question: How?

I told the story to Thilo Deckersbach, a Harvard psychologist who both did research and treated patients, and he thought it made perfect sense. "His treatment was brilliant!" Deckersbach said. "State of the art."

Anxiety, Deckersbach thought, was the key. He was quick to add that he was convinced that mold really did cause direct physiological problems—it wasn't "all in my head." But after so many experiences of mold sickening me, Deckersbach argued, I couldn't help but be anxious when I felt exposed. The anxiety itself further drove the reaction, and Timmy's treatment had helped with that component of the problem.

Deckersbach also thought he knew how Timmy did it: It was a variation of a treatment Deckersbach used with his anxiety patients called exposure and response prevention, which had strong scientific backing.

Suppose, Deckersbach explained, that a patient is terrified of flying. On a plane, he experiences extreme physical symptoms—heart palpitations, sweating, difficulty breathing. His fear feeds the symptoms, and the symptoms feed his fear. He avoids flying, and the few times he's tried it, he's fled the plane. Deckersbach would arrange for such a patient to sit on an airplane separate from a flight. The patient would feel his terror but not allow himself to flee, and eventually, the terror would begin to fade. He'd do it again and find himself not quite as frightened, with fewer physical symptoms. Eventually, he'd fly, and the experience of surviving it would further decrease the fear.

Deckersbach's theory was that Timmy had given me the courage to stay in the moldy hotel lobby longer than I would have otherwise. I had discovered that the mold didn't harm me as I expected, and that had decreased my anxiety and hence my future reactions.

In this understanding, most of what Timmy did was irrelevant. Timmy's theory that my sensitivity to mold was rooted in childhood trauma was likely bunk, and neither the reading nor the energy work had made the difference directly. Instead, it had provided an elaborate illusion that had inspired me to break my own cycle of anxiety.

Much as I loved having my bizarre experience put into a scientifically respectable framework, an objection niggled at my mind: I didn't decide to stay in the hotel lobby. I was fleeing, just as I would have if I'd wandered into that room unsuspecting. The only reason I didn't turn around was that I thought I could get across the room about as quickly. And the only reason I didn't continue to flee was because the reaction had already started to fade, before my behavior changed. Plus, I'd stayed in other moldy places for longer than that plenty of times before without the reaction abating—say, the time I collapsed paralyzed in a movie theater. Furthermore, my experience in the hotel lobby hadn't changed my long-term response to exposures, since I still got the hell out of there. And yet the improvement from Timmy held up: I didn't get paralyzed, my brain didn't fuzz over, I didn't lose the power to talk.

Still, I found Deckersbach's idea useful, with some modification. It seemed to me Timmy had done something to reset me, putting me lower down on the reactivity spiral. I imagined this as a sort of psychic version of a beta-blocker, the drug that people with stage fright often use to prevent racing hearts and sweaty palms when performing.

But after Timmy had reduced my initial reaction, I could imagine that the analogy with the patient who's afraid of flying might apply: Each time I reacted less than I expected, I grew more confident and less anxious, further reducing the component of the reaction due to anxiety. That got rid of the extreme reactions like getting crippled or going into convulsions. My assumption was that the milder responses, like the feeling of compression of my nervous system or my teeth chattering, were direct impacts of the mold on my neurological and immune systems. Since they weren't mediated by anxiety (I presumed), Timmy's "treatment" didn't affect them.

Like Deckersbach, I had a hard time accepting Timmy's view that my vulnerability to mold was directly caused by my early traumas. I couldn't disprove it, but I didn't feel like I had any strong evidence to support it either, despite the success of his treatment.

What made more sense to me is that mold attacked my body, and it would have even if I'd had the easiest of childhoods. But whatever our inner vulnerabilities, they may end up relevant in a situation like this. When my body was under attack, it felt like an even bigger attack because I felt unprotected and profoundly alone, based on my childhood experiences. And it seemed reasonable to me that internalizing a sense of protection and connection helped reset my body, reducing the physiological perception of threat. This reduction, I thought, was the essence of Timmy's "psychic beta-blocker."

I couldn't prove all those connections scientifically, but they also didn't require anything supernatural or woo-woo, despite Timmy's credentials. Nor did that theory make the reactions my fault, or make my illness a psychological one, or put me in a different category from any other ill person. My feeling of unprotectedness would likely have exacerbated any illness I might have gotten, whether ME/CFS or multiple sclerosis or lupus. And we already had good evidence that psychology could impact many illnesses whose physiological basis was clearly understood: People are more likely to have heart attacks, for example, at moments of great anger. Furthermore, having a psychological treatment help didn't make it a fundamentally psychological disease. If I'd had multiple sclerosis and a hormone treatment improved my symptoms, that wouldn't make my disease fundamentally hormonal—the immune system dysregulation and breakdown of myelin sheaths would still be at the root of it.

Still, it was painful to have a psychological intervention like this have such a helpful impact on me when the mental health profession had had such a vicious impact on patients with ME/CFS. I couldn't help but feel like I was betraying my fellow patients. I also felt extremely vulnerable: If I allowed any crack in the imagined door separating mind from body, I worried that I (and the entire illness) would get shoved through it, locked onto the wacko side. And I felt uncomfortable arguing, "I am not a wacko!" It had an uncomfortable resonance with "I am not a crook!"— once I started defending myself from that accusation, I'd already lost.

Ultimately, I simply didn't believe in this division of mind and body. I considered that whole model deeply unscientific. It makes no sense to imagine our minds floating freely outside our bodies, occasionally screwing up and creating illness. The mind and body aren't just connected, they're aspects of the same thing, heads and tails, yin and yang, utterly inextricable.

Dealing with illness skillfully, I thought, required analyzing that yin-yang relationship in a nuanced way. Psychology and physiology weren't opponents in a winner-take-all game. They were partners in a dance. And it was my job to help them move to the music with more connection and grace.

ABOUT A MONTH AFTER Timmy's bewitchment, I got a call from Troy, one of my half sisters on my father's side, saying that she was going to be in Denver. Would John and I like to meet for dinner? I of course said yes.

She looked the same as she had when I'd first met her and my other half siblings a decade earlier, dressed in a crisp white shirt and pearls, with platinum blond hair and a soft Texas drawl. She embraced us warmly, and we talked about our lives. I told her about my health, and she told me she'd been dealing with similar health issues, though she was convinced that mold wasn't at the root of it. She cooed over the story of our courtship.

I wasn't sure that we would talk about our father. I didn't know what to ask—I'd asked all the questions I could think of a decade earlier, and my half siblings had each been generous in sharing him with me. Still, my knowledge of him felt flat, two-dimensional. It made me feel like a bad journalist. Shouldn't I be better at coming up with questions?

When we finished our food, she asked me if I'd like to hear about our dad, and then stories poured out of her. Most of them were familiar from before, but I felt the stories clicking together in my mind for the first time.

Like me, our father, Don, had grown up without a dad. He was the youngest of seven kids, deserted by their father during the Depression in tiny Palestine, Texas. At eight years old, he was working in the fields to help support his family.

After a few hard-earned years of college, he started the first of a long string of businesses: a burger stand, then billboards, then insurance.

In the early 1960s, he moved to a bigger stage when the Federal Communications Commission decided to release the last AM radio frequency in Texas, KEYH, to the person who would use it to best serve the public interest. He beat out the richest families in Houston to get it, selling himself on his then-unheard-of vision of an all-news radio station (despite his complete lack of experience in news). His reporters won awards for their investigations, but all-news radio was so novel that the station never made much money.

In the meantime, he'd become deeply involved with minority communities in Houston, starting an Optimist Club for black people and a chapter of the Special Olympics. Houston had hundreds of thousands of Hispanic residents, with no citywide radio station to serve them. He converted his to all-Spanish language, and it became the number-one radio station in Houston.

But his greatest successes were followed by great failures. Though he loved inventing businesses, the daily work of running them bored him. He got in trouble with the Internal Revenue Service when he traded radio advertising for goods and didn't count the trades as income. His insurance company did well until a series of natural disasters in Texas in the early 1980s. He won the legal battle that ensued when the bankruptcy liquidator claimed he'd used money from that business to prop up another, but it exhausted him.

He looked like a typical Texas man with his 10-gallon Stetson, Cadillac, and cowboy boots, but he lacked a taste for hunting or golf and remained on the outside of the good-ol'-boy clubs. The Christian Science church was his only community—as a smart, ambitious, penniless boy, he had loved both its intellectualism and the wealth of its members—and he became one of its leaders.

Before I came along, Don and his wife would see my mother and her husband at church every Sunday. Don and my mother worked together to establish a new branch of the church in Texas City, walking from house to house as they passionately discussed how to appeal to its poor black population—all the while, falling in love.

Don had, of course, never told Troy what the secret relationship meant to him, but she said that from her memories of the two of them, she thought they were well suited, perhaps even sharing a great love.

Here, I jumped in to tell Troy the small bits my mother had told me about their relationship. During the three years of their affair, she'd reworked her life, intensely seeking God. Before meeting Don, she had dropped out of college to marry at 18, working as a secretary until my sister, Robin, was born. When she couldn't get pregnant a second time, she adopted my brother, Ty. She kept house and tended to the children. The confines of her proper life cut deep, and she was convinced that a clear-sighted, principled search for God was the way out.

Don was the first person she'd met who thought as deeply as she did, who believed as passionately that principle and spirit underlay the world. She longed to become a Christian Science healer, guiding the sick to health through prayer. My father promised to use his influence to help her succeed. When my mother became pregnant with me, she felt I was her "answer," the outcome of all her seeking and prayer.

Troy told me that after my birth in 1972, she would come to our house with her parents and assorted siblings to play with "the baby"— me, who, unbeknownst to the rest of them, was Don's baby. Troy babysat me and made pralines with my mother, awestruck by how my tall, dark, glamorous mom resembled Jackie O. During that time, my father spotted a cradle at an antique auction with his wife. "That would be the perfect gift for Susan Rehmeyer!" he cried, and bought it, stunning his poor wife. (The story brought a shock of recognition for me: I had loved that cradle so much that long after I outgrew it, I would oust its stuffed-animal occupants and climb in, my legs splaying over its wooden sides.)

When I was six months old, my mother left her husband. But my father stayed with his wife, who learned of the affair a couple of years later. Don denied I was his child, and she believed him. Still, she insisted that they move a distance from my mother to a ranch in the country. When I was almost five, we moved to San Diego, after my mother's relationship with both the church and her family had become strained when she refused to hide my origins (especially, rumor held, as I grew to look more and more like my half sister Tricia).

Halfway across the country from us, my father was always working on projects at his ranch, hauling his kids up at seven each Saturday morning, crying: "Time's a-wasting! We've got lots to do!" He'd sit on the porch swing with Troy for hours and talk, planting ideas. "Ever thought of holding a horse show?" he asked her when she was a teenager. "What steps would it take to start one?" And then a couple of weeks later: "Thought any more about that horse show? What about a series of horse shows? What about putting together a brochure for them and selling advertising?" Troy ended up doing all of that, running horse shows at 16. This story left me looking down at the table blinking hard, imagining an alternative reality with my own young legs swaying on that porch swing, my voice singing out answers to my father's questions.

I told Troy about how I had talked to Don exactly once that I remember, when I was 18 and my mother was dying. I'd called Information, and the operator had rattled off my father's number. My hand shook as I wrote it down.

I dialed it over and over, hanging up two digits short, then one digit short, then just after finishing the number. Finally, I allowed the phone to ring.

"Hello?" a man's voice answered.

"Is this Don?" I asked.

"Yes."

"This is Julie Rehmeyer."

"Unnnh-huh," my father said. I wasn't sure what kind of response I'd expected, but it wasn't that.

"I'm, uh, Susan Rehmeyer's daughter."

"Unnnh-huh," he said, his voice as flat and closed as the first time.

I struggled for something to say next. Then, to my relief, he asked me a couple of questions, banal things like where we were living. I mentioned that my mother was sick, maybe dying.

Silence. I worked up my gumption. "I was just wondering, if you might like to . . . um . . . have some kind of relationship?"

"No," he said.

"Okay, bye!" I squeaked, hanging up the phone as fast as I could.

A few months later, I heard that he'd died. He was 61.

Troy told me that around the time I'd called, his life was falling apart. His latest businesses had failed and he was trying to win back his wife, who had finally left him. Still, he had new business ideas that were, as usual, ahead of their time: For one, he unsuccessfully tried to sell the idea of cogeneration power plants to Kenneth Lay at Enron, a decade before they made Enron millions upon millions of dollars. He also had a non-paying project, a plan for businesses to provide at-risk kids with mentors throughout their school careers.

In December 1990, my father remarked to Troy's husband, "If I die now, I'll die a happy man. I've already lived the life of seven men." A week later, he had a seizure, and he insisted on no doctors, no ambulance, no hospital. He was ready, he said, and he died that night. He might have felt complete, Troy told me, but he was also just tired.

Of course, that meant he felt complete without having ever known me. Troy's view was that my father had an impossible problem: He saw himself as an upright man, but he had fathered a child from a long, intense affair. He was committed to his five previous children and his wife who had stuck by him for decades, but she could neither connect with the parts of him that my mother had nor handle my existence. What was the moral thing to do? He made his choice.

Had he lived longer, Troy said, she was certain he would have gotten in contact with me. When I called him, his desire to reunite with his wife made my very existence dangerous for him—but Troy's mother was done, not coming back. And if we had gotten to know one another, Troy said, my father and I would have taken great pleasure in one another. "You have the same kind of mind."

When Troy wrapped her arms around me at the end of the evening, I felt as though the hug were being transmitted across death and time and space from my father.

A FEW WEEKS LATER, when we next returned to Boulder, I woke up in the middle of the night feeling poisoned, unable even to sit up in bed. John had to help me get to the shower. I hadn't felt like that since before Timmy's bewitchment. We resumed our familiar routine: John pulled off the sheets while I showered, and then I made the bed with fresh sheets. But even while making the bed, I started feeling poisoned again. The bed, it seemed, was contaminated.

Even worse, we'd left our camping pads in Santa Fe. I'd been doing so much better that we'd gotten less careful about such things. We ended up squishing together to sleep, rather miserably, on the couch (John refused to sleep apart from me). A friend from Berkeley—Berkeley of the dreaded ick—had stayed in the house while we'd been gone, and I figured that the extensive precautions we'd given her must not have been enough.

I managed to get in to see Timmy the next day, hoping for a repeat performance of his miracle cure.

He had me lie once more on the single bed in his office, and this time, he asked me to think back to the first time I'd felt sick. I told him the story about the day after our plaster party, when we were building the house and Geoff was falling apart and I could barely walk up the path to the house. That was when I thought for the first time, "Maybe I'm not just tired. Maybe I'm sick."

He asked me detailed questions about it, reimmersing me in that moment. I again felt as though I were losing everything—my husband, my life, and most of all, my sense of my own potency. I again felt that desperate, disoriented incomprehension closing in on me, the sense that I could no longer hear God's voice, that the currents I'd oriented myself to my whole life had dried up. I felt all alone in this impossible situation, determined to save my husband and get my house built but slowly recognizing that the task was way beyond my capabilities. I could feel my poor exhausted body sagging against Geoff's arm as I looked up the path, fighting the urge to dissolve into the pine needles at my feet.

"Now bring in your higher spirits," Timmy said. "What would they say to you? What would they do?"

I felt those spirits pulling me out of my leaden body, raising me up to hover above the scene with them. All the stress and difficulty stayed down in that poor exhausted body, and I was free to float above the lush stripe of the valley that swept down the mountain and out across the desert, a miracle of green and plenty amongst the dryness. The straw of my house gleamed golden against the brown patches of mud plaster, as if the house were the love child of the sun and the earth. I felt as though I were seeing the house for the first time, no longer obscured by the miasma of the endless list of tasks it represented. It took my breath away, gorgeous even in its incompleteness.

Next, the image came into my mind of the spirits of my parents joining us, floating above the valley. My mother looked at me with a love I'd forgotten in all those years since she'd died, a love that had vanished from my understanding of the world. Even my father wrapped his arms around me, claiming me as his own. In my mind, I stayed in his arms a long time, feeling his hard, round belly against my own, my head resting on his shoulder.

A long line of ancestors joined us, a huge tribe of people whose blood and lives and loves flowed through me, many of whom had devoted their lives to ensuring that I might live. I felt as though I had an invisible army standing behind me, not just at that moment but all the time.

The idea that I was alone suddenly seemed laughable.

This whole clan lifted that poor heavy dead body of mine up from its heap on the ground, whooshing and glowing all the death and heaviness out of it, suffusing it once more with my spirit. I was restored to my body, but I knew I could choose which of my burdens to pick up along with it. None were mandatory. I didn't have to build this house. I didn't have to stay with Geoff. I didn't have to be a professor. I didn't have to redeem my mother or be a success at anything.

I returned to my house, bouncing up and down the temporary staircase made of straw bales, spinning around the great open upstairs, which felt like a big dance floor with its internal walls still unbuilt. *I can't know, at this moment, if I'll be able to finish this house. But it doesn't really matter. It's beautiful, just as it is.*

I would keep working on it, but only with a sense of ease and pleasure. If I was lucky, those unburdened labors would lead to its completion. But that, I accepted, was beyond my control. Nor could I know what would happen to Geoff. *I can't save him, no more than I could save my mother. All I can do is love him and let him find his way.*

A rush of something like joy filled me, an awe at the beauty of my life at that very moment, living in those moldy trailers with my crazy husband, breaking body, and half-built house. I felt as though I had been clutching on to him, my hand exhausted. I let go, I turned to him, and I bowed.

As we wrapped up the session, my body felt purified, light, spacious. Timmy told me that before bed, I should visualize a force field of protection around myself. I should remember my parents and all those ancestors surrounding me, supporting me, defending me. I should think of the man who had molested me in the park and again say "No!" from deep in my belly, imagining my family saying it with me. *I am connected. I am supported. I am protected.*

That night, I slept through the night in the bedroom. The next morning, I felt better than I had in ages.

As much as I appreciated Timmy's help, I didn't want to be dependent on a psychic every time I had a nasty reaction. Plus, the problem with a bizarre, incomprehensible cure is that it wouldn't be especially bizarre or incomprehensible for it to just stop working. So I began to think about more direct ways that I could, on my own, convince my nervous system that mild exposures to mold were not a catastrophic threat and to teach it to respond calmly.

And that made my thoughts drift back to training Frances.

When I taught Frances to get along with John's cat, Lao, the precise thing I was doing was rewiring her nervous system so that she responded to him calmly. When she first met Lao, her excitement so overwhelmed her that she couldn't take in any information. Her brain had exploded. When she was frantically scrabbling and whining to get at the cat, her nervous system was overloaded—just like mine when I was screaming and convulsing. The first step in training her had less to do with teaching and more to do with reducing her brain overload.

The tool I had employed in this neurological intervention had been cheese. When I'd crammed cheese into Frances's mouth as Lao appeared, I'd sent her brain firing along a different neural pathway, focused on the amazing windfall that was raining down upon her taste buds. So then the question was, what was my version of cheese? What would my neurological system find sufficiently compelling to distract it from a freak-out? I didn't know, but I figured I'd just try everything I could think of.

I decided to undergo "training sessions" like I'd given Frances by going into my trailers. When I walked in, I definitely felt the mold: I felt a sense of pressure in my nervous system, a creepy-crawly feeling on my skin. The trailers were not as bad as many buildings in town, and I was glad—just as we'd kept Lao far enough away from Frances to not overwhelm her, I figured I needed to start with a building that didn't have mold sliming across the walls. And I kept my first session short, just a few minutes, for the same reason.

I started by talking to myself, out loud. "Thank you, nervous system, for letting me know about the mold in here. I hear you. You've been doing me such a service in alerting me to mold—I've really needed that, so that I had a chance to heal. But we're doing so incredibly well now! Remember how okay we were in that moldy hotel lobby? No way could we have handled that months ago. So I'm confident that you can handle a few minutes of being in here now. You can trust me—I'm listening to you, and I promise I won't let you get hurt. But for a few minutes, we're going to be fine."

After that, I got inventive. Sometimes I meditated or did yoga. Sometimes I stroked my skin soothingly. Often I put on raucous music and danced. Sometimes I walked around congratulating myself for how well I was doing, throwing my arms in the air in a victory sign, giving myself hugs, jumping up and down in glee. Sometimes I visualized the mold bouncing off a force field around me, or entering my lungs and then being breathed right out. Sometimes I thought of that man in the park and practiced shouting "No!" as loud as I could, thrusting my arm up in a stop signal. Sometimes I thought of my tribe of ancestors surrounding me, keeping that bad man at a distance, and I mimed hugging them, one after another. My theory was that I wanted to do things that would reach my body and not just my mind, things that would convince my body that it was safe. Each time I noticed the mold, I acknowledged it, thanked my nervous system for the information, and told myself that at this level, it was just fine.

Day by day, I stretched my time in the trailers longer or waited longer to shower afterward. And day by day, I felt the strength of my reaction diminishing. Not only that, but I found that other moldy buildings were bothering me less as well. I didn't manage to end the reactions completely, but I did reduce them substantially.

Just as I didn't think that the success of my work with Timmy showed that my body's response to mold was purely an overreaction of my brain to an otherwise harmless substance, I didn't think this did either. Mold had to have hurt me before my brain could have learned to overreact.

But it made sense to me that once mold had sickened me, an exposure set off a characteristic firing pattern in my brain, over and over again. And that alone is enough to change a brain: An old saying in neuroscience is "Neurons that fire together, wire together." With each reaction, I was essentially practicing a particular response, as if I were playing a musical passage again and again on the piano, burning a pattern of finger movements into the wiring of my brain. Just as practicing piano allowed my fingers to flow more fluidly over the scales, "practicing" reactivity allowed my body to respond more quickly and powerfully to the presence of mold.

My ridiculous antics in the trailer were a way of unlearning that response. It was as if I'd made the same mistake over and over as I'd learned a new piece on the piano—the way to get rid of it was to start from the beginning and play the passage slowly, carefully, and accurately, as many times as necessary, rewiring that neural pathway in my brain, teaching it a new pattern of response.

I became convinced that I'd learned how to hack my own nervous system.

CHAPTER 24

A SHAKESPEAREAN ENDING

Six weeks after John and I first met, we were driving back to Santa Fe to meet up with my sister Robin and her husband, Kevin, who were driving in from Arkansas. It was the first time John would meet any of my family.

We'd just entered New Mexico and were driving past the smooth, round hump of San Antonio Mountain in companionable silence when a thought flitted through my mind so naturally I almost didn't even notice it: *One of these days, we'll have to get around to getting married.*

I reported the thought to John, commenting on my surprise both to have thought it and to have had it seem so self-evident. He responded intently: "Do you want to?"

"Yeah, at some point," I said, carefully keeping my voice light and casual.

"So . . . shall we tell people we're engaged?" John asked.

Oh my god! I thought. *That's not what I meant. I'm not ready for that. We haven't even had a fight yet. Maybe you turn into a monster!*

I couldn't figure out what to say. The silence stretched.

John reached for my hand. "That scared you, huh?" I gave a tight little nod.

"We don't have to do anything that scares you," he said. "We can take as much time as you want." I almost wept with relief.

THE WEEKEND WITH ROBIN AND KEVIN was perfectly comfortable, the four of us settling into an easy rhythm of chatting and cooking and hanging out and walking and fishing. The person I was with John and the person I was with Robin felt entirely compatible with one another, and when I talked with Robin about him, I felt a relaxed pleasure and pride in him I'd never felt about a previous partner.

John was training for a 31-mile trail race in the Rockies, no biggie by his hundred-mile, 15,000-foot-elevation-gain standards, and Kevin asked to join John on a run. "Okay," John said, "but I'm going to be running for five hours in the mountains. You up for that?"

"Sure!" Kevin said. Kevin ran fast road marathons with his buddies in Arkansas, and he calculated that the distance John was planning wouldn't be more than he was used to. He was well groomed and tightly muscled, a salesman for a pet-supply company to Walmart, with an extremely positive, can-do attitude perfectly suited for a soccer coach. As the two of them talked about the run, I could see male bonding in action.

Kevin arrived for the run with a fanny pack carrying two vials of water that held approximately one thimbleful apiece. John and I exchanged a look: *This guy has no idea what he's getting into.* But we got him supplied with extra water and off they went, out the door and up the trail.

Robin and I luxuriated in vicarious pleasure in their run. I described the route they'd be running through to her, starting at our house at 7,200 feet, going past waterfall after waterfall, up a rocky cliff, across an aspen-studded meadow, past the ski basin, up through dark ponderosas, and then above tree line at 11,600 feet, where they'd have views across the whole Rio Grande Valley. My favorite land in all the world.

We rushed out when we heard Kevin running up the driveway: "How was it? How was it?"

He stopped, spread his arms wide, looked up at the sky, and gave an exclamation I never heard from him before or since: "That was a spiritual experience!"

John ran in a half hour later, having added a side trip. He and Kevin gleefully recounted nearly every step of the run as they drank their beers and ate green chile stew and cornbread. John had coached him through it, teaching him form tricks, encouraging him to take energy from the landscape, helping him keep going when he thought he couldn't make it. The next day, on John's suggestion, the two of us bought a topographic map, drew the route on it, and framed it for Kevin as a gift.

As we drove to meet Robin and Kevin for dinner in town and give them the framed map, I told John that I'd changed my mind in the last few days. Holding back felt silly. "Let's tell them we're engaged."

"Are you sure?" he asked. "Like I said, there's no hurry. I'll wait for you as long as I need to." I just smiled and squeezed his hand in response.

Robin screamed and hugged us when we told her.

WE DECIDED TO HAVE the wedding in June of 2013, a year after we met. John, who had never been married, had clear ideas about it: He wanted to invite all his friends, he wanted music, he wanted dancing. A big shindig.

Oof. I thought. *I'm not sure I can do that.* I'd already had one wedding that was a big shindig. I was thinking instead of a few friends, a quiet ceremony, dinner afterward. But John was already waxing on about the songs he wanted on the wedding playlist, and I could see that no small, quiet ceremony would cut it. I was going to have to come around.

Over the year, as my health varied, the wedding felt like a goal line. By then, I wanted to be all better. I felt as though I were on a treasure hunt, finding the clues I needed to repair my health: mold avoidance, showers, laundry, ozone, coffee enemas, saunas, supplements, Timmy, connecting with my family, brain retraining. Each one seemed like a piece of a puzzle, and once I assembled them all, I would once more be whole—or at least I hoped so. I could feel a tension in myself around that, a sense of pressure, but I couldn't entirely let go of that expectation and ambition either.

Since we were going big on this wedding, I naturally invited all seven of my assorted siblings. I was sure Robin would come, but I hadn't seen

Ty in many years, and I had no idea how many of my half siblings on my father's side would make the trek—especially because they didn't all get along with one another. Two of them, Troy and Carol, hadn't spoken in years, driven apart by family history and clashing personalities. But one by one, I heard back from each one that they'd come. I held my breath: What would happen when Troy and Carol realized the other was also planning to come?

A little while later I heard from each of them, saying the same thing: "I'm coming for you, Julie. The rest will just have to work itself out."

Ty also said he was coming and bringing his seven-year-old son with him. But at the last moment, he told me he couldn't afford the airfare. A cousin of mine had given me a gift of $1,000 to spend on the wedding, "for something you wouldn't do otherwise," she said. I bought Ty and his son plane tickets with great satisfaction.

Never before had all eight of us siblings been together.

I WALKED DOWN the aisle on the arm of a dear friend. John was looking extremely dapper in white tails, with the continental divide providing a backdrop, its peaks still topped with the tiniest bit of white. We were in the meadow outside the house John owned in the mountains. He'd bought it years before I met him, the fulfillment of his Colorado mountain man dreams. After he'd lived there a couple of years, though, he grew so lonely—he was single then and didn't want to be—that he moved to a rented house in town and rented out his mountain house. John had sadly accepted that the mountain house was too moldy for me when I staggered out of it the first time. Having our wedding here felt like a way of pulling the potent energies the house contained forward into our life together.

John took my hand and helped me up onto our little stage in front of the audience. I looked out over everyone assembled: Not only were all seven of my siblings there, but also Geoff, cousins, and aunts and uncles of mine, John's family, old friends, joint friends, new friends, Frances— more than a hundred people who loved us (plus a dog). In the front row, we'd set aside chairs for our three parents who had died, with pictures and flowers. My mother's also had her gold watch; my father's had his cowboy boots and bolo tie. It seemed unimaginable that a year and a half earlier, I was lying in my trailers feeling utterly, profoundly alone, unsure whether I'd ever have much of a life again.

During the ceremony, John and I each spoke about why we loved each other. I started: "Being with John has opened me wide to the world . . ." Then I had to stop because I was already crying. I looked at John and he wiped a tear from my cheek. I buried my face in his neck, breathing him in and feeling his arm around my waist. I felt the seconds stretching as I worked to smooth my breathing.

Then I tried again. "Being with John has opened me wide to the world, infused every aspect of my life with meaning, and softened me. He's contributed to an amazing transformation in my life that began before I met him, helped to prepare me for him, and has only accelerated in the time I've known him."

I gave a quick sketch of my illness and described how generously and gracefully John responded to it. Then I talked about the spaciousness and ease and abundance he'd brought into my life, and to illustrate that, I told a story from the previous weekend, when we went for a hike with a couple of John's relatives. Early in the hike, I found myself feeling tired, and I told him that I needed to stop and rest but that they should continue. We were both disappointed—we'd hoped I'd be able to gambol up the trail like a mountain goat with him, as I sometimes could. But John immediately didn't just accept my decision; he embraced it, hugging me, equipping me with everything I might need, and continuing on with a bounce in his step.

After they disappeared up the trail, I lay on a rock, listening to the roar of the white water next to me, feeling the support of the earth and the cleansing power of that water, and all the while I felt as though John were right with me, holding me and cheering me on. I had the space I needed for myself because I knew I could trust him to enjoy himself without me. Eventually, I found myself up for walking on to rejoin them, and soon I saw John running down the trail toward me, his face aglow and his arms open wide.

"Over and over," I said during the ceremony, "my illness has presented John opportunities to feel resentful and constrained, but he's embraced the challenge every time, offering me his faith in my body's ability to heal. Most of the time, we've managed to make the whole thing feel like a crazy adventure, but there have been moments when we've both felt overwhelmed, worried that I'd never get better. Then John has embraced even that, his love burning through his fear, and he's told me that . . ." Here, I choked up again, and then spoke through my tears: "He's told me that even then he would be thrilled to be with me. I am quite awed by that."

When it was John's turn, I listened eagerly, not having heard in advance what he was going to say. He began by describing my lack of victimization and my courage in dealing with my illness and with life in general. "This has made it so easy for me to show up and be helpful," he said, "and to be a way I love to be, which is to feel needed. It's given me so much joy to be able to make a difference. I love to be able to help you." I'd long felt that from him, but still, I soaked in his words.

He went on to describe my combination of strength and softness; the comfort, ease, and spaciousness of our relationship; how our relationship supported him. He wrapped his comments up with this: "When I look into your rich brown eyes, I see an invitation and a reward at the same time—to be all that I am, to forgive all that I'm not, to heal all that's broken." My eyes filled with tears once more.

We didn't exchange vows. When we'd met with our officiant (a dear friend) to plan the ceremony, he'd crinkled his nose in disgust when we mentioned them. "You don't need that," he said. "Vows set you up for failure. They're heavy. Make offerings instead. Offer your partner only what you can easily, joyfully give." I had smiled when he'd said that— lightness and ease had filled our relationship from the beginning, so offerings felt just right.

So in the ceremony, I started off by offering John my deep joy in life, pointing out that the previous couple of years had taught me what an incredible gift it is to be alive and showed me that I could feel joy even when things were difficult, indeed even in the difficulties themselves. I offered him my commitment to keep myself aligned to that joy. I offered him my attention; my commitment to ask for what I wanted; my belief that there was plenty of space for both of us to have what we want, together and separately. And I offered my support in allowing his creative work to unfold and be central in his life, along with my certainty that this world needed the best, fullest expression of him and would provide him what he needed to bring it that.

John started, "I offer you my warmth and love and affection, in their endless supply. Because they come from a love larger than mine that is endless, I have a large love to share with you." That got me right away: *I'll take it!* Just as I had, he offered to let me know what he needed, and to help figure out how to get my needs met. He offered his communication skills, his peace, his support for my writing and emotional development, his sense of humor, his family and friends. When he added, "I offer you . . . a running companion," everyone laughed.

"I offer you a bond with me that will be family, and to add to that family in whatever form it takes. I know we will have offspring that will be love manifested, through home projects, writing projects, endless projects. And perhaps we will be so lucky"—here it was his turn to choke up—"to have offspring in the form of a child."

After we walked back down the aisle together, we wrapped each other up in a hug. Everyone else fell away, and our two bodies became an entire universe we inhabited together. I felt as though a channel had opened between the earth and the heavens, and a giant flow of energy was pouring down through us and out into the world, encompassing this beautiful place and all these people we loved. We stayed there for many long minutes, swaying gently together and kissing one another, as everyone got up and laughed and chatted and moved toward the drinks.

We finally let go, and I suddenly became aware that I was exhausted. We'd been pushing for weeks organizing the wedding, and suddenly, my energy was running dry. We'd known this might happen, so we'd set up Maxine in an out-of-the-way corner as a retreat. I let John know where I was going, and as I slid her metal door open and climbed inside, I felt so grateful for this little bubble of quiet. I laid down on her bench seat and let every muscle release, my mind pulling in, following the energy traveling through my bones and sinews. I pushed away my niggling fear that I wouldn't be strong enough to be at my own wedding.

One thing John had said when he was describing why he loved me floated back into my mind: "You even had the audacity to say you would be well by this wedding, and compared to where you've been, I'd say you're pretty damn near well!"

He was right—"pretty damn near." But I was not well, not as I'd imagined I'd be. I was in a different world than I'd been when I was unable to turn over in bed, alone, but my body still felt a bit like a toddler, to be managed and planned around, its needs coming first. I couldn't speak of the illness in the past tense—it was still with me, and it might always be. I couldn't know.

I tuned in to the leaden heaviness in my bones, and I stopped resisting it. I imagined it as my child-self, and I pulled it into my lap, feeling that wild, strong, frightened little being leaning into me. *You've been working hard, body, getting ready for this wedding on top of working to heal. Thank you, thank you, thank you. And I've been putting pressure on you on top of that, demanding that you be all the way well. I'm sorry. I take it back. You don't have to be any stronger or more healed than you are. Just rest, and absorb all this loving energy that surrounds you.* I closed my eyes, listened to the strains of music filtering down to me, and let my mind fall blank.

Maxine's door slid open, and John appeared with two plates of food, smiling. I sat up and kissed him, and thighs touching, we ate our food.

I REJOINED THE FESTIVITIES in time for socializing and then toasts, sitting as much as possible to preserve my energy. When I found myself flagging, I took a moment to look at that amazing view that John so loved, following the jagged ridgeline, feeling all that space that lay between me and it, drawing in the immense capacity of the earth. It didn't make the tiredness vanish, but it eased me back each time from its sharp edge, allowed me to stand beside it rather than jab against it.

Geoff came over and wrapped his arms around me. "I'm so happy to see you so happy," he said, and I felt a rush of love for him and gratitude for that day 20 years earlier when I'd seen him in that MIT classroom and thought, *Now there's a good-looking man.* Illness had nearly destroyed each of us, and it had destroyed our marriage, but throughout the whole thing our love had stayed intact. "Thank you," I said, hugging him again, feeling his solidity. "Thank you."

Later, I stood up and toasted my mother, commenting that she felt very present to me that evening even though she had died 22 years earlier. I told a story about how when I was 15, my mother and I were out shopping together, and I saw a beautiful white lace dress on the rack. I checked the price, and it was $262. My mother came over and remarked on how beautiful it was, and I said, "Yeah, but it's way too expensive," showing her the price tag.

My mother said with impish glee, "Oh, but you can try it on!" It looked so gorgeous that she bought it for me, even though it was far too pricey for a 15-year-old girl and even though I had no place to wear it. It was just too beautiful on me to pass up, she said.

The dress sat unworn in my closet for 25 years. It didn't go to Berkeley, so it survived the Great Purge. And it became the wedding dress I was wearing right then. John had cut off the price tag that morning.

The crowd offered up a big "awwww" and clinked their glasses.

Then I offered a toast to my father. I described how even though I'd never known him directly, I felt like I was having a chance to get to know him through his other children, all of whom were there, along with my siblings on my mother's side. Then all seven of them came up: Robin, the one I'd grown up with most, who had spent days at my service helping us get ready for the wedding—including by making the caramel brownies my mother baked and my father loved; Ty, who reached past terrible abuse and rejection to join me on that day and to build a loving relationship with his own son; Carol, the oldest of my father's kids, who had been friends with my mother around the time that I was born and seen the whole drama unfold; Troy, who had inherited my father's business drive and who had shared him with me so generously; Wes, who had initially welcomed me into the family and who pulled John aside during the wedding to say, "Julie's father would be so proud of her"; Cindy, who had created a joyful life with her husband driving around the country in an RV with their sign-making business and who had kept reaching out to me over the years; and Patricia, who had so resembled me as a child and who told me, "Seeing how wonderful you two are together gives me hope I might find a partner I really want to be with too!"

We formed a tribe, the eight of us standing there with interlinked arms. A family. My family.

WHEN THE MUSIC STARTED ("Let's Stay Together" by Al Green), John wrapped his arm around my waist and we moved together with total comfort. I caught glimpses of people's smiles and tapping feet. At the next song ("Barbie Girl," which we'd chosen for its silliness and infectious dance beat), friends piled onto the dance floor, and I tossed all reserve aside and danced with abandon. I knew that unlike in years past, my incaution wouldn't come back to bite me.

The sun set over the Rockies and the stars began twinkling into life above us. The pine trees surrounded us like guardians, protecting this bubble of joy and love and wholeness. The music played on, and I danced and danced.

EPILOGUE

As I finish this book, John and I have celebrated our third wedding anniversary together. The realization that this relationship is for real is seeping into my bones. Morning after morning, I feel a bit less incredulous to wake up next to him, but no less appreciative. We continue living primarily in our house (not just "my house" now) outside Santa Fe, which has come to bear John's stamp in a thousand ways. The yard, which was mostly dirt and weeds when we met, now blooms.

My health continues to be generally good. At times, I'm close to 100 percent well—consistently feeling good, able to exercise as much as I want, and reactive only to the worst buildings—but other times are more difficult. During those difficult times, caring for my body requires significant effort and caution, but even then I'm able to live a full life, and I no longer would consider myself disabled. I continue to experiment on all levels—avoidance, detox, medications, psychological work, woo-woo experiments—to figure out what will restore me.

I also continue to dig into scientific hypotheses that may be relevant to my experiences. The most recent idea I've been exploring is that a type of immune cell called a "mast cell" may be overeager in me, going mad and releasing histamine in response to tiny quantities of mold. One could think of it as an especially severe type of allergy that doesn't show up in ordinary allergy tests. It's an exciting idea both because it gives a plausible explanation for what's going on inside my body and it offers a possible treatment, a combination of antihistamines and drugs that calm the mast cells. As this book goes to press, I'm completely unclear whether this applies to me. We'll see.

Frances and Lao are now buddies. Lao will crouch on a chair, paw extended in menacing invitation, and Frances will run up, biting at him with an open mouth while he whacks her with claws retracted. If Lao is outside and comes running back to the house bushy-tailed, Frances runs past him to find whatever scared him. When Lao catches a mouse, Frances steals it, and Lao accepts that with resignation. While they don't seek one another out to cuddle, they do occasionally end up butt-to-butt when they join us for a morning snuggle in bed.

I gave up on training Frances to be a service dog after I met John. I didn't need her help so much with John in my life, plus I was coming to realize that Frances's exuberant personality made training her as a service dog a struggle. Also, training her required that I devote a significant portion of my attention to her whenever she was with me, and I wanted the freedom to focus all on John.

Over the years, I have finally come to claim the ME/CFS community as my own. I now feel ashamed that, early in my illness, I allowed my unrecognized fear of the severity of my fellow patients' illness to curdle into disdain. I bought into a narrative of victim-blaming that my fellow patients didn't deserve and that didn't serve me. I had to myself descend into frightening levels of illness before I realized the kinship I had with my fellow sufferers.

I've now become deeply attached to my patient friends. They did, of course, more or less save my life, and so many of them are very impressive people, carving out meaningful lives for themselves despite enormous suffering and tight limitations. The devotion and commitment of ME/CFS activists particularly inspire me, especially because they've persisted in spite of such enormous obstacles and in the face of so little apparent progress. I am one of the many beneficiaries of their efforts.

As my own health improved, I began to feel responsible for helping to improve the situation for ME/CFS patients as a whole. Writing, I figured, was my most powerful tool. In 2014, the Department of Health and Human Services announced that the National Academy of Medicine* was going to be writing a report on chronic fatigue syndrome, and I used that as an opportunity to describe the overall situation for ME/CFS in the *Washington Post*. In February 2015, when the report appeared, it turned out to be a significant step forward: It summarized much of the research, decried the lack of research funding and the limited research that has resulted, pointed out the hostility of many doctors, and stated that any doubts about whether ME/CFS is a "real" illness should be laid to rest. I

---

*   Then called the Institute of Medicine.

wrote an op-ed for the *New York Times* about it, arguing that the only way that would happen is if the National Institutes of Health started making serious investments into research on the disease. The article was the most popular story on the entire Web site for 24 hours.

That report is just one of several major steps of progress for the ME/CFS community in the last couple of years. In late 2015, the PACE trial empire at last began to crumble. A 14,000-word exposé by David Tuller, academic coordinator of the joint master's program in public health and journalism at the University of California, Berkeley, finally revealed the scientific flaws of the study to the world. It was a remarkable act of public service: Tuller, who is neither a patient nor a relative of a patient, spent a year investigating the trial on his own, without institutional support, legal backing, or remuneration. He exposed the problems I learned of back in 2011 along with more, publishing his piece in *Virology Blog*, hosted by the influential Columbia University microbiologist Vincent Racaniello. I wrote a piece for *Slate*, describing his investigation in condensed form.

Tuller's heroic effort finally got outside scientists to examine the problems in the trial. Forty-two researchers and clinicians signed an open letter to the *Lancet* demanding an independent investigation of the trial.

At the same time, a Freedom of Information request from a patient for a portion of the data from the trial was making its way through the British court system. The patient, Alem Matthees, asked for the anonymized data necessary to assess how the researchers' weakening of their standards of success had impacted the outcomes of the trial. Queen Mary University of London, the institution of the lead researcher, refused Matthees's request on the grounds that malicious patients, it asserted, would use the data to identify participants in the trial and publish their names.

In court, the university's key security witness admitted that such identification was impossible with the given data alone, but he suggested a scenario in which "borderline sociopathic or psychopathic" patients stole records from the National Health Service and combined that information with the PACE trial data to identify participants. The researchers presented the news reports about the death threats to support this notion. During questioning in court, however, one of the researchers admitted that none of the PACE researchers nor the participants had ever received a death threat—an astonishing admission after so many public accusations.

The court rejected the university's claims as "wild speculations," cited the open letter to the *Lancet*, and ordered the data to be released to Matthees. In September 2016, the university complied.

By this point, I decided to abandon any pretense of journalistic detachment, and I got involved behind the scenes in the efforts to debunk the trial. I had the joy of watching Matthees and other patients analyze the data with the help of statisticians I linked them to. They exercised a degree of scientific care and caution that I rarely observe even among scientists.

Their findings were shocking, though hardly surprising. The PACE researchers had claimed that 60 percent of patients who received CBT or graded exercise improved and 22 percent recovered. Had they not changed their definitions of "improvement" and "recovery," they would have had to say that only 20 percent of CBT or exercise patients improved, half of whom would have done so without the treatments. And virtually no patients recovered. Recovery rates were in the mid-single digits for all arms of the trial, with no statistically significant differences.

In other words, CBT and graded exercise are, at best, about as effective for ME/CFS as for other physical illnesses, and they do not lead to recovery.

I broke the news about the reanalysis in an essay in *STAT News*. It became their most-read article for a week, news stories and blog posts based on my article spread, and the patient community celebrated wildly. Scientific vindication was complete.

However, many public health organizations continue to recommend graded exercise and CBT, and patients continue to be at risk of harm from inappropriate treatments. Much work remains to be done.

And of course, what's needed isn't just to get rid of bad research—it's to get much more of the good kind. There, too, things seem to be changing. In late 2015, the NIH at last promised it would make a real investment in the disease, including by significantly increasing research funding. The NIH quickly began working on an in-house study of ME/CFS. In early 2017, however, it announced that it expected its funding for research in 2017 to be only $13 million, an improvement over $7 million in 2016, but still chump change.

Even if the NIH fails to fulfill its promise to transform research in the disease, I see signs that research on the illness will burgeon. For example, Ron Davis, a giant in genetics research at Stanford University whose son has a severe case of the illness, has become determined to decode the basic physiology of the disease. Despite being rejected repeatedly for NIH funding, he's plowing ahead by raising private funds through a private foundation, the Open Medicine Foundation. He and collaborators are analyzing bodily fluids from severely ill patients in thousands of different ways using big-data techniques. Before his work, severely ill patients had been almost entirely ignored in medical research. Davis and his colleagues have found some remarkable abnormalities in metabolism and mitochondrial function.

Other high-powered researchers have also become fascinated by the disease. Ian Lipkin, the famous "virus hunter" at Columbia University, Robert Naviaux of the University of California, San Diego, Øystein Fluge and Olav Mella of the University of Bergen in Norway, and Maureen Hanson of Cornell University have all started producing top-notch research on it. Several of these groups have independently discovered metabolic abnormalities, which increases the likelihood that these abnormalities are consistent across patients and central to the disease process.

Furthermore, the patient community has revolutionized itself. For decades, advocates have worked to expose the political problems in our medical research and clinical training systems that have hamstrung ME/CFS research and treatment, but recently, they've become more organized and active. A group called #MEAction, cofounded by patient and filmmaker Jennifer Brea, collaborated with other organizations to begin a series of worldwide protests called Millions Missing, highlighting the millions of people missing from their lives along with the millions of dollars missing from research and medical education. In late 2016, #MEAction persuaded 55 members of the US Congress to sign a letter to the NIH asking for increased investment in ME/CFS research. And Brea's documentary about the disease, *Unrest,* premiered at Sundance days after her TED talk went up online.

All of this leaves me optimistic about the future for this disease. But until major research findings come through and doctors become far more educated about the illness, patients will continue to be substantially on their own, coming up with ad hoc solutions like mold avoidance.

My experience obviously doesn't establish that ME/CFS as a whole is caused by mold or related contaminants, and I strongly doubt that's true. Accurately assessing how many ME/CFS patients are affected by mold is impossible at this point. Only a small percentage of patients have tried extreme mold avoidance, and we have no statistics about how many of them have found benefit.

Based on my personal observations and what I hear on Facebook and other patient communities, my guess is that it's a significant component of the illness for many patients—but that's only a guess, and I wouldn't be shocked if it turned out to be 10 percent or 90 percent. I also recognize that having benefited from mold avoidance myself, I inevitably see the world through mold-tinted glasses and may well be inclined to overestimate its relevance.

But here are my observations, for what they're worth. I have intensively counseled around 10 ME/CFS patients who have tried mold avoidance, and all became persuaded that mold exposures contribute to their symptoms at least somewhat. Some have experienced remarkable improvements, though none have improved as much as I have.* Some have found it to be a valuable tool, but it hasn't been transformative. Others have concluded that while mold indeed worsens their symptoms, the benefits they experience from extreme mold avoidance aren't sufficient to justify the extreme effort and disruption it requires. One about lost her mind trying it. I also counseled two patients who didn't have ME/CFS but had related issues that seemed plausibly related to mold, and neither found that mold avoidance had a clear effect.

Many, many more patients have experimented with mold avoidance under the influence of Erik the Mold Warrior and other moldies. Among this larger group, my improvement is far from unique. This kind of success story is quite rare in the ME/CFS community (the notable exception being those who receive treatment with the drug Ampligen, which has languished in patient-paid clinical trials for decades without FDA

---

* The best information about mold avoidance is available at paradigmchange.me. Be sure to check out Lisa Petrison's book *A Beginner's Guide to Mold Avoidance*, which is currently available for free if you sign up for the Rabbit Hole mailing list at paradigmchange.me. In addition, I recommend Sara Riley Mattson's *Camp Like a Girl*.

approval). A very active Facebook group devoted to the nuts and bolts of mold avoidance now has more than 6,000 members,* and many of them are profiting—sometimes enormously—from the methods. It's become a bit of a movement within the ME/CFS community.

There are also patients who have tried extreme mold avoidance without success at all. Of course, because avoiding mold is so difficult, it's impossible to be certain that mold or related environmental contaminants aren't contributing to their illness, despite their unsuccessful efforts. This is exactly what worried me so much when I set out on my Death Valley experiment: No matter how careful I was, it was always possible that I wouldn't manage to steer clear of the particular mold that had sickened me, hence hindering my ability to draw any conclusions. Had my experiment been unsuccessful, I certainly would not have taken well to strident assertions that I simply hadn't done it correctly. Unsurprisingly, neither do others. Extreme mold avoidance has thus become controversial in the patient community.

The overwhelming difficulty of extreme mold avoidance is far more problematic for those who commit to it. I was lucky that when I tried, I didn't require a caregiver or medical interventions, my health outside my ME/CFS was good, I had few responsibilities, I didn't have kids, my mental state was solid, and I experienced upswings I could seize for my trip. Without these advantages, it can be next to impossible, even dangerous.

This was brought home for me after I befriended a British woman named Katie Steward on Facebook who was severely ill and bedbound. She went to Spain to try extreme mold avoidance—an unimaginably difficult task in that state of illness. As far as I know, she was the most ill patient to ever try it, and I was so moved by her determination that I became deeply involved in helping her, eventually doing everything I could, short of flying to Spain. She's received clear indications that her body can come back astonishingly quickly when the conditions are right, but she's found that she is reactive not only to mold but also to fungicides and pesticides that are in widespread use in Spain. After two years of trying to find a location in Spain that would allow her to heal and undergoing horrendous suffering along the way, she's now trying to get to Death

---

* The Mold Avoiders group

Valley. Every step of her journey has required a fortitude and determination that has awed me, and even so, it's not clear whether she'll succeed. It breaks my heart that all I've learned isn't enough to make this process anything close to manageable for her.

All of this means that extreme mold avoidance is one hell of a lousy treatment, as grateful as I am for it personally. Even if mold plays a major role for all ME/CFS patients—an unlikely speculation—we're not going to cure it by shipping millions of them to the desert.

While extreme mold avoidance doesn't offer an effective, large-scale treatment for this illness, it does strongly suggest that serious research on the connection between mold and ME/CFS is urgent. We need to find out how big a role mold plays in the disease. We need to know the full range of health impacts that exposure to water-damaged buildings can have, since there are patients outside the ME/CFS community who are also benefiting from extreme mold avoidance. We need to find out how many people are affected. We need treatments that work without upending patients' lives or requiring impossible feats of endurance. We need the serious risks of mold exposure to be far more widely understood so that people can avoid getting sick in the first place. And all of that is in addition, of course, to the critically needed research that can unravel the basic physiology of this disease and develop non-mold-related treatments.

Nancy Klimas, the ME/CFS doctor who treated me, has now started studying mold in ME/CFS as well as treating patients for it, and she told me that she was convinced to do that in part because of my work. That made my heart swell.

A couple of years ago, I visited Berkeley to see if the "ick" theory held up. The experience was utterly bizarre: It felt as though there were an invisible patchy fog throughout Berkeley, and when we drove into it, my nervous system got crushed. It seemed incredible to me that everyone else around was proceeding normally. I kept asking John, "You don't feel that???" but of course, he didn't. Then, a couple of blocks later, I'd feel fine—until the next batch of it. But I was strong enough that the exposure had no lasting consequences.

That experience sheds little light, though, on what I was reacting to, and when I've talked to scientists who specialize in the impact of air quality on human health, none of them have reported any special problems in Berkeley. I won't be moving back there anytime soon, though.

Several fellow patients have gone to see Timmy the Wood Elf. All of them have reported to me that they've had remarkable experiences, but as far as I know, the work didn't bring anyone else significant health improvements. That's part of the problem with treatments that lie far outside of scientific understanding: They are rarely repeatable or reliable. Interestingly, Timmy gave varying explanations to each mold patient who came to him—his idea that the hypersensitivity was caused by childhood trauma was, apparently, individual to me.

I do continue to focus on my own psychology at times when my health is problematic, as one approach among many. "Psychology" means a lot of different things for me: thinking about my immediate experience in a way that keeps me from feeling victimized and helps me create richness and meaning in my life; revisiting old trauma to see if there are ways to shift my relationship to it and perhaps improve my physical health as a result; working to calm my nervous system's response to exposure.

I find this work valuable, but it seems to have far less direct effect on my health than avoiding mold does. And when I can't successfully avoid mold—for example, the skylight in our bedroom in Santa Fe developed a leak in the spring of 2016—it still has a devastating impact. I suspect that my body will always require an unusual level of care and attention.

Although I've certainly worked hard to improve my health as I have, I also want to be clear: I got lucky. I could have done everything I did and still be desperately ill. I think I get some credit for my improvement, but only some. A big part of it is simple good fortune.

That also means that I see my relatively good health as a blessing that might be revoked at any time. I have won no exemption from suffering, physical or emotional. This experience has honed my ability to create meaning for myself in any situation, not to resist my suffering, and to appreciate the present moment, whether I'm getting what I want or not. Those skills are ones I treasure, but I also recognize that their powers are limited. I don't hold myself above any of the desperately ill ME/CFS patients who have been driven to take their lives, including Vanessa Li, Jodi Bassett, Tom Hennessy, Louise Ramage, Tom Jarrett, and many more. I'm terribly sorry to have lost them.

One of the costs of my illness is that it seems indeed too late for me to have a child. I haven't given up hope completely, but I've accepted that if I do get pregnant, it will be a kind of miracle, something outside my control. I'm sad about it, and at times, very sad. Going for a walk up our stream with John and watching him bounce with excitement at the glowing fall aspens as we revel in Frances's athletic leaps and dashes, I so wish we had a kid to share it all with. And perhaps a child will come into our lives another way, through adoption or just through building a strong relationship with someone else's child. But I also know that we simply don't always get what we want, and I'm okay with that. After all, I died out there in the desert. This is all extra, all bonus.

That sense of acceptance is far easier to attain because my life is truly wonderful. Not only do I have a husband I delight in, a dog and cat who bring me joy, a beautiful house I created with my own hands in a magical place, and pretty good health, I am also able to do work that uses my skills and talents and is impacting people's lives.

I am wildly blessed.

A NOTE ON ACCURACY

The standards for accuracy in memoir are hotly debated, so I wanted to tell you about the standards I applied in writing this book.

I made it as factual as I could. There are no composite characters, no changes in timeline, no intentional embellishments. I was also scrupulous to report my emotions accurately, even when they seemed inappropriate or strange.

At the same time, memory is a soft material from which to sculpt a book. The shocking unreliability of memory has been thoroughly scientifically documented. So I have little doubt but that there are errors of many kinds, large and small, in this book. All I can say is that I've done my best.

Also, memory is a fundamentally different thing from a story. For one thing, memory is often indefinite where stories need specificity. I was willing, when necessary, to accept minor details that were likely but not certain. For example, I cannot swear that there were two large brown circles on my white T-shirt the day of the plaster party in Chapter 1, though I can say with confidence that I often had such circles at the end of a day of plastering.

Furthermore, turning memories into a story requires selection. I've had to omit many experiences that were important to me but that I decided didn't serve the book.

I used pseudonyms for a number of people in the book and changed some identifying details. In one case, I obscured the role of an individual at that person's request.

I relied on both documents and the memories of others to prop up my memories. Although I've never managed to sustain a journal for more than a few weeks, I very much enjoy writing long, detailed e-mails to friends, and I relied extensively on such correspondence as the raw material for the book. I checked financial records for dates when I could. I also interviewed friends about their memories of events in the book.

ACKNOWLEDGMENTS

An army of people and institutions have stood behind me in creating this book, and I can hardly describe my gratitude.

Two online communities played a huge role in the development of the book: the WELL and the Posse. The WELL is one of the oldest online communities, and the smart, deep, thoughtful people there have been following my life for nearly a decade, supporting me, brainstorming, commiserating, you name it. The Posse is a small science-writers' group I started with some friends.

Both groups helped me develop the book starting when it was a distant dream in my Berkeley days and the huge hurdle of daily survival stood in its way. I felt as though I had a cadre of invisible friends behind me all the time, ones that occasionally manifested themselves in the three-dimensional world. My e-mails and posts to them formed the backbone of a large part of this book.

Specific Posse members gave me particular support. George Johnson wrote me an e-mail in 2011 that essentially outlined my book for me. Siri Carpenter was my personal cheerleader through the project, offering incredibly skillful editing of chapter after chapter, listening to me whine, reminding me of my authority at times I felt small and powerless, and just all-around being an amazing friend. Jennie Dusheck read and commented on many drafts and offered her wise, compassionate presence over and over again. Mason Inman was an extraordinarily careful, dedicated, and thoughtful reader, and Jeanne Erdmann offered boundless encouragement and support.

From the WELL, Erin Bow offered clarity and direction at a moment of despair. David Kline helpfully and aggravatingly demanded that I rewrite the stuff about my mother over and over and over, and Tiffany Lee Brown offered me a high vision for my work.

I also received great support from fellow patients and advocates. Tom Kindlon, Simon McGrath, and their crew of merry PACE-destroying men and women were fantastically helpful with the chapter on PACE. Jennifer Spotila and Mary Dimmock offered expertise on the history and politics of the disease along with general wisdom. Eva Fisher's exclamations and all-caps enthusiasms brought me both smiles and comfort, and Jennifer Lunden was a comrade-in-arms.

The Mapleton Hill book group read the book when it was a not-quite-complete manuscript, and for the first time, I could see the book come to life in the minds of readers who barely knew me. It was a huge thrill that powered me through the rest of the book-writing process. They also gave very useful guidance in polishing the book.

Naomi Lubick patiently read many chapters at the early, "vomit" stage and helped me figure out what the heck to do with them. Lynda Myers helped me reckon with deficiencies in the manuscript. Geoff's sister made suggestions that deepened my portrayal of Geoff. David Tuller fact-checked the PACE chapter, helped on others, and offered camaraderie. Helge Dascher assured me at a late stage that the book could stand up to an astute reader.

I of course owe a huge debt to the ME/CFS and moldie communities, without whom I wouldn't have had this book to write. One patient played an especially big role in introducing me to mold avoidance and helping me learn how to do it. I have respected her request not to be included in the book, but my gratitude to her is overwhelming.

My thanks to Erik Johnson, who was an awfully good sport. As much as he annoyed the hell out of me when I visited him in Reno, he also pretty well saved my life—plus, as I got to know him better, I discovered that at heart, he's a very sweet human being. I promised him that I'd let him read the manuscript before publication, and when I did, he corrected some minor errors but didn't object to a thing. "I WAS annoying," he told me. "Knew it at the time."

I also owe a debt to Ritchie Shoemaker. Though I didn't pursue his treatments or rely on his scientific claims, he did a tremendous amount to raise public awareness that mold could cause serious, non-respiratory health problems like mine. I also know many patients who have benefited from his treatments.

I couldn't have sorted out the science without the generous help of many, many scientists. I'm especially grateful to Harriet Ammann, who proved an invaluable guide to the science of mold and was unstintingly generous with her time and knowledge. In addition, Jonathan Lee Wright and Sharon Noonan Kramer provided invaluable guidance as I worked to unravel the history of mold research. Wright made a tremendous effort to bring the issue of mold's health dangers to congressional attention, and Kramer has worked tirelessly for many, many years to expose the fraud in how the science of mold has been marketed, at great personal expense.

Through the Shadowlands is also the title of a beautiful biography of C. S. Lewis written by Brian Sibley. The story of Lewis's love for his wife and his spiritual maturation following her death was an inspiration for me in writing this book.

I wrote much of the book while I was a Ted Scripps Environmental Journalism Fellow at the University of Colorado, Boulder. That gave me the time and financial support to write and put the riches of the university at my disposal. Tom Yulsman and Michael Kodas offered tremendous support, ideas, and resources.

My agent, David Doerrer, ably guided me through the whole process, and my editor, Marisa Vigilante, gave sharp, thorough, and thoughtful edits that greatly improved the book.

Portions of the book appeared previously in *High Country News, Slate, Aeon,* and *STAT News,* in altered form.

I describe in the book how I felt both orphaned and abandoned during much of my illness, but many people stepped up to support me in all kinds of ways, far beyond obligation. Leonard Miller and Geoff's parents supported me financially when I needed it. My dear friend Dan eased some of the most difficult moments of my illness and enriched my life for two decades. William loved me during hard times. Patients offered wise counsel, friendship, and critical practical advice. Nancy Klimas and Erica Elliott gave me skillful medical care. William's brother Gary was remarkably generous and kind. I don't know how I would have gotten home to Santa Fe when I was at my sickest without my friend Sheila. My former tenant and current friend Bruce heard my groans and helped me into the kitchen trailer many times, among other ways that he supported me.

And then there were all the people who weren't so close but nonetheless stepped up in moments I needed them: the neighbor in Berkeley who gave me a ride home when I was stuck; the passersby who helped me up the stairs to the YMCA so I could swim when I'd gotten crippled; the employees at the Fort Marcy gym who would bring a wheelchair out to my car; the neighbor in Santa Fe who got me groceries; and many more.

I thank Llewellyn Vaughan-Lee for his wisdom, inspiration, and energy.

My mother's love during my childhood has provided a kind of rocket fuel that has powered me throughout my life and has been key to finding my way through my illness. I'm grateful for the support I feel from her—and from my father, though I didn't know him—to this day.

In telling my story, I inevitably had to tell a tiny bit of my siblings' stories too. Similarly, I had to describe some of the worst, most vulnerable moments of my ex-husband Geoff's life. I revealed all kinds of stuff about John. I'm grateful to all of them for their gracious acceptance of this.

My biggest debt of all, of course, is to John, who tirelessly read draft after draft, cheer-led throughout the entire process, cared for me in every way he could, created the most wonderful part of the story, and gives me joy that animates my life. This book is one of the fruits of our love.

ENDNOTES

CHAPTER 3

27 **"yuppie flu"**: "Chronic Fatigue Syndrome," *Newsweek*, November 11, 1990, www.newsweek.com/chronic-fatigue-syndrome-205712.

CHAPTER 5

58 **"I would rather have HIV"**: "Readers Ask: A Virus Linked to Chronic Fatigue Syndrome," *New York Times*, October 15, 2009, http://consults.blogs.nytimes.com/2009 /10/15/readers-ask-a-virus-linked-to-chronic-fatigue-syndrome/.

58 **"Psychotherapy Eases Chronic Fatigue Syndrome, Study Finds"**: David Tuller, "Psychotherapy Eases Chronic Fatigue Syndrome, Study Finds," *New York Times*, February 17, 2011, www.nytimes.com/2011/02/18/health/research/18fatigue.html.

59 **"nicknamed the PACE trial"**: P. D. White, et al., "Comparison of adaptive pacing therapy, cognitive behaviour therapy, graded exercise therapy, and specialist medical care for chronic fatigue syndrome (PACE): A randomised trial," *Lancet* 377, no. 9768 (March 2011): 823–36.

59 **"641 subjects, $8 million"**: It was 5 million British pounds, which converts to $8 million in 2011 dollars. See Section 2.1.4 of www.rae.ac.uk/submissions/ra5a.aspx?id=176& type=hei&subid=3181. "The PACE trial (7 UK centres) of chronic fatigue syndrome (CFS) treatments (MRC; £5.0M)."

60 **"CNN"**: Tom Watkins, "Study supports use of 2 controversial treatments for chronic fatigue," CNN.com, February 18, 2011, www.cnn.com/2011/HEALTH/02/17/chronic .fatigue/.

60 **"NPR"**: Richard Know, "Psychotherapy and Exercise Look Best to Treat Chronic Fatigue Syndrome," WBUR.org, February 18, 2011, www.wbur.org/npr/133865482 /psychotherapy-and-exercise-look-best-to-treat-chronic-fatigue-syndrome/.

60 **"the BBC"**: "Brain and body training treats ME, UK study says," BBC.com, February 18, 2011, www.bbc.com/news/health-12493009.

60 **"*Reuters*"**: Kate Kelland, "Pushing limits can help chronic fatigue patients," *Reuters*, February 17, 2011, www.reuters.com/article/2011/02/18/ us-fatigue-me-idUSTRE71H0320110218.

60 **"the *Independent*"**: Jeremy Laurance, "Got ME? Just get out and exercise, say scientists," *Independent,* February 17, 2011, www.independent.co.uk/life-style/health-and -families/health-news/got-me-just-get-out-and-exercise-say-scientists-2218377.html.

60 **"the *Times of London*"**: Chris Smyth, "ME sufferers 'better pushing their limits'," *Times,* February 18, 2011, www.thetimes.co.uk/tto/health/news/article2917876.ece.

60 **"had a full recovery"**: "Got ME? Fatigued patients who go out and exercise have best hope of recovery, finds study," *Daily Mail,* February 18, 2011, www.dailymail.co.uk/health /article-1358269/Chronic-fatigue-syndrome-ME-patients-exercise- best-hope-recovery-finds -study.html. See also notes 9 and 10.

60 **"refused these treatments"**: "Insurance Industry Practices Which Discriminate Against People with ME," (presentation, All Party Parliamentary Group, London, December 14, 2004). www.roydsrdw.com/pdf/APPG%20minutes%20241204.pdf.

60 **"against their will"**: Criona Wilson, "The Story of Sophia and ME," Invest in ME, www.investinme.org/Article-050%20Sophia%20Wilson%2001.htm.

60 "online patient forum": http://forums.phoenixrising.me/index.php.

61 "got out of shape": Mary Burgess and Trudie Chalder, "Manual for Therapists: Cognitive Behaviour Therapy for CFS/ME," December 8, 2004: 17–18. www.wolfson.qmul .ac.uk/images/pdfs/3.cbt-therapist-manual.pdf.

61 "remained unfit": Ibid.

61 "a vicious spiral": Ibid.

61 "lacking a stable social environment": U.M. Nater, J.F. Jones, J.M. Lin, E. Maloney, W.C. Reeves, and C. Heim, "Personality features and personality disorders in chronic fatigue syndrome: A population-based study," *Psychotherapy and Psychosomatics* 79, no. 5 (July 2010): 312–18. doi: 10.1159/000319312.

62 "*Journal of Psychosomatic Research*": S.S. Taillefer, L.J. Kirmayer, J.M. Robbins, and J.C. Lasry, "Correlates of illness worry in chronic fatigue syndrome," *Journal of Psychosomatic Research* 54, no. 4 (April 2003): 331–37.

CHAPTER 6

64 "psychotherapist Larry LeShan": Lawrence LeShan, *Cancer As a Turning Point: A Handbook for People with Cancer, Their Families, and Health Professionals*, Revised ed. (New York: Plume, 1994).

68 "known as XMRV": Vincent C. Lombardi, et al., "Detection of an infectious retrovirus, XMRV, in blood cells of patients with chronic fatigue syndrome," *Science* 326, no. 5952 (October 2009): 585–89.

68 "embroiled in controversy": Martin Enserink, "Conflicting Papers on Hold as XMRV Frenzy Reaches New Heights," *Science* 329, no. 5987 (July 2010): 18–19.

75 "how to exercise safely": This video provides a guide to Klimas's exercise recommendations: https://vimeo.com/ondemand/klimasexercise.

75 "before she could recommend it": At the time this book goes to print, research results on rituximab, the drug in question, continued to look promising. It is in phase three clinic trials in Norway.

Miriam E. Tucker, "Immune-Modulating Agents Eyed for 'Chronic Fatigue Syndrome'," Medscape, November 11, 2016, www.medscape.com/viewarticle/871787.

CHAPTER 7

79 "in seven dimensions": Robert Siegel, "American Mathematician Wins Abel Prize," NPR, March 24, 2011, www.npr.org/2011/03/24/134832727/American-Mathematician -Wins-Abel-Prize.

CHAPTER 8

91 "only proven treatments for ME/CFS": These websites recommended CBT and graded exercise before the PACE trial as well, based on previous, smaller studies by the same group of British mental health professionals, which had similar flaws. The PACE trial reinforced the belief in these treatments.

"Chronic Fatigue Syndrome: Managing Activities and Exercise," CDC.gov, February 14, 2013, https://www.cdc.gov/cfs/management/managing-activities.html.

"Chronic Fatigue Syndrome: Treatments and Drugs," Mayoclinic.com, August 30, 2016, www.mayoclinic.org/diseases-conditions/chronic-fatigue-syndrome/basics/treatment /con-20022009.

Stephen J. Gluckman, "Treatment of Systemic Exertion Intolerance Disease (Chronic Fatigue Syndrome)," UpToDate.com, December 2016, www.uptodate.com/contents /treatment-of-systemic-exertion-intolerance-disease-chronic-fatigue-syndrome.

"Chronic Fatigue Syndrome: Using Graded Exercise to Get More Energy," Healthwise, March 29, 2016, http://bit.ly/kaiser-cbt-get.

92 "evil": Phoenix Rising forums, "CAA is Listening," February 18, 2011, http://forums .phoenixrising.me/index.php?threads/caa-is-listening.2280/page-16#post-54877.

92 **"warped"**: Phoenix Rising forums, "Simon Wessely's Warped Mind Strike Again," September 24, 2011, http://forums.phoenixrising.me/index.php?threads/simon-wesselys -warped-mind-strikes-again.12370/.

92 **"morally bankrupt"**: Ibid.

92 **"association with psychiatry"**: You can gorge on quotations (with citations) from Wessely's work here: http://forums.phoenixrising.me/index.php?attachments/wessely-board1-pdf.4279/. This particular quote comes from The National Archives of the UK: Public Record Office (PRO) BN 141/1, 1 October 1993, Wessely to Aylward, 17–18.

92 **"benefits, etc."**: Simon Wessely, "Chronic Fatigue Syndrome: Current Issues," *Reviews in Medical Microbiology* 3 (1992): 211–16.

92 **"preserves self-esteem"**: S. Butler, T. Chalder, M. Ron, and S. Wessely, "Cognitive Behaviour Therapy in Chronic Fatigue Syndrome," *Journal of Neurology, Neurosurgery, & Psychiatry* 54 (1991): 153–58. doi:10.1136/jnnp.54.2.153.

92 **"make patients worse"**: The National Archives of the UK: Public Record Office (PRO) BN 141/1, October or November 1993, McGrath Summarizing Talk by Thomas and Wessely, 6–8, 10. http://forums.phoenixrising.me/index.php?attachments/wessely-board1-pdf.4279/.

92 **"like mental illnesses are"**: Stephen T. Holgate, Anthony L. Komaroff, Dennis Mangan, and Simon Wessely, "Chronic Fatigue Syndrome: Understanding a Complex Illness," *Nature Reviews Neuroscience* 12, no. 9 (September 2011): 539–44. doi: 10.1038/nrn3087.

92 **"power to change them"**: "...[CFS] symptoms are perpetuated by a cycle of inactivity, deterioration in exercise tolerance and further symptoms. This is compounded by the depressive illness that is often part of the syndrome. The result is a self-perpetuating cycle of exercise avoidance."

S. Wessely, A. David, S. Butler, and T. Chalder, "Management of chronic (post-viral) fatigue syndrome," *Journal of the Royal College of General Practitioners* 39, no. 318 (January 1989): 26–29.

92 **"less likely they are to recover"**: "Attributing fatigue to social reasons appears to be most protective."

T. Chalder, M. J. Power, and S. Wessely, "Chronic Fatigue in the Community: 'A Question of Attribution'," *Psychological Medicine* 26, no.4 (July 1996): 791–800.

92 **"seeing problems as catastrophes"**: "The most important starting point is to promote a consistent pattern of activity, rest, and sleep, followed by a gradual return to normal activity; ongoing review of any 'catastrophic' misinterpretation of symptoms and the problem solving of current life difficulties."

Michael Sharpe, Trudie Chalder, Ian Palmer, and Simon Wessely, "Chronic Fatigue Syndrome: A practical guide to assessment and management," *General Hospital Psychiatry* 19, no. 3 (June 1997): 185–99. doi: 10.1016/S0163-8343(97)80315-5.

92 **"focusing on their symptoms"**: "Diagnosis elicits the belief the patient has a serious disease, leading to symptom focusing that becomes self-validating and self-reinforcing and that renders worse outcomes, a self-fulfilling prophecy, especially if the label is a biomedical one like ME."

M.J. Huibers and S. Wessely, "The act of diagnosis: pros and cons of labelling chronic fatigue syndrome," *Psychological Medicine* 36, no. 7 (July 2006): 895–900.

92 **"search for physiological treatments"**: "Many patients referred to a specialized hospital with chronic fatigue syndrome have embarked on a struggle. This may take the form of trying to find an acceptable diagnosis, or indeed any diagnosis, and may involve reading the scientific literature concerned with the condition—health professionals appear to be over-represented among those seen in hospital practice with this condition. One of the principal functions of therapy at this stage is to allow the patient to call a halt without loss of face."

S. Wessely, A. David, S. Butler, and T. Chalder, "Management of chronic (post-viral) fatigue syndrome," *Journal of the Royal College of General Practitioners* 39, no. 318 (January 1989): 26–29.

92 **"search for physiological problems"**: "However, the simple combination of history, examination and basic tests will establish those who require further investigation. In the majority this simple screen will be normal, and over investigation should be avoided. Not only is it a waste of resources, it may not be in the patients' interest, and may reinforce maladaptive behaviour in a variety of ways."

Simon Wessely, "Chronic fatigue syndrome," *Journal of Neurology, Neurosurgery, & Psychiatry* 54 (1991): 669–671.

93 **"medical science had to offer"**: Wessely continued to maintain this for years. For example, he posted this comment on a blog post: "I do believe that the studies of CBT and GET for CFS (including but certainly not restricted to the PACE trial) . . . remain the best evidence that we have for anything that can offer at least some help for sufferers."

Steven Lubet, "An Open Letter to Dr. Simon Wessely, Defender of the PACE Study," The Faculty Lounge, November 14, 2016, www.thefacultylounge.org/2016/11/an-open-letter -to-dr-simon-wessely-defender-of-the-pace-study.html.

93 **"the brain for that"**: In later correspondence, Wessely told me that the reason we haven't "cracked the problem yet" is "because the brain is bloody difficult, mate—if this was just immunology or muscle pathology, we would have it sorted. But it's not."

93 **"2002 article in the *Guardian*"**: Jerome Burne, "Battle Fatigue," *Guardian,* March 29, 2002, www.theguardian.com/society/2002/mar/30/health.lifeandhealth.

95 **"back to normal"**: Sarah Boseley, "Study Finds Therapy and Exercise Best for ME," *Guardian,* February 18, 2011, www.theguardian.com/society/2011/feb/18/ study-exercise-therapy-me-treatment.

95 **"an 80-year-old"**: Ann Bowling, Matthew Bond, Crispin Jenkinson, and Donna L. Lamping, "Short Form 36 (SF-36) Health Survey Questionnaire: Which normative data should be used? Comparisons between the norms Provided by the Omnibus Survey in Britain, the Health Survey for England and the Oxford Healthy Life Survey," Journal *of* Public Health Medicine 21, no. 3 (September 1999): 255–70.

96 **"qualify as 'recovered'"**: A few technical details: The extensive press coverage about recovery came from two places. At the press conference when the *Lancet* study was first announced, one of the PACE researchers claimed that twice as many patients had gotten "back to normal" with CBT or exercise than without. In addition, a commentary accompanying the *Lancet* paper said that 30 percent met "a strict criterion for recovery."

The *Lancet* paper itself, however, didn't discuss recovery. Instead, it described the percentage of patients who were "within the normal range" on their fatigue and physical function scores. The "normal range," however, is a statistical term that is unrelated to being "back to normal" or "recovered." Nevertheless, that analysis was the basis for the claims in the press conference and commentary, and it provided the thresholds for fatigue and physical function scores I discuss.

Two years later, the researchers published their full analysis of recovery, in *Psychological Medicine.*

P. D. White, et al., "Recovery from chronic fatigue syndrome after treatments given in the PACE trial," *Psychological Medicine* 43, no. 10 (October 2013): 2,227–35.

That paper's claims were slightly more modest, reporting a 22 percent recovery rate for patients who received exercise or CBT, rather than 30 percent.

To be "recovered," patients had to meet the same thresholds for fatigue and for physical function as in the "normal range" analysis in *the Lancet.* In addition, they had to meet two other criteria: Patients had to say they overall felt "much" or "very much" better, and they had to no longer qualify as having chronic fatigue syndrome. The latter sounds very impressive, but it excluded almost no participants who met the first three criteria.

All four of these criteria were much looser than the researchers had proposed before they started the trial.

96 "an accompanying commentary": Gijs Bleijenberg and Hans Knoop, "Chronic fatigue syndrome: Where to PACE from here?" *Lancet* 377, no. 9768 (March 2011): 786–88. doi: 10.1016/S0140-6736(11)60172-4.

96 "hadn't done these treatments": Michael Sharpe, "Functional Symptoms and Syndromes," *Trends in Health and Disability 2002* (February 2012): 15–22.

96 "25 years earlier": Anthony S. David, Simon Wessely, and Anthony J. Pelosi, "Postviral fatigue syndrome: time for a new approach," *British Medical Journal* 296, no. 6623 (March 1988): 696–99.

96 "ideas about the illness": Mary Dimmock's *Thirty Years of Disdain* chronicles this history thoroughly. It's available for free here: http://bit.ly/30-years-of-disdain.

96 "carefully argued letters": Andrew James Kewley, "The PACE trial in chronic fatigue syndrome," *Lancet* 377, no. 9780 (May 2011): 1832.

96 "and commentaries": Alem Matthees, "Assessment of recovery status in chronic fatigue syndrome using normative data," *Quality of Life Research* 24, no. 4 (April 2015): 905–7. doi: 10.1007/s11136-014-0819-0.

96 "in peer-reviewed journals": For example, Tom Kindlon, "Reporting of Harms Associated with Graded Exercise Therapy and Cognitive Behavioural Therapy in Myalgic Encephalomyelitis/Chronic Fatigue Syndrome," *Bulletin of the IACFS/ME* 19, no. 2 (2011): 59–111 and Mark Vink, "The PACE Trial Invalidates the Use of Cognitive Behavioral and Graded Exercise Therapy in Myalgic Encephalomyelitis/Chronic Fatigue Syndrome: A Review," *Journal of Neurology and Neurobiology* 2, no. 3 (March 2016): 1–12.

97 "greatest number of patients": Wolfson Institute of Preventive Medicine, PACE trial frequently asked questions, 2011, www.wolfson.qmul.ac.uk/images/pdfs/pace/faq2.pdf.

97 "overwhelming majority of patients": "Comparison of treatments for chronic fatigue syndrome—the PACE trial," *Health Report,* April 18, 2011, www.abc.net.au/radionational /programs/healthreport/comparison-of-treatments-for-chronic-fatigue/2993296.

97 "majority of the requests": www.whatdotheyknow.com/search/pace%20Trial/all.

97 "qualified as harassment": This is one request from a patient who was denied on the grounds that it was "vexatious:" www.whatdotheyknow.com/request/fitness_data_for _pace_trial #outgoing-464451.

Later, the data request from psychologist James Coyne of the University Medical Center, Groningen, was denied on the same grounds: Alex Anderssen, "'Vexatious': King's College London Dismisses James Coyne's Request for PLOS ONE PACE Data," December 12, 2015, www.meaction.net/2015/12/12/ vexatious-kings-college-london-dismisses-james-coynes-request-for-plos-one-pace-data/.

97 "death threats to researchers": Jenny Hope, "Scientists investigating ME get 'death threats' for investigating psychological causes," *Daily Mail,* July 29, 2011, www.dailymail .co.uk/health/article 2020241/Scientists investigating ME-death-threats-investigating -psychological-causes.html.

Nigel Hawkes, "Dangers of research into chronic fatigue syndrome," *BMJ* 342 (June 2011): d3780.

Michael Hanlon, "This man faced death threats and abuse. His crime? He suggested that ME was a mental illness," *Sunday Times,* May 5, 2013, www.thesundaytimes.co.uk/sto /Magazine/Features/article1252529.ece.

97 "feel a lot safer": Stefanie Marsh, "Interview with Professor Simon Wessely," ME Association, August 6, 2011, www.meassociation.org.uk/2011/08/ interview-with-professor-simon-wessely-the-times-6-august-2011/.

98 "research they agree with": Nigel Hawkes, "Dangers of research into chronic fatigue syndrome," *BMJ* 342 (June 2011): d3780.

99 "mistreating him": Ean's story: www.youtube.com/watch?v=cDeu_OlMivU.

Professional investigation: Caroline Richmond, "Isle of Man provides unique forum for presenting health care grievances," *Canadian Medical Association Journal* 150, no. 1 (January 1994): 66–67.

Document showing Wessely's involvement: Malcolm Hooper, "The Mental Health Movement: Persecution of Patients? A Consideration of the Role of Professor Simon Wessely and Other Members of the 'Wessely School' in the Perception of Myalgic Encephalomyelitis (ME) in the UK," Background Briefing for the House of Commons Select Health Committee, December 2, 2003, www.mcs-international.org/downloads/009_mental_health_movement.pdf.

100 **"kidney failure":** Criona Wilson, "The Story of Sophia and ME," Invest in ME, www.investinme.org/Article-050%20Sophia%20Wilson%2001.htm.

101 **"didn't always work":** Kelvin Lord, "Interview with Dr. Lapp—A Pioneer and Patriarch," October 1, 2010, http://ampligen-treatment.blogspot.mx/2010/10/interview-with-dr-lapp-pioneer-and.html.

101 **"National Institutes of Health":** "Estimates of Funding for Various Research, Condition, and Disease Categories (RCDC)," National Institutes of Health, February 10, 2016, https://report.nih.gov/categorical_spending.aspx.

CHAPTER 9

108 **"how to behave in public":** These instructions are called *Training Levels,* and they're amazing: http://sue-eh.ca/.

CHAPTER 10

115 **"was going on":** Julie Rehmeyer, "Stolen Notebooks and a Biochemist in Chains," *Slate,* December 2, 2011, www.slate.com/articles/health_and_science/medical_examiner/2011/12/judy_mikovits_in_prison_what_does_it_mean_for_research_on_chronic_fatigue_syndrome_.html.

115 **"*Osler's Web*":** Hillary Johnson, *Osler's Web: Inside the Labyrinth of the Chronic Fatigue Syndrome Epidemic,* 1st ed. (New York: Crown, 1996).

116 **"reported in her book":** Hillary Johnson, *Osler's Web: Inside the Labyrinth of the Chronic Fatigue Syndrome Epidemic,* 1st ed. (New York: Crown, 1996): 140.

117 **"even vaguely like it":** *Ibid.,* 135.

117 **"twenty-nine years old":** *Ibid.,* 154.

118 **"London in 1955; and more":** Nathaniel C. Briggs and Paul H. Levine, "A comparative review of systemic and neurological symptomatology in 12 outbreaks collectively described as chronic fatigue syndrome, epidemic neuromyasthenia, and myalgic encephalomyelitis," *Clinical Infectious Disease* 18, supplement 1 (1994): S32–42.

118 **"getting more active":** S. Wessely, A. David, S. Butler, and T. Chalder, "Management of chronic (post-viral) fatigue syndrome," *Journal of the Royal College of General Practitioners* 39, no. 318 (January 1989): 26–29.

119 **"misrepresent the data":** Hillary Johnson, *Osler's Web: Inside the Labyrinth of the Chronic Fatigue Syndrome Epidemic,* 1st ed. (New York: Crown, 1996): 319.

119 **"definition of the disease":** William C. Reeves, et al., "Chronic Fatigue Syndrome—A clinically empirical approach to its definition and study," *BMC Medicine* 3 (2005): 19. doi: 10.1186/1741-7015-3-19.

119 **"as having ME/CFS":** Leonard A. Jason, Nicole Porter, Molly Brown, Abigail Brown, and Meredyth Evans, "A Constructive Debate with the CDC on the Empirical Case Definition of Chronic Fatigue Syndrome," *Journal of Disability Policy Studies* 20, no. 4 (2010): 251–56.

119 **"money to other diseases":** United States General Accounting Office, "Chronic Fatigue Syndrome: CDC and NIH Research Activities Are Diverse, but Agency Coordination Is Limited," Report to the Honorable Harry Reid, US Senate, June 2000, www.gao.gov/new.items/he00098.pdf.

119 **"General Accounting Office":** Hillary Johnson, *Osler's Web: Inside the Labyrinth of the Chronic Fatigue Syndrome Epidemic,* 1st ed. (New York: Crown, 1996): 483, 587, and 591.

United States General Accounting Office, "Chronic Fatigue Syndrome: CDC and NIH Research Activities Are Diverse, but Agency Coordination Is Limited," Report to the Honorable Harry Reid, US Senate, June 2000, www.gao.gov/new.items/he00098.pdf.

120 **"$5 million a year on ME/CFS research"**: "Estimates of Funding for Various Research, Condition, and Disease Categories (RCDC)," National Institutes of Health, February 10, 2016, https://report.nih.gov/categorical_spending.aspx.

122 **"the finding in *Science*"**: Vincent C. Lombardi, et al., "Detection of an Infectious Retrovirus, XMRV, in Blood Cells of Patients with Chronic Fatigue Syndrome," *Science* 326, no. 5952 (October 2009): 585–89.

123 **"A Wired article"**: John Timmer, "How a Collapsing Scientific Hypothesis Ended in an Arrest," *Wired*, November 30, 2011, www.wired.com/2011/11/xmrv-lawsuit-arrest/.

CHAPTER 16

192 **"undergo these treatments"**: Scott Gavura, "Ask the (Science-Based) Pharmacist: What are the benefits of coffee enemas?" Science-Based Medicine, July 11, 2013, https://science basedmedicine.org/ask-the-science-based-pharmacist-what-are-the-benefits-of-coffee-enemas/.

CHAPTER 18

215 **"story on assignment"**: Julie Rehmeyer, "Fatal Cancer Threatens Tasmanian Devil Populations," *Discover*, March 31, 2014, http://discovermagazine.com/2014/may/13-the -immortal-devil.

CHAPTER 19

228 **"to an unclean place"**: Leviticus 14:45.

228 **"moldy wine cellar"**: Alex Sakula, "Sir John Floyer's *A Treatise of the Asthma* (1698)," *Thorax* 39, no. 4 (April 1984): 248–54.

229 **"infested the straw"**: J. D. Miller, T. G. Rand, and B. B. Jarvis, "Stachybotrys chartarum: cause of human disease or media darling?" Medical Mycology 41, no. 4 (August 2003): 271–91.

V. G. Drobotko, "Stachybotryotoxicosis: A New Disease of Horses and Humans," American *Review of* Soviet Medicine 2, no. 3 (1945): 238–42.

229 **"$1.4 billion per year"**: De-Wei Li, ed., *Biology of Microfungi* (Switzerland: Springer International Publishing AG): 495–524.

229 **"death within minutes"**: George P. Shultz, "Chemical Warfare in Southeast Asia and Afghanistan: An Update," United States Department of State Special Report No. 104, November 1982.

229 **"in the late 1980s"**: Zygmunt F. Dembek, ed., *USAMRIID's Medical Management of Biological Casualties Handbook*, 7th ed. (Washington, DC: US Government Printing Office, 2011): 8.

230 **"Baby-Killing Fungus"**. July 31, 1997

231 **"an anonymous panel"**: "Reports of Members of the CDC External Expert Panel on Acute Idiopathic Pulmonary Hemorrhage in Infants: A Synthesis," Centers for Disease Control and Prevention, December 1999, www.cdc.gov/mold/pdfs/aiphi_report.pdf.

231 ***"Carpet Monsters and Killer Spores: A Natural History of Toxic Mold"***: Nicholas P. Money, *Carpet Monsters and Killer Spores: A Natural History of Toxic Mold* (London: Oxford University Press, 2004). I highly recommend this book despite its rather overheated title—it manages to simultaneously be scientifically sober and quite entertaining.

231 **"want to throw up"**: Lisa Belkin, "Haunted by Mold," *New York Times*, August 12, 2001, www.nytimes.com/2001/08/12/magazine/haunted-by-mold.html.

232 **"it handled 15,000"**: Jordan Smith, "The 'Mold Queen' Fights Back: The woman the insurance companies love to hate says they ain't seen nothin' yet," *Austin Chronicle*, March 21, 2003, www.austinchronicle.com/news/2003-03-21/150675/.

232 **"cost $275 billion"**: James R. Copland, "Asbestos," Point of Law, May 21, 2004, www.pointoflaw.com/asbestos/overview.php.

232 **"protecting industry from mold claims"**: W. Stephen Benesh, "Life after Ballard: Mold Litigation in the New Millennium," FDCC Quarterly 56, no. 4 (2006): 525–44.

232 **"from an official statement"**: B. D. Hardin, B. J. Kelman, and A. Saxon, "Adverse human health effects associated with molds in the indoor environment," *Journal of Occupational and Environmental Medicine* 45, no. 5 (May 2003): 470–78.

233 **"unsupported by actual scientific study"**: Cliff Hutchinson and Robert Powell, "A New Plague–Mold Litigation: How Junk Science and Hysteria Built an Industry," paper commissioned by the US Chamber Institute for Legal Reform and the Center for Legal Policy at The Manhattan Institute, July 17, 2003, www.uschamber.com/sites/default/files/legacy /press/ilr_mold.pdf.

234 **"water-damaged buildings"**: D. Mudarri and W. J. Fisk, "Public health and economic impact of dampness and mold," *Indoor Air* 17, no. 3 (June 2007): 226–35.

234 **"meddling scientists down in Ohio"**: Nicholas P. Money, *Carpet Monsters and Killer Spores: A Natural History of Toxic Mold* (London: Oxford University Press, 2004).

234 **"large insurance company"**: "Biography: Jeffery P. Koplan, MD, MPH: Vice President for Global Health," Emory University Woodruff Health Sciences Center, http://whsc.emory .edu/home/about/leadership/bio-jeffrey-koplan.html.

234 **"respiratory dangers of mold in 2016"**: The May and June 2016 issues of the *Journal of Allergy and Clinical Immunology* contain a series of articles from the AAAAI panel on environmental allergens.

CHAPTER 20

238 **"than intact spores"**: Tiina Reponen, et al., "Fungal Fragments in Moldy Houses: A Field Study in Homes in New Orleans and Southern Ohio," *Atmospheric Environment* 41, no. 37 (December 2007): 8140–49.

239 **"without known mold exposure"**: K. H. Kilburn, "Neurobehavioral and pulmonary impairment in 105 adults with indoor exposure to molds compared to 100 exposed to chemicals," *Toxicology & Industrial Health* 25, no. 9-10 (October-November 2009): 681–92.

239 **"controlling for other factors"**: W. Jedrychowski, et al., "Cognitive function of 6-year-old children exposed to mold-contaminated homes in early postnatal period. Prospective birth cohort study in Poland," *Physiology & Behavior* 104, no. 5 (October 2011): 989–95. doi: 10.1016/j.physbeh.2011.06.019.

239 **"linked to diabetes"**: Salynn Boyles, "Air Pollution Linked to Risk of Diabetes: Study Suggests a Diabetes Risk Even at 'Acceptable' Exposure Levels," WebMD, October 1, 2010, www.webmd.com/diabetes/news/20101001/air-pollution-linked-to-diabetes-risk.

239 **"heart disease"**: Ibid.

239 **"and dementia"**: Clayton Aldern, "Meet the scientist connecting the dots between air pollution and dementia," *Grist*, February 17, 2016, http://grist.org/climate-energy/meet-the -scientist-connecting-the-dots-between-air-pollution-and-dementia/.

240 **"20 micrograms at once"**: S. A. Carey, et al., "Satratoxin-G from the black mold Stachybotrys chartarum induces rhinitis and apoptosis of olfactory sensory neurons in the nasal airways of rhesus monkeys," *Toxicologic Pathology* 40, no. 6 (August 2012): 887–98. doi: 10.1177/0192623312444028.

240 **"too big a stretch"**: M. Nishiyama and T. Kuga, "Central effects of the neurotropic mycotoxin fumitremorgin A in the rabbit. (II). Effects on the brain stem," *Japanese Journal of Pharmacology* 52, no. 2 (February 1990): 201–8.

241 **"inflammation in their brains"**: C. F. Harding, et al., "Environmental mold exposure, brain inflammation, and spatial memory deficits," *Brain, Behavior, and Immunity* 49, supplement (October 2015): e42.

241 **"human cells in a petri dish"**: Arati A. Inamdar, et al., "Fungal-derived semiochemical 1-octen-3-ol disrupts dopamine packaging and causes neurodegeneration," *PNAS* 110, no. 48 (November 2013): 19,561–66. doi: 10.1073/pnas.1318830110.

I also wrote a news story about this for *Discover*: Julie Rehmeyer, "How the Smell of Your Home Could Be Making You Sick," *Discover,* January 14, 2014, http://blogs.discovermagazine .com/crux/2014/01/14/how-the-smell-of-your-home-could-be-making-you-sick.

243 **"breathed right in"**: He discusses all this, and much more, in an episode of IAQ radio: http://recordings.talkshoe.com/TC-1547/TS-1105904.mp3. I really recommend a listen, especially if you're interested in environmental contributors to asthma, on which Miller is truly a world authority. You'll also hear that he's quite an affable guy, even though I couldn't make sense of his positions on mycotoxins.

243 **"mycotoxins could contribute to asthma"**: Thomas G. Rand, J. DiPenta, C. Robbins, and J. D. Miller, "Effects of low molecular weight fungal compounds on inflammatory gene transcription and expression in mouse alveolar macrophages," *Chemico-Biological Interactions* 190, no. 2-3 (April 2011): 139–47. doi: 10.1016/j.cbi.2011.02.017.

246 **"including schools"**: K. Fog Nielsen, "Mycotoxin production by indoor molds," *Fungal Genetics and Biology* 39, no. 2 (July 2003): 103–17.

EPILOGUE

300 **"in the *Washington Post*"**: Julie Rehmeyer, "What is chronic fatigue syndrome, and why aren't we doing more to treat the illness?" *Washington Post,* October 6, 2014, www.washingtonpost.com/national/health-science/what-is-chronic-fatigue-syndrome -and-why-arent-we-doing-more-to-treat-the-illness/2014/10/06/4cfff312-d458-11e3-8a78 -8fe50322a72c_story.html.

Julie Rehmeyer, "How the definition of chronic fatigue syndrome keeps changing," *Washington Post,* October 6, 2014, www.washingtonpost.com/national/health-science /how-the-definition-of-chronic-fatigue-syndrome-keeps-changing/2014/10/06/def05db4 -0d1c-11e4-b8e5-d0de80767fc2_story.html.

301 **"14,000-word exposé"**: David Tuller, "Trial by Error: The Troubling Case of the PACE Chronic Fatigue Syndrome Study," Virology Blog, October 21, 2015, www.virology .ws/2015/10/21/trial-by-error-i.

301 **"I wrote a piece for *Slate*"**: Julie Rehmeyer, "Hope for Chronic Fatigue Syndrome: The debate over this mysterious disease is suddenly shifting," *Slate,* November 13, 2015, www.slate.com/articles/health_and_science/medical_examiner/2015/11/chronic_fatigue _pace_trial_is_flawed_should_be_reanalyzed.single.html.

301 **"investigation of the trial"**: Ronald W. Davis, et al., "An open letter to Dr. Richard Horton and the *Lancet*," Virology Blog, November 13, 2015, www.virology.ws/2015/11/13 /an-open-letter-to-dr-richard-horton-and-the-lancet/.

302 **"released to Matthees"**: Queen Mary University of London v. The Information Commissioner, (2015) A. C. EA/2015/0269 (H. L.) (Eng.), http://bit.ly/pace-tribunal.

302 **"without the treatments"**: K.A. Goldsmith, P.D. White, T. Chalder, A.L. Johnson, and M. Sharpe, "The PACE Trial: Analysis of Primary Outcomes Using Composite Measures of Improvement," September 8, 2016, www.wolfson.qmul.ac.uk/images/pdfs/pace/PACE _published_protocol_based_analysis_final_8th_Sept_2016.pdf.

Note that this portion of the reanalysis was performed by the PACE researchers themselves, and its findings were spun in the most positive possible light. But the bottom line is that 20 percent of patients who received medical care plus either cognitive behavioral therapy or exercise "improved" by the original protocol, while 10 percent who received only medical care improved. Thus, 10 percent of patients who received cognitive behavioral therapy or exercise improved when they wouldn't have otherwise.

302 **"no patients recovered"**: Vincent Racaniello, "No 'Recovery' in PACE Trial, New Analysis Finds," Virology Blog, September 21, 2016, www.virology.ws/2016/09/21 /no-recovery-in-pace-trial-new-analysis-finds/.

302 **"essay in *STAT News*"**: Julie Rehmeyer, "Bad science misled millions with chronic fatigue syndrome. Here's how we fought back," *STAT,* September 21, 2016, www.statnews .com/2016/09/21/chronic-fatigue-syndrome-pace-trial/.

302 **"graded exercise and CBT"**: The Mayo Clinic, WebMD, Kaiser Permanente, UptoDate, Healthwise, and the CDC, among others, promote at least one of the therapies on their Web sites. The American Academy of Family Physicians and the American College of Physicians endorse them.

302 **"increasing research funding"**: Miriam E. Tucker, "Chronic Fatigue Syndrome Research Gains Funding, and Controversy," NPR, November 4, 2015, www.npr.org/sections /health-shots/2015/11/04/454335755/chronic-fatigue-syndrome-research-gains-funding-and -controversy/.

302 **"still chump change"**: Ibid.

303 **"physiology of the disease"**: Miriam E. Tucker, "With his son terribly ill, a top scientist takes on chronic fatigue syndrome," *Washington Post*, October 5, 2015, www.washingtonpost.com/national/health-science/with-his-son-terribly-ill-a-top-scientist -takes-on-chronic-fatigue-syndrome/2015/10/05/c5d6189c-4041-11e5-8d45-d815146f81fa _story.html.

303 **"the Open Medicine Foundation"**: "End ME/CFS Project," Open Medicine Foundation, www.openmedicinefoundation.org/the-end-mecfs-project/.

303 **"and mitochondrial function"**: Cort Johnson, "Fuel Shortage: Norwegian Study Expands on Energy Problem in Chronic Fatigue Syndrome (ME/CFS)," *Health Rising*, December 27, 2016, www.healthrising.org/blog/2016/12/27/ chronic-fatigue-syndrome-energy-problems-fluge-mella-study/.

303 **"at Columbia University"**: "Scientists Discover Robust Evidence That Chronic Fatigue Syndrome is a Biological Illness," Columbia University, February 27, 2015, www.mailman .columbia.edu/public-health-now/news/ scientists-discover-robust-evidence-chronic-fatigue-syndrome-biological.

303 **"the University of California, San Diego"**: Ariana Eunjung Cha, "Chronic fatigue syndrome may be a human version of 'hibernation'," *Washington Post*, September 6, 2016, www.washingtonpost.com/news/to-your-health/wp/2016/09/06/ chronic-fatigue-syndrome-may-be-a-human-version-of-hibernation/.

303 **"of Cornell University"**: Krishna Ramanujan, "Indicator of chronic fatigue syndrome found in gut bacteria," Cornell University, June 24, 2016, www.news.cornell.edu/stories /2016/06/indicator-chronic-fatigue-syndrome-found-gut-bacteria.

303 **"Millions Missing"**: http://millionsmissing.org

303 **"investment in ME/CFS research"**: "Dozens of US Representatives Support Letter to NIH for ME/CFS Research," MeAction.net, September 9, 2016, www.meaction.net/2016 /09/09/us-congress-letter-to-nih/.

303 **"went up online"**: Jennifer Brea, "What happens when you have a disease doctors can't diagnose," TEDSummit, June 2016, www.ted.com/talks/jen_brea_what_happens _when_you_have_a_disease_doctors_can_t_diagnose